D1601673

# THE LINK BETWEEN INFLAMMATION AND CANCER

# Wounds that do not heal

# Cancer Treatment and Research

## Steven T. Rosen, M.D., *Series Editor*

Sugarbaker, P. (ed): *Peritoneal Carcinomatosis: Principles of Management*. 1995. ISBN 0-7923-3727-1.
Dickson, R.B., Lippman, M.E. (eds): *Mammary Tumor Cell Cycle, Differentiation and Metastasis*. 1995. ISBN 0-7923-3905-3.
Freireich, E.J, Kantarjian, H. (eds): *Molecular Genetics and Therapy of Leukemia*. 1995. ISBN 0-7923-3912-
Cabanillas, F., Rodriguez, M.A. (eds): *Advances in Lymphoma Research*. 1996. ISBN 0-7923-3929-0.
Miller, A.B. (ed.): *Advances in Cancer Screening*. 1996. ISBN 0-7923-4019-1.
Hait , W.N. (ed.): *Drug Resistance*. 1996. ISBN 0-7923-4022-1.
Pienta, K.J. (ed.): *Diagnosis and Treatment of Genitourinary Malignancies*. 1996. ISBN 0-7923-4164-3.
Arnold, A.J. (ed.): *Endocrine Neoplasms*. 1997. ISBN 0-7923-4354-9.
Pollock, R.E. (ed.): *Surgical Oncology*. 1997. ISBN 0-7923-9900-5.
Verweij, J., Pinedo, H.M., Suit, H.D. (eds): *Soft Tissue Sarcomas: Present Achievements and Future Prospects*. 1997. ISBN 0-7923-9913-7.
Walterhouse, D.O., Cohn, S. L. (eds): *Diagnostic and Therapeutic Advances in Pediatric Oncology*. 1997. ISBN 0-7923-9978-1.
Mittal, B.B., Purdy, J.A., Ang, K.K. (eds): *Radiation Therapy*. 1998. ISBN 0-7923-9981-1.
Foon, K.A., Muss, H.B. (eds): *Biological and Hormonal Therapies of Cancer*. 1998. ISBN 0-7923-9997-8.
Ozols, R.F. (ed.): *Gynecologic Oncology*. 1998. ISBN 0-7923-8070-3.
Noskin, G. A. (ed.): *Management of Infectious Complications in Cancer Patients*. 1998. ISBN 0-7923-8150-5.
Bennett, C. L. (ed.): *Cancer Policy*. 1998. ISBN 0-7923-8203-X.
Benson, A. B. (ed.): *Gastrointestinal Oncology*. 1998. ISBN 0-7923-8205-6.
Tallman, M.S., Gordon, L.I. (eds): *Diagnostic and Therapeutic Advances in Hematologic Malignancies*. 1998. ISBN 0-7923-8206-4.
von Gunten, C.F. (ed.): *Palliative Care and Rehabilitation of Cancer Patients*. 1999. ISBN 0-7923-8525-X
Burt, R.K., Brush, M.M. (eds): *Advances in Allogeneic Hematopoietic Stem Cell Transplantation*. 1999. ISBN 0-7923-7714-1.
Angelos, P. (ed.): *Ethical Issues in Cancer Patient Care* 2000. ISBN 0-7923-7726-5.
Gradishar, W.J., Wood, W.C. (eds): *Advances in Breast Cancer Management*. 2000. ISBN 0-7923-7890-3.
Sparano, J. A. (ed.): *HIV & HTLV-I Associated Malignancies*. 2001. ISBN 0-7923-7220-4.
Ettinger, D. S. (ed.): *Thoracic Oncology*. 2001. ISBN 0-7923-7248-4.
Bergan, R. C. (ed.): *Cancer Chemoprevention*. 2001. ISBN 0-7923-7259-X.
Raza, A., Mundle, S.D. (eds): *Myelodysplastic Syndromes & Secondary Acute Myelogenous Leukemia* 2001. ISBN: 0-7923-7396.
Talamonti, M. S. (ed.): *Liver Directed Therapy for Primary and Metastatic Liver Tumors*. 2001. ISBN 0-7923-7523-8.
Stack, M.S., Fishman, D.A. (eds): *Ovarian Cancer*. 2001. ISBN 0-7923-7530-0.
Bashey, A., Ball, E.D. (eds): *Non-Myeloablative Allogeneic Transplantation*. 2002. ISBN 0-7923-7646-3.
Leong, S. P.L. (ed.): *Atlas of Selective Sentinel Lymphadenectomy for Melanoma, Breast Cancer and Colon Cancer*. 2002. ISBN 1-4020-7013-6.
Andersson , B., Murray D. (eds): *Clinically Relevant Resistance in Cancer Chemotherapy*. 2002. ISBN 1-4020-7200-7.
Beam, C. (ed.): *Biostatistical Applications in Cancer Research*. 2002. ISBN 1-4020-7226-0.
Brockstein, B., Masters, G. (eds): *Head and Neck Cancer*. 2003. ISBN 1-4020-7336-4.
Frank, D.A. (ed.): *Signal Transduction in Cancer*. 2003. ISBN 1-4020-7340-2.
Figlin, R. A. (ed.): *Kidney Cancer*. 2003. ISBN 1-4020-7457-3.
Kirsch, M.; Black, P. McL. (ed.): *Angiogenesis in Brain Tumors*. 2003. ISBN 1-4020-7704-1.
Keller, E.T., Chung, L.W.K. (eds): *The Biology of Skeletal Metastases*. 2004. ISBN 1-4020-7749-1.
Kumar, R. (ed.): *Molecular Targeting and Signal Transduction*. 2004. ISBN 1-4020-7822-6.
Verweij, J., Pinedo, H.M. (eds): *Targeting Treatment of Soft Tissue Sarcomas*. 2004. ISBN 1-4020-7808-0.
Finn, W.G., Peterson, L.C. (eds.): *Hematopathology in Oncology*. 2004. ISBN 1-4020-7919-2.
Farid, N. (ed.): *Molecular Basis of Thyroid Cancer*. 2004. ISBN 1-4020-8106-5.
Khleif, S. (ed.): *Tumor Immunology and Cancer Vaccines*. 2004. ISBN 1-4020-8119-7.
Balducci, L., Extermann, M. (eds): *Biological Basis of Geriatric Oncology*. 2004. ISBN
Abrey, L.E., Chamberlain, M.C., Engelhard, H.H. (eds): *Leptomeningeal Metastases*. 2005. ISBN 0-387-24
Platanias, L.C. (ed.): *Cytokines and Cancer*. 2005. ISBN 0-387-24360-7.
Leong, S. P.L., Kitagawa, Y., Kitajima, M. (eds): *Selective Sentinel Lymphadenectomy for Human Solid Cancer*. 2005. ISBN 0-387-23603-1.
Small, Jr. W., Woloschak, G. (eds): *Radiation Toxicity: A Practical Guide*. 2005. ISBN 1-4020-8053-0.
Haefner, B., Dalgleish, A. (eds): *The Link Between Inflammation and Cancer*. 2006. ISBN 0-387-26282-2.

# THE LINK BETWEEN INFLAMMATION AND CANCER

## Wounds that do not heal

edited by

**ANGUS G. DALGLEISH, MD**
*Division of Oncology*
*St. George's Hospital Medical School*
*London, UK*

**BURKHARD HAEFNER, PhD**
*Department of Oncology*
*Johnson & Johnson Pharmaceutical*
*Research and Development*
*Beerse, Belgium*

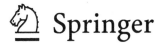 Springer

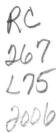

Burkhard Haefner, PhD
Department of Oncology
Johnson and Johnson Pharmaceutical
Research and Development
Turnhoutseweg 30, Box 6423
2340 Beerse, Belgium

Angus G. Dalgleish, MD
Division of Oncology
St. George's Hospital Medical School
Cranmer Terrace
London SW17 0RE, United Kingdom

THE LINK BETWEEN INFLAMMATION AND CANCER
Wounds that do not heal

Library of Congress Control Number: 2005934590

ISBN-10: 0-387-26282-2        e-ISBN-10: 0-387-26283-0
ISBN-13: 978-0387-26282-6     e-ISBN-13: 978-0387-26283-3

Printed on acid-free paper.

Printed in the United States of America.

9 8 7 6 5 4 3 2 1        SPIN  11053699

springeronline.com

# CONTENTS

vi

# FOREWORD

A link between inflammation and cancer has been established many years ago, yet it is only recently that the potential significance of this connection has become apparent. Although several examples of chronic inflammatory conditions, often induced by persistent irritation and/or infection, developing into cancer have been known for some time, there has been a notable resistance to contemplate the possibility that this association may apply in a causative way to other cancers. Examples for such progression from chronic inflammation to cancer are colon carcinoma developing with increased frequency in patients with ulcerative colitis, and the increased incidence of bladder cancer in patients suffering from chronic Schistosoma infection. Inflammation and cancer have been recognized to be linked in another context for many years, i.e., with regards to pathologies resembling chronic lacerations or 'wounds that do not heal.' More recently, the immunology of wound healing has given us clues as to the mechanistic link between inflammation and cancer, in as much as wounds and chronic inflammation turn off local cell-mediated immune responses and switch on growth factor release as well the growth of new blood vessels – angiogenesis. Both of these are features of most types of tumours, which suggest that tumours may require an immunologically shielded milieu and a growth factor-rich environment.

The discovery that some cancers are associated with viral infections and that these viruses only cause cancer in a small percentage of infected individuals has served to highlight that these 'oncogenic' viruses are extremely 'mild' with regard to the time it takes to induce cancer and that other factors must be involved. Examples of these viruses include human papilloma viruses (HPV), Epstein Barr Virus (EBV) and the two hepatitis viruses, HBV and HCV. HPV causes cervical cancer in only a small percentage of infected women, most of whom eventually become clear of infection. Chronic infection with HPV would appear to be more likely in the presence of additional infectious agents leading to established infection and chronic cervicitis. EBV only rarely causes cancer in

Western populations, but where it is clearly linked with cancers in a causative sense, e.g. Burkitt's Lymphoma (BL) in Africa and nasopharyngeal carcinoma (NPC) in China, there are other chronic co-factors involved. In the case of BL, there is a strong link to malaria and with NPC, salted fish acting as an irritant/carcinogen is required. However, HBV (and HCV) infection, over decades, will induce chronic hepatitis which evolves into cirrhotic changes from which hepatomas develop. Although co-factors may be involved, they do not appear necessary. These examples emphasize that these are extremely weak oncogenic viruses contained for years by an effective immune response (the only clear link between EBV and tumours (lymphomas) in the West are seen in immunosuppressed patients and the tumours often resolve upon reversal of immunosuppression). The bottom line is that all these viruses usually only cause malignant transformation after many years of inflammatory infection.

The rapid growth in our understanding of molecular signaling pathways in the past decades has taught us that some of these regulatory cascades appear to be key to the development of cancer from chronic inflammatory conditions. Pivotal among these signaling circuits appears to be the NF-κB pathway, crucial for the regulation of immune and inflammatory responses, and linked to non-inflammatory core pathways in oncogenesis, such as the p53 pathway. A major focus of this book, therefore, is the NF-κB pathway as well as the interaction between the tumour and its microenvironment involving the immune response, apoptotic pathways, cytokines and the selectins. In this volume we have tried to highlight the complexity of these processes, yet at the same time show just how fundamental the basic link is. Inevitably this means looking at the same scene from different angles, and hence, there is some degree of overlap. However, the detail is so impressive that we feel this helps enforce the clarity of the overall picture, which only goes to raise the question: 'Why has the link been denied for so long?' The major impact of this book, however, should be to emphasize the obvious dramatic therapeutic and preventative implications. Chronic viral infections, for example, can be vaccinated against. For instance, the widespread availability of a HBV vaccine for several decades has greatly reduced the incidence of hepatoma and, as such, can claim to be the first effective preventative cancer vaccine. The common 'non-infection'-related tumours such as colon, lung, breast, and prostate cancer, may be 'preventable' by regular administration of anti-inflammatories such as aspirin. More specific drugs may be derived from studies included in this book which will lead to more effective preventative strategies as well as treatments. The link between an inflammatory environment and more rapid progression has been recognized for a number of tumours, including breast cancer, clearly suggesting that anti-inflammatory agents may have a major role in therapy. Unfortunately, several studies using the new COX-2 inhibitors have had to be halted because of the association with increased heart attack risk. Aspirin of course is a COX inhibitor which protects against heart attacks and is an obvious candidate. Unfortunately, gastritis and increased gastric bleeding tendency have reduced enthusiasm for such studies even though aspirin has been reported to be preventative for a number of solid tumours, including breast cancer as well as colorectal cancer. Clearly, there still is plenty of scope for the development of improved anti-inflammatory drugs which can be used in cancer prevention as well as treatment.

The recognition of the link with chronic inflammation allows for new ways of understanding how cancers progress and how different types of cancer can show similar responsiveness to drug treatment, which is already being seen for Avastin, a monoclonal antibody which targets vascular endothelial growth factor and is active in disparate tumour types. Another example of how this approach can influence cancer treatment is Revlimid, a Thalidomide analogue developed by Celgene. It was selected for its anti-TNF and thus anti-inflammatory activity but was found to also have strong anti-angiogenic properties and to stimulate the cell-mediated immune response. This compound may thus deliver an ideal three-way blow to tumours and has recently been shown to be highly active against multiple myeloma. It would be surprising if it did not act against other tumour types as well. Thus, we feel confident in proclaiming that this book does not merely cover a speculative theory, but rather the basis for a therapeutical revolution in the treatment of cancer.

*Angus G. Dalgleish, MD*
*Burkhard Haefner, PhD*

# CONTRIBUTORS

*Josep M. Argilés,* PhD, Professor, Department of Biochemistry and Molecular Biology, Faculty of Biology, University of Barcelona, Barcelona, Spain

*Jessica Bertout,* Center for Research on Reproduction and Women's Health, University of Pennsylvania Medical Center, Philadelphia, PA

*Sílvia Busquets,* MD, Department of Biochemistry and Molecular Biology, Faculty of Biology, University of Barcelona, Barcelona, Spain

*Angus G. Dalgleish,* MD, Professor, Division of Oncology, St. George's Hospital Medical School, London, UK

*Harald Dinter,* PhD, Scientific Director of Oncology Research, Berlex Biosciences, Richmond, CA

*B. Mark Evers,* MD, Professor and Robertson-Poth Distinguished Chair in General Surgery, Department of Surgery and Director, The Sealy Center for Cancer Cell Biology, The University of Texas Medical Branch, Galveston, TX

*Burkhard Haefner,* PhD, Department of Oncology, Johnson & Johnson Pharmaceutical Research and Development, Beerse, Belgium

*Guy Haegeman,* PhD, Professor, Laboratory for Eukaryotic Gene Expression and Signal Transduction (LEGEST), Department of Molecular Biology, Ghent University, Gent, Belgium

*Lindsey N. Jackson,* MD, Department of Surgery, The University of Texas Medical Branch, Galveston, TX

*Francisco J. López-Soriano,* MD, Department of Biochemistry and Molecular Biology, Faculty of Biology, University of Barcelona, Barcelona, Spain

*Ken O'Byrne,* MD, Consultant and Clinical Lecturer in Medical Oncology, St James's Hospital and Trinity College, Dublin Ireland

*Arndt J. Schottelius*, MD, Director, Non-Clinical Immunology Drug Development, Development Sciences, Genentech, Inc., South San Francisco, CA

*Andrei Thomas-Tikhonenko,* PhD, Associate Professor, Department of Pathobiology, University of Pennsylvania, Philadelphia, PA

*Wim Vanden Berghe,* PhD, Laboratory for Eukaryotic Gene Expression and Signal Transduction (LEGEST), Department of Molecular Biology, Ghent University, Gent, Belgium

*Linda Vermeulen,* PhD, Laboratory for Eukaryotic Gene Expression and Signal Transduction (LEGEST), Department of Molecular Biology, Ghent University, Gent, Belgium

*Harald Wajant,* PhD, Professor, Department of Molecular Internal Medicine, Medical Clinic and Polyclinic II, University of Wuerzburg, Wuerzburg, Germany

*Theresa L. Whiteside,* PhD, Professor, University of Pittsburgh Cancer Institute, Hillman Cancer Center, Pittsburgh, PA

*Issac P. Witz,* PhD, Professor, Department of Cell Research and Immunology, The George S. Wise Faculty of Life Sciences, Tel Aviv University, Tel Aviv, Israel

# Chapter 1

# INFLAMMATION AND CANCER:

*The role of the.immune response and angiogenesis*

Angus G. Dalgleish[1] and Ken O'Byrne[2]

[1]*Division of Oncology, St. George's Hospital Medical School, London, UK*
[2]*Medical Oncology, St James's Hospital and Trinity College, Dublin, Ireland*

Abstract:     The link with chronic inflammation and cancer has been recognized for certain
              cancers for several decades. However, only recently has the biology of chronic
              inflammation begun to be understood, to the point that it may play a major role
              in tumour development. The biology of chronic inflammation has many
              similarities with that of wound healing. In particular, local cell mediated
              immunity is attenuated and angiogenesis is increased along with other growth
              factors. When present long term, this provides the ideal environment for
              mutated cells to be nurtured and escape immune surveillance. It is of note that
              this process still appears to take two or three decades, as witnessed by the
              close association between chronic ulcerative colitis and colon cancer as well as
              chronic hepatitis and hepatocellular carcinoma. Closer study of the
              inflammatory pathways show the close interaction with apoptosis and anti-
              apoptotic pathways, as well as the main tumour suppressor genes, such as p53,
              as well as a number of growth factors, such as the insulin-like growth factor. A
              full study of these processes reveals that there are key molecules in these
              pathways which may provide therapeutic as well as anti-inflammatory targets.

## 1. INTRODUCTION

The association between chronic inflammation and cancer is not new. However, the previously recognized associations had limited practical implications and it is only the relatively recent understanding of molecular mechanisms of cancer and the interaction of the immune system and angiogenesis that have led to the potential for targeted intervention to both prevent and treat a number of different cancers.

It was recognized in the nineteenth century that certain cancers were due to chronic irritation, notably the scrotal cancer of chimney sweeps where the irritant was the coal dust and male breast cancer associated with chronic irritation by braces. It was Virchow in 1863 who wrote about the possibilities of cancers arising from sites of chronic inflammation, noting that cancers are similar to wounds that failed to heal. The striking similarities between wound healing and tumour stroma have been reviewed more recently by Dvorak. (Dvorak 1986) Other chronic inflammatory conditions that are recognized as being associated with an increased risk of cancer include schistosomiasis (bladder) and ulcerative colitis (colon).

## 2. INFECTIOUS CAUSES

The relatively recent realization that many chronic bacterial and viral infections are also associated with tumour formation provides the most compelling examples. In addition to schistosomiasis and bladder cancer, the more recently discovered *Helicobacter pylori*, originally associated with chronic gastritis, is now recognized as a causative agent for gastric adenocarcinoma and gastric mucosal-associated lymphoid tissue lymphomas (Williams and Pounder, 1999).

### 2.1 Virus association

Perhaps the strongest association between chronic infection and the development of cancer is that between chronic viral infections and tumour induction. (Dalgleish, 1991). The best examples are those of chronic hepatitis B and hepatitis C virus infection, both of which cause chronic hepatitis from which primary liver cancers evolve, often decades later. Similarly, chronic human papilloma virus infection is clearly associated with inflammatory changes in the cervix leading to cervical cancer and cancers of the perineal region. Epstein Barr Virus (EBV), which exists in a dormant state in the vast majority of the Western population, is able to cause Burkitt's lymphoma in Africa, where the additional stimulus is chronic immune activation, probably by malaria. Similarly, it is associated with nasopharyngeal carcinoma, particularly in the Far East where chronic irritation/inflammation/immune activation by salted fish stimulates EBV replication leading to these unusual tumours. EBV is largely asymptomatic but is clearly able to cause lymphomas, particularly in immunosuppressed patients, such as post transplant patients or acquired immune deficiency syndrome (AIDS) patients.

The most recent example of a virus causing a tumour is the discovery of the new herpes sarcoma virus or human herpesvirus 8 (HHV-8), which is the causative agent of Kaposi's sarcoma (Brooks *et al.*, 1997). There is a strong association with HIV and this cancer may undergo spontaneous resolution with treatment leading to a reduction of HIV load. HIV is associated with chronic immune activation, which is reduced when the viral load is lowered.

## 2.2    The requirement for chronic inflammation

Although the viruses above have well described oncogenic properties, they rarely cause disease in the absence of chronic immune activation or inflammation. The fact that chronic irritation/inflammation does not need to be caused by an infectious agent in order to increase the propensity for cancer to develop is clearly shown by tobacco-related cancers. Lung cancer, for instance, is clearly associated with smoking and it is dependent on the amount smoked (packs per day) as well as the number of years smoked. Many of the patients suffer from chronic bronchitis for a number of years and even in those patients who do not have overt bronchitis, histology of non macroscopically tumour-free bronchi show chronic inflammatory changes. Other chronic irritants also lead to inflammation and subsequent tumours, such as asbestos in mesothelioma. Inappropriate enzymatic exposure can also result in chronic inflammation. For example, reflux esophagitis and Barratt's esophagitis are both associated with the development of esophageal adenocarcinoma. For a full list of associations of cancer or recognized associations of cancer and chronic infection/irritation/inflammation see Table 1.

The association between chronic inflammation and tumour formation strongly suggests that sites of chronic inflammation are ideal microenvironments for cancer to evolve (Table 1). Here, the similarity with wound healing is pertinent as in wounds, cell-mediated immunity is suppressed, presumably to prevent breaking of tolerance of "self" tissue as it is being repaired. The second component is the induction of angiogenesis, being new blood vessel formation which in itself is associated with increased

Table 1. Relationship between known causes of Chronic Inflammation and Cancer

| Causative inflammatory stimulus | Cancer | Mechanism of action and precursor states |
|---|---|---|
| EBV | Burkitts Lymphoma (BL) Nasopharyngeal (NPL) Post transplant lymphoma Immunosuppression associated lymphoma NHL Breast cancer | Associated with chromic immune activation such as malaria in BL and smoked food in NPC  Immune suppression post transplantation |
| HBV/HCV | Viruses induce hepatitis followed by cirrhosis (angiogenesis) followed by oncogenic transformation - hepatic cancer | Aflatoxin may enhance the degree of inflammation |
| HPV | Cervix/anal/perineum/?upper aerodigestive track | May require extra exogenous causative agent of cervicitis to progress, e.g. chlymidia, and/or immunosuppression |
| HHV-8 | Kaposi's Sarcoma | Only in presence of immunosuppression due to age (mild) or HIV infection (aggressive) which causes marked immune activation |
| HIV | • Lymphoma (EBV driven) • Kaposi's Sarcoma (HHV-8 driven) • Cervix (HPV driven) • (HIV is not oncogenic directly in contrast to the above) | HIV induces immunosuppression as well as chronic immune activation which appears dependant on the immunogenetics of host |
| HTVL-1 | • T-cell lymphomas and leukaemia | Causes chronic T-cell activation |
| *Helicobacter pylori* | • Stomach cancer • Lymphoma of gut (MALT) | Gastritis/ulcers |
| Schistosomiasis | Bladder | Chronic cystitis |
| Tobacco smoke Nicotine Infections | Lung cancer | Chronic bronchitis Inflammation of tunica medica |
| Asbestos | Mesothelioma | Asbestos, fibrotic, plaques |
| Ulcerative colitis Crohn's ? bile salts | Colorectal cancer | Causes of inflammatory bowel disease including polyps and adenomas |
| Reflux +? | Oesophageal cancer | Oesophagitis/obesity/tobacco/ nicotine |
| Prostatitis ?cause | Prostate cancer | ?infectious cause |
| Chronic pancreatis ?cause | Pancreatic cancer | Causative agent unclear |
| UV light | Melanoma | Skin inflammation and immunosuppression |
| Chronic tar/soot irritation | Scrotum | Common in chimney sweeps in Victorian era |

amounts of growth factors. If continued indefinitely, as in chronic inflammation, this environment would be ideal for cancer to develop. It is broadly recognized that cancer is a sequence of stochastic events involving permanent activation of oncogene pathways and deletion of tumour suppressor genes and their pathways. On average, six such events are required to occur for cancer to develop. It has been shown that single mutations in oncogenes can be recognized by cytotoxic T lymphocytes suggesting that in the absence of suppression of the immune system, a cell developing such a mutation would induce an immune response against this new epitope and the cell would be killed. In a background of chronic inflammation, immune induction does not occur and the cell is able to survive long enough to develop the next random event. When the tumour does start to develop, it has an environment full of growth factors and the ability to establish new vasculature.

The most important impact of the association between chronic inflammation and cancer is that treatment of chronic inflammation should lead to a lower incidence of cancer. This is one of the most convincing aspects of the association as there are numerous studies showing that the daily use of anti-inflammatories, such as aspirin, other NSAIDS, and cyclooxygenase (COX)-2 inhibitors, are able to reduce the incidence of colorectal cancer by up to half. In addition, the incidence of other solid tumours are also reduced by a significant amount (Harris *et al.*, 2005).

## 3. CANCER AND THE IMMUNE RESPONSE

T cells produce (at least) two major cytokine patterns. The first is generated by Th-1 cells, which produce interleukin (IL)-2, interferon (IFN)-γ, and IL-12 and affect the cell mediated immune (CMI) response, and the second by Th-2 cells, which release IL-4, IL-5, IL-6, and IL-10 and affect the hormonal response (HIR). This discovery, initially in mice but later also in humans, has had a major impact on understanding the complex changes and interactions between an infectious agent and the immune system (Mosman and Coffman, 1989). Th-1 cytokines are required for a strong CMI response and are decreased in many chronic infectious diseases, including AIDS, tuberculosis (TB), and many tropical infections. In what might appear a compensatory response, Th-2 cytokines are associated with humoral immunity (HI) and often increase as is the case in diseases where CMI is suppressed, e.g., AIDS and tuberculosis.

Many malignancies are associated with some degree of suppression of CMI responses (Lee *et al.* 1997; Maraveyas *et al.*, 2000; Pettit *et al.*, 2000). Cancers use a wide variety of methods to evade an immune response including downregulation of molecules of the major histocompatibility complex (MHC, HLA in humans) and upregulation of ligands that kill engaging killer T-cells, i.e. CD95L and DC178. The production of immunosuppressive cytokines by tumours, such as TGFβ and IL-10 could account for much of the inhibition of CMI (Doherty *et al.*, 1994; Ganss and Hanahan, 1998; Garrido *et al.*, 1993; Gorter and Meri, 1999; Melief and Kast, 1991; Strand and Galle, 1998; Pettit *et al.*, 2000).

The suppression of local CMI responses has been reported in a number of studies evaluating inflammatory cellular infiltrates in tumours from patients with malignant cancers including non-small cell lung cancer (NSCLC), head and neck, oesophagus, breast and genitourinary cancers, lymphomas and sarcomas (Asselin-Paturel *et al.*, 1998; O'Sullivan *et al.*, 1996; Hildesheim *et al.*, 1997; Lee *et al.*, 1997; Aziz *et al.*, 1998; O'Hara *et al.*, 1998) as well as carcinoma *in situ* including Barrett's oesophagus and cervical intraepithelial neoplasia (CIN) (Hildesheim, *et al.* 1997; Oka, *et al.* 1992; Sonnex, 1998). Systemic immunosuppression can be documented by looking at intracellular cytokine production following stimulation of lymphocytes *in vitro* and has been shown in several cancer types including melanoma and colorectal cancer (Maraveyas *et al.*, 1999; Heriot *et al.*, 2000). The presence of a dominant Th-2 immune response in potentially curable tumours, such as lymphomas, is associated with a fatal outcome (Lee *et al.*, 1997). Absent or reduced delayed hypersensitivity reactions to common T-cell recall antigens are a manifestation of CMI. These responses are either reduced or absent in many pre-malignant and malignant tumours including CIN, Hodgkin's disease, gastric carcinoma, small cell lung cancer, and malignant melanoma (Roses *et al.*, 1979; Lang *et al.*, 1980; Johnston-Early *et al.*, 1983; Richtsmeier and Eisele, 1986; Cainzos, 1989; Hopfl *et al.* 2000).

T-cell anergy is commonly seen in malignant disease. A number of processes may be responsible for this. T-cells from cancer patients have abnormalities in their signal transduction pathways. The T-cell receptor (TCR)-αβ or -γδ chains bind the peptide ligand while, in turn, the TCR is coupled to intracellular signal transduction components by TCR-ζ subunits. The TCR-associated signalling molecule CD3 is made up of a number of components which stabilize surface expression of the TCR and are essential for interaction with MHC-antigen complexes. The T-cell alterations found in *in vivo* models of malignant disease include complete absence of CD3-ζ which is replaced by the Fc εγ-chain and a reduction in the ability of T lymphocytes to produce the Th-1 cytokines IL-2 and IFN-γ (Mizoguchi *et al.*, 1992; Salvadori *et al.*, 1994; Zea *et al.*, 1995).

In malignant mesothelioma, the relative CDδ, CDγ and CDζ mRNA levels expressed by tumour infiltrating lymphocytes (TILs) decrease. In addition, transforming growth factor-β (TGFβ), a potent tumour cell growth and immunosuppressive factor, is produced. (A feature which is not limited to mesothelioma.) In this disease, however, the suppression of CD3 subunit expression with resultant functional impairment of TILs is reversed *in vivo* by inducing TGFβ antisense RNA. This indicates that TILs are deactivated by tumour-associated immunosuppressive factors upon infiltration of the tumour microenvironment (Jarnicki *et al.*, 1996).

COX enzymes are responsible for the synthesis of prostaglandins, the precise prostaglandin synthesized depending on the prostaglandin synthase enzyme present in the cell. COX-2, the inducible form of the enzyme, is constitutively expressed in virtually all premalignant and malignant cancers, including colorectal, upper gastrointestinal tract, pancreatic, head and neck, lung and breast cancers (Murata *et al.*, 1999; Koshiba *et al.*, 1999; Mestre *et al.*, 1999; Molina *et al.*, 1999; Wolff *et al.*, 1998; Huang *et al.*, 1998; Taketo, 1998; Tsujii *et al.*, 1997; Uotila, 1996; Vainio and Morgan, 1998; Vane *et al.*, 1998). More recently, COX-2 expression has been shown to correlate with local chronic inflammation and tumour neovascularisation in human prostate cancer (Wang, *et al.* 2005). It is particularly associated with prostaglandin E2 (PGE$_2$). On binding to its receptor on T-cells, PGE$_2$ induces cyclic adenosine monophosphate (cAMP) which inhibits the proliferation of Th-1/CMI-associated CD4$^+$ lymphocytes while stimulating the proliferation of Th-2 CD4$^+$ lymphocytes resulting in avoidance of immunesurveillance. The importance of the Th-1/CMI response in both tumour regression and rejection underscores the significance of these changes. Tumour-specific cytotoxic T-cells represent a major effector arm of theTh-1/CMI response as demonstrated by studies of adoptive T-cell transfer (Greenberg, 1991; Papadopoulos *et al.*, 1994; Rooney *et al.*, 1995). However, the presence of such effector cells is only seen in a small minority of cases in the setting of tumour progression. Both Th-1 and Th-2 cytokine gene transduction experiments in animal tumour cell lines have resulted in CMI responses capable of inhibiting a subsequent challenge with parental tumour cells. Moreover, in order to induce established tumour regression, Th-1 cytokine secreting effector cells are required (Forni and Foa, 1996), and where tumour rejection occurs, the induction of tumour-specific CMI responses is generally seen. Collectively these findings indicate that tumour growth either fails to stimulate an effective CMI response or evades immunesurveillance at least in part through inhibition of TIL CMI functions both locally and systemically (Browning and Bodmer, 1992; Jarnicki *et al.*, 1996).

Malignant melanoma is a highly metastatic cancer of the melatonin-producing cells of the skin and is notoriously resistant to classical treatments such as chemotherapy and radiotherapy. Employing the same fluorescence-activated cell sorting (FACS) techniques used to detect intracellular cytokines in AIDS patients, a significant reduction in Th-1 cytokine production can be found in these patients (Maraveyas *et al.*, 1999). For many years, however, it has been recognised that this cancer is sensitive to a variety of immunology-based therapies which act by boosting CMI responses. Skin lesions often disappear following direct intralesional administration of Bacillus Calmette-Guerin (BCG) vaccine. Similar responses have been seen with cell-based vaccines or lysates, melanoma specific peptides, either given alone or pulsed onto dendritic cells. Successful treatment with immunotherapy, resulting in either stable disease or an objective tumour response has been found to be associated with a switch from a Th-2/HI dominant profile to a Th-1/CMI dominant one (Grange *et al.*, 1995; Sredni *et al.*, 1996; Hu *et al.*, 1998; Hrouda *et al.*, 1998; Dalgleish, 1999).

The impact of a reduced CMI response being induced by a tumour is illustrated by colorectal cancer in which even in patients with early small volume (Duke's A and B) tumours, a reduction in systemic Th-1-like responses is seen compared to age- and sex-matched controls without disease (Heriot *et al.*, 2000). In the latter case, the observation that these responses return to normal following surgery strongly supports the deduction that it is the tumour that causes the reduction in CMI responses. More recently, the same patients have been reanalysed and the level of Th-1 responses have been found to correlate with survival irrespective of subsequent treatment (Charles Evans and co-workers, unpublished data).

In NSCLC malignant pleural effusions, the majority of lymphocytes are T-cells with a Th-2 phenotype whilst less than 1% are natural killer cells. Following Th-1 cytokine therapy with IL-2 and IL-12, the T-helper lymphocytes shift to a Th-1 phenotype. The specific anti-tumour cytotoxic property of these T-lymphocytes can be restored by the use of IL-2 treatment and TCR-CD3 engagement. IL-2 and IL-12 act synergistically in this setting (Chen *et al.*, 1998; Chen *et al.*, 1997b).

Gene knockout experiments have provided the most conclusive evidence for an association between deficient Th-1 responses and a predisposition to cancer. An increased incidence of solid tumours is seen in IFN-γ, IFN-γ receptor or signal transducer and activator of transcription (STAT) 1 (a component of the IFN signalling pathway) knockout mice (Chen *et al.*, 1998; Kaplan *et al.*, 1998). Therefore CMI suppression may provide the ideal environment for cancer cells to develop and grow. A single mutation in an oncogene would probably be identified by a cytotoxic T lymphocyte in a normal environment but cells carrying such a mutation are able to survive in a privileged, depressed CMI immune response site. As a result, the mutation may persist leaving the cells' DNA primed for another stochastic event to occur, such as a p53 mutation.

As the neoplastic lesion grows, it becomes progressively hypoxic. Hypoxia is associated with suppression of CMI responses (Lee *et al.*, 1998; Sairam *et al.*, 1998) which in turn would allow escape of the malignant process from immunesurveillance. Collectively these findings indicate that effective reversion of immune tolerance may have a role to play not only in the treatment of established malignant disease but also in chemoprevention.

Exposure to a foreign antigen results in upregulation of the non-specific pro-inflammatory cytokines IL-1$\alpha$ and $\beta$ and the Th-1 cytokines in inflammatory cells. COX-1 and -2 are among the most important enzymes in the regulation of the immune response and play a key role in angiogenesis, the inhibition of apoptosis, cell proliferation and motility. COX-1 is constitutively expressed by many cells. In contrast COX-2 is produced by epithelial, mesenchymal and inflammatory cells following exposure to pro-inflammatory cytokines (Taketo, 1998; Uotila, 1996; Vane *et al.*, 1998), which are induced by infective agents and environmental factors known to be associated with the development of malignant disease including *Helicobacter pylori* infection (Sawaoka *et al.*, 1998a), nicotine (Schror *et al.*, 1998), and tobacco-specific nitrosamine 4-(methylnitrosamino)-4-(3-pyridyl)-1-butanone (NNK) (El-Bayoumy *et al.*, 1999). Overexpression of COX-2 is sufficient to induce tumorigenesis in the mammary glands of transgenic mice derived using the murine mammary tumour virus promoter (Liu *et al.*, 2001). Th2 cytokines, such as IL-4 and IL-10, which can inhibit the synthesis of Th-1 cytokines by CD4$^+$ T-helper lymphocytes, are produced in COX-2 expressing environments. These Th-2 cytokines not only downregulate both pro-inflammatory/Th-1 cytokines but also COX-2 expression itself (Della Bella *et al.*, 1997; Subbaramaiah *et al.*, 1997; Uotila, 1996; Vane *et al.*, 1998) (Fig. 1). Chronic antigen exposure may drive a continuous cycle in which induced pro-inflammatory and Th-1 cytokines upregulate COX-2 leading to chronic HI/Th-2 cytokine production and subsequent impairment of the CMI response. In predisposed individuals, this cycle may eventually lead to a predominant HI response environment. The importance of pro-inflammatory cytokines driving the HI response is underpinned by the observation that TNF-deficient mice are resistant to skin carcinogenesis (Moore *et al.*, 1999).

The results of these studies consistently demonstrate that not only is cancer itself associated with a shift from a Th-1 to a Th-2 dominant phenotype but that conditions predisposing to malignant disease likewise induce similar changes. This suggests that in many cases, the immune response shift precedes the development of the neoplastic process and may play a key role in carcinogenesis.

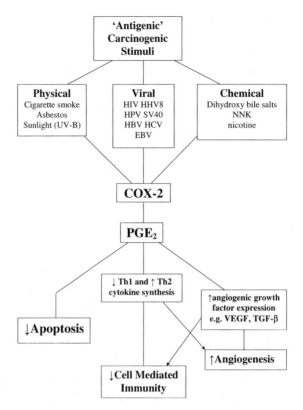

Figure 1. Exposure to carcinogenic stimuli results in upregulation of cell survival factors in affected cells including cyclooxygenase (COX)-2. COX-2 plays a key role in the conversion of arachidonic acid to prostaglandins including PGE2. PGE2 downregulates the synthesis of Th1 cytokines and upregulates Th-2 cytokines in inflammatory and/or affected epithelial, mesenchymal or haematopoietic cells resulting in suppressed cell mediated immune responses (CMI), increased angiogenesis and inhibition of apoptosis. In an acute exposure situation the feedback between the initial pro-inflammatory response and the anti-inflammatory Th2 cytokines is self-limiting. However in the case of cancer associated chronic immune activation conditions sustained exposure to the antigen/chemical drives the cycle continuously resulting in a sustained pre-dominant Th2 immune response, angiogenesis and inhibition of apoptosis facilitating the development of cancer in a pre-disposed individual.

## 4.      INITIAL INFLAMMATION RESPONSE: KILL OR CURE

The difference between a pro-inflammatory response to an antigen or irritant and the type of immune response established is crucial as to whether the cancer is fed by inflammation or is rejected by it. There are numerous factors which can determine whether an immune response favours cancer progression or its elimination. There are several studies showing that tumour infiltrating lymphocytes are a good prognostic factor. Indeed, reculturing these lymphocytes and expanding them *ex vivo* before re-infusion with IL-2 was reported as being capable of inducing clinical responses (Rosenberg *et al.*, 1986). However, it is now apparent that non-infiltrating immune cells are exhibiting anti-tumour activity. Tumour-associated macrophages (TAMs) have been shown to correlate with vessel density in a number of malignancies and the associated expression of epidermal growth factor (EGF) and EGF receptor (EGFR) in cancer cells. This is associated with reduced patient survival. Co-culture of cancer cells with macrophages can actually enhance cancer cell invasive potential and matrix degrading activity and upregulate pro-tumorigenic genes. Chen *et al.* have shown that this activity can be reduced with anti-inflammatory drugs, including Thalidomide (Chen *et al.*, 2005). Whether the macrophages have a positive or negative effect on tumour growth clearly depends on the tumour microenvironment and the stroma involved. Indeed, different results reported in the literature would appear to be dependent on whether the macrophages are predominantly in the tumour islets or in the stroma. Thus, it would appear that macrophages predominantly in the stroma are pro-tumorigenic, whereas macrophages predominant in the tumour islet are associated with a significant survival time. Indeed, Tomas Walsh and colleagues (personal communication) have noted that patients with a high islet macrophage density but incomplete resection have an overall longer survival than patients with low islet macrophage density but complete resection.

What determines the result of this interaction is unclear but would appear to involve chemokines and their receptors as most cancers express an extensive network of these. Tumour-associated chemokines are thought to control leukocyte infiltration into the tumour, the immune response against it, the regulation of angiogenesis and the control of metastatic spread. Chemokines can influence the distribution of the immune response, including lymphocytes, monocytes/macrophages and pre-dendritic cells. They are also able to promote angiogenesis and may also contribute directly to the transformation of cells by acting as growth and survival factors. Moreover, they are crucial to the spread of cells. Indeed, in mouse models, the level of expressed tumour-derived chemokines determines whether macrophage infiltration is pro-tumorigenic or capable of destroying tumour cells. Manipulating chemokine levels and their receptors clearly could have a major role in the treatment of cancer. In order to reject a tumour, an acute, as opposed to a chronic inflammatory state needs to be introduced. Here, it is clear that the interplay between innate and adaptive immunity and, in particular, the interactions between NK and dendritic cells are of vital importance for effective tumour control (de Visser and Coussens, 2005). The importance of the immune response in controlling the development of cancer can only be fully appreciated when considering the numerous methods employed by tumours to escape immune control (reviewed by Igney and Krammer, 2005).

## 5. THE INTER-RELATIONSIP BETWEEN THE IMMUNE RESPONSE AND ANGIOGENESIS

The relationship between the immune response and angiogenesis (O'Byrne *et al.*, 2000a) is important in its own right with regard to fostering tumour growth. Angiogenesis, the formation of a new blood supply from an existing vasculature, is necessary for the development of early neoplastic lesions and the growth of invasive and metastatic disease. This process occurs in all tumours and is under the regulation of pro-angiogenic factors including Th-2 cytokines such as IL-6 and vascular endothelial growth factor (VEGF). The intensity of the angiogenic process, as assessed by microvessel counting methods, correlates with primary tumour growth, invasiveness, and metastatic spread of the disease (Folkman, 1995; O'Byrne *et al.*, 2000b). Furthermore, there is a strong correlation between tumour cell expression of angiogenic growth factors, such as VEGF and angiogenesis, and patient outcome (O'Byrne *et al.*, 2000b).

Recent research indicates that normal physiological processes which require angiogenesis, such as ovulation, implantation into the ovary and wound healing, occur in a HI-predominant environment (Folkman, 1995; Richards *et al.*, 1995; Kodelja *et al.*, 1997; Piccini *et al.*, 1998; Schaffer and Barbul, 1998; Singer and Clark, 1999). HI-stimulated macrophages induce endothelial cell proliferation 3 to 3.5 times more than CMI stimulated macrophages in coculture experiments (Kodelja *et al.*, 1997). These findings are supported by work in IL-6 knockout mice where the capacity to heal wounds and regenerate normal hepatic tissue, both processes which require angiogenesis, is impaired (Gallucci *et al.* 2000; Wallenius *et al.*, 2000). In contrast to the upregulated HI immune response seen, CMI responses are suppressed during ovulation, implantation, and wound healing. This prevents rejection of sperm and embryo, and presentation of damaged tissues to the immune system as non-self, which might induce an autoimmune response to healing or healed tissues (Richards *et al.*, 1995; Piccini *et al.*, 1998; Schaffer and Barbul, 1998; Singer and Clark, 1999). In contrast to HI immune response-induced angiogenesis, CMI immune responses tend to inhibit angiogenesis (Watanabe *et al.*, 1997). B lymphocytes, which are synonomous with HI have been shown to be vital in promoting chronic inflammation-dependent *de novo* carcinogenesis (de Visser *et al.*, 2005).

Unlike normal physiological processes, the factors that suppress CMI and switch on angiogenesis persist in many established chronic infectious/inflammatory states, particularly conditions associated with the subsequent development of malignant disease (Fig. 2). These include chronic viral infections (see below), asbestos (Bielefeldt-Ohmann *et al.*, 1996) and cigarette smoke (Mayne *et al.*, 1999). Chronic exposure to cigarette smoke leads to chronic obstructive pulmonary disease (COPD) in predisposed individuals. COPD is an independent predictor for the development of lung cancer (Mayne *et al.*, 1999). In keeping with this, inflamed lung mucosa has increased vascularity compared with uninflamed mucosa (Fisseler-Eckhoff *et al.*, 1996). Furthermore, bronchial dysplasia and carcinoma *in situ*, precursors to the development of malignant disease, have increased vascularity compared to normal bronchial epithelium (Fontanini *et al.*, 1996; Fisseler-Eckhoff *et al.*, 1996). Using fluoroscent bronchoscopy, angiogenic squamous dysplastic lesions have been identified in 34 percent of high risk smokers without carcinomas and in 60 percent of patients with squamous cell lung carcinoma (Keith *et al.*, 2000). Cigarettes contain a number of factors, including nicotine, which may predispose to the development of malignant disease. Nicotine induces angiogenesis and reduces CMI which would facilitate the survival and proliferation of a cell transformed by carcinogens such as NNK (Heeschen *et al.*, 2001).

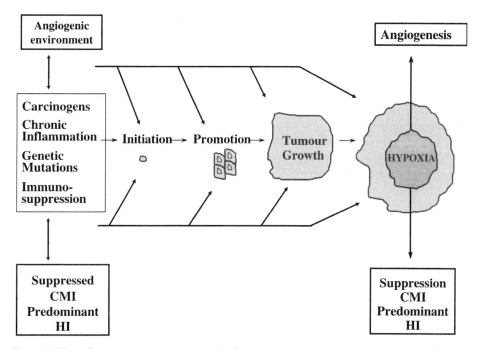

Figure 2. The inflammatory environment resulting in angiogenesis and growth factors, as well as reduced cell mediated immune surveillance, provides the ideal environment for a mutant cell to evolve through the six or more minimum changes required for metastatic cancer to develop. These features help both initiation and promotion resulting in a tumour that tries to replicate this favourable environment by secreting angiogenetic and immunosuppressive factors.

If this state occurs for several years, then random mutations in the cells of the affected tissues, caused by carcinogens or unregulated proliferation, would occur not only in an immunologically tolerant, but also a microvessel-rich environment. Phenotypic changes, e.g. proteins resulting from mutations in the *ras* oncogene, which would normally be detected by cytotoxic lymphocytes, may escape immune surveillance. At the same time, these cells would have an adequate supply of oxygen and nutrients as well as clearance of waste metabolic products allowing another step in the stochastic progression towards malignancy to occur (Gjertsen *et al.*, 1997). Indeed, it is so important to maintain this environment that developing neoplastic cell clones evolve to mimic this state in order to progress and metastasise. This contention is supported by the fact that tumours secrete CMI immunosuppressive cytokines such as TGFβ and IL-10 (Kiessling *et al.*, 2000).

Again, induction of COX-2 may be central to the development of an angiogenic environment in many of the conditions leading to the subsequent development of malignancy. COX-2 expressing tumour cells are associated with the production of a number of angiogenic growth factors and the synthesis and activation of matrix metalloproteinases (MMPs), both of which favour tumour invasion and angiogenesis (Tsujii *et al.*, 1997; Tsujii *et al.*, 1998; Takahashi *et al.*, 1999). Cigarette smoke carcinogens, including the tobacco-specific carcinogen NNK (which reproducibly induces pulmonary adenocarcinomas in laboratory rodents) and nicotine are associated with COX-2 upregulation. NNK, which is a beta-adrenergic receptor agonist, does so by releasing arachidonate and nicotine acts through nicotinic acetylcholine receptors (Saareks *et al.*, 1998). Inhibition of COX-2 activity reduces IL-6 and IL-8 levels secreted by human cell lines further supporting the strong link between inflammation, HI cytokine expression and angiogenesis (Luca *et al.*, 1997; Salgado *et al.*, 1999; Hong *et al.*, 2000).

## 6. INFLAMMATION AND APOPTOSIS

Chronic inflammation also gives rise to the production of growth factors and cytokines, and the activation of intracellular cell survival pathways that would result in inhibition of apoptosis. An example of such a factor released during inflammatory states is macrophage inhibitory factor (MIF), which has recently been shown to repress the transcription activity of p53 and its downstream targets *p21* and *bax*, thereby having a marked anti-apoptotic effect (Cordon-Cardo and Prives, 1999; Hudson *et al.*, 1999). Experimental evidence indicates that p53 plays an important role in the mediation of Th-1 cytokine-induced cytotoxicity (Yeung and Lau, 1998; Das *et al.*, 1999; Kano *et al.*, 1999; Um *et al.*, 2000; Takagi *et al.*, 2000). p53 induces Transporter Associated with Antigen Processing (TAP) 1 expression through a p53-

responsive element. TAP1 is required for the MHC class I antigen presentation pathway. p73, which is homologous to p53, also induces TAP1 and cooperates with p53 to activate TAP1. Through the induction of TAP1, p53 enhances the transport of MHC class I peptides and expression of surface MHC-peptide complexes. p53 cooperates with IFN-$\gamma$ to activate the MHC class I pathway. These results indicate that, as part of their function as tumour suppressors, p53 and its homologue p73 may play a role in tumour surveillance (Zhu *et al.*, 1999). Therefore, inflammation is capable of inactivating one of the most important cell regulatory pathways controlling cancer development, reducing the effectiveness of the body's own cellular defense reaction to a mutation. p53 also has a key role in the regulation of angiogenesis, in part through induction of the anti-angiogenic factor thrombospondin (Dameron, 1994). Furthermore, mutations of p53 may result in induction of the synthesis of the most potent angiogenic agent known, VEGF, leading to increased angiogenesis (Kieser *et al.*, 1994; Volpert *et al.*, 1997). Therefore, loss of p53 would also result in an impaired CMI response, facilitate angiogenesis, and result in a loss of apoptotic activity. Mutations of the *ras* oncogene can induce IL-8 and induce stromal inflammation that can lead to cancer progression (Sparmann and Bar-Sagi, 2004).

There is thus increasing evidence that exposure to carcinogens, such as ultraviolet light (UV) (Athar *et al.*, 1989), the tobacco-specific carcinogen NNK (El-Bayoumy *et al.*, 1999), nicotine (Saareks *et al.*, 1998), *Helicobacter pylori* (Konturek *et al.*, 2000; Sawaoka *et al.*, 1998a) and colonic luminal contents, in particular the dihydroxy bile acids deoxycholate and chemodeoxycholate (Zhang *et al.*, 2000; Glinhammar *et al.*, 2001) all upregulate COX-2 in the affected tissue. In both non-neoplastic and neoplastic cells, COX-2 is associated with cell proliferation (Tsuji *et al.*, 1996; McGinty *et al.*, 2000) and inhibition of apoptosis, at least in part through the induction of *bcl-2* (Tsujii and DuBois, 1995).

The serine/threonine kinase Akt (protein kinase B) is activated in response to a variety of stimuli. This factor provides a survival signal that protects cells from apoptosis induced by growth factor withdrawal. Through the phosphorylation of specific targets such as Bad (del Peso *et al.*, 1997) and procaspase-9 (Cardone *et al.*, 1998), the Akt cell survival signalling pathway inhibits apoptosis. Some carcinogens act, at least in part, by inducing oxidative stress in exposed cells. Oxidative stress results in the activation of intracellular survival cell signalling pathways. In a variety of cell types, $H_2O_2$, an inducer of oxidative stress, has been shown to induce elevated Akt activity in a time- and dose-dependent manner by a mechanism involving phosphoinositide 3-kinase (PI3K). Inhibitors of PI3K activity, including wortmannin and LY294002, and expression of a dominant negative mutant of p85, a regulatory component of PI3K, inhibited $H_2O_2$

induced Akt activation. $H_2O_2$ treatment led to EGFR phosphorylation. Inhibition of EGFR activation blocked Akt activation suggesting that activation of the Akt pathway by $H_2O_2$ is dependent on EGFR activation. $H_2O_2$ induces apoptosis of HeLa cells, which is significantly enhanced by the Akt inhibitors wortmannin and LY294002. In contrast, expression of exogenous myristoylation-activated Akt, and constitutive expression of v-Akt, inhibit apoptosis of $H_2O_2$-treated NIH3T3 cells. These results suggest that $H_2O_2$ activates Akt via an EGFR/PI3-K-dependent pathway and that elevated Akt activity confers protection against oxidative stress-induced apoptosis (Wang *et al.*, 2000). In keeping with these observations, UV light exposure, which results in EGFR phosphorylation and activation of the Akt pathway in a variety of cell types, including keratinocytes, NIH fibroblasts and HC11 mouse mammary cells, has recently been demonstrated to induce $H_2O_2$ (Huang *et al.*, 1996; Peus *et al.*, 2000). Likewise, carcinogenic asbestos fibres have been demonstrated to induce EGFR phosphorylation, an effect blocked by N-acetyl cysteine (Faux *et al.*, 2000). A recent report suggests that EGF vaccinations in mice can decrease chronic inflammation with improving tissue healing (Casaco *et al.*, 2004).

EGFR activation may also result in COX-2 expression (Coffey *et al.*, 1997; Mestre *et al.*, 1999), although the pathways linking EGFR to induction remain to be fully elucidated. However, evidence is increasing for an important role for the transcription factor NF-κB. This transcription factor plays an important role in the regulation of a number of genes intrinsic to inflammation and cell proliferation (Thanos and Maniatis, 1995). EGFR phosphorylation activates the extracellular regulated kinase 1 and 2 (ERK1/2) and p38 signalling pathways (Peus *et al.*, 2000). PI3K/Akt activates the transcription factor NF-κB (Beraud *et al.*, 1999; Madrid *et al.*, 2001). Akt has recently been shown to target the transactivation function of NF-κB by stimulating the transactivation domain of the RelA/p65 subunit of the transcription factor. This appears to depend on IκB kinase β (IKKβ) activity. p38 is required for NF-κB transcriptional activity. Consistent with this, activated Akt has been shown to induce p38 activity (Madrid *et al.*, 2001). Carcinogenic asbestos fibres induce NF-κB activation in pleural mesothelial cells and this is linked to cell proliferation (Janssen *et al.*, 1997; Faux *et al.*, 2000). The selective EGFR tyrosine kinase inhibitor PKI166 (Novartis Pharmaceuticals) inhibits the DNA binding of NF-κB. PKI166 and NF-κB decoy proteins reduce cell viability thus showing the importance of this pathway in mesothelial cell survival following asbestos exposure (Faux *et al.*, 2001). A second member of the Erb family of type 1 tyrosine kinase receptors, HER-2/neu/c-ErbB-2, has also been demonstrated to induce NF-κB. HER-2 overexpression induces the transcription factor by a PI3K/Akt pathway which involves calpain-mediated IκBα degradation (Pianetti *et al.*,

2001). The NF-κB binding motif is found in the promoter region of the COX-2 gene (Du Bois *et al.*, 1998). In keeping with the important role of pro-inflammatory cytokines and angiogenic growth factors in the carcinogenic process, IL-1β and bFGF, combined with EGF, have been shown to enhance the induction of COX-2 (Majima *et al.* 1997; Yucel-Lindberg *et al.*, 1999). IL-1β induces p38 activity and this is dependent on Akt and IKK activation (Madrid *et al.*, 2001). Likewise, akin to HER-2 overexpression in breast cancer, NF-κB activation by IFN-α and -β involves degradation of IκBα (Yang *et al.*, 2001). Finally, Akt activation of NF-κB is involved in cell survival and resistance to apoptosis induced following exposure to TNF, similar to the situation seen with IL-1β and IFN-α and -β (Zhou *et al.*, 2000). These findings are in keeping with the observation that pro-inflammatory and Th-1 cytokines induce COX-2 expression.

Growth factors such as EGFR may protect against apoptosis through a number of other mechanisms. For example, in keratinocytes EGFR upregulates the expression of the anti-apoptotic factor Bcl-xL through the activation of a MEK-dependent pathway. Furthermore, activation of the PI3K/Akt and phospholipase Cγ/protein kinase Cα pathways is required for keratinocyte survival independent of EGFR activation or Bcl-xL expression (Jost *et al.*, 2001). In keeping with this are the observations that dihydroxy bile acids, promoters of gastrointestinal tract cancer, induce COX-2 transcription and a 10-fold increase in $PGE_2$ expression in human esophageal adenocarcinoma cells which is blocked by inhibitors of PKC. Furthermore, increased binding of the transcription factor AP-1, an inducer of COX-2 transcription, to DNA is also seen (Zhang *et al.*, 1999).

Therefore, as well as inducing a HI predominant immune response and angiogenesis, chronic immune activation may lead to inhibition of apoptosis in the affected cells. Carcinogen-induced reactive oxygen species and the formation of carcinogenic metabolites produced by the inflammatory process, e.g. malondialdehyde resulting from the metabolism of arachidonic acid by COX-2 (Subbaramaiah *et al.*, 1997), may lead directly to DNA damage and subsequent mutations. Under these circumstances, cells may transform, acquire mutations, proliferate and, through microenvironmental selection pressures (Pettit *et al.*, 2000), eventually take on a malignant phenotype through the development of cell clones, which themselves are capable of resisting apoptosis, suppressing CMI responses and inducing angiogenesis.

## 7.    THE BIOLOGY OF ONCOGENIC VIRUSES: IMPACT ON THE IMMUNE RESPONSE, ANGIOGENESIS AND APOPTOSIS

The data presented indicate that chronic immune activation may give rise to the prerequisite environment necessary for the development of malignant disease in predisposed individuals. This environment includes the presence of suppressed CMI, angiogenesis and growth factors which inhibit apoptosis. If such a postulate is true, one would expect that from a biological standpoint oncogenic viruses would have the capacity to induce identical environmental features.

As mentioned earlier, human papilloma virus (HPV) infection predisposes to cervical carcinoma and to a number of other malignancies, including anal, head and neck, and possibly oesophageal and lung cancer (Markham, 1996). HPV16 and 18 are the principal HPV subtypes associated with neoplastic disease. These produce the E6 and E7 proteins which inactivate the p53 and retinoblastoma (Rb) tumour suppressor proteins, respectively (Dalgleish, 1991). CMI responses are crucial to the pathogenesis of HPV infection. Regression of genital warts is characterised by a pronounced increase in Th-1 cells and macrophages associated with a localised delayed hypersensitivity response. A number of cytokines are secreted with IL-12 being present at very high levels. However, only recently has clear evidence accumulated that persistent HPV infection is associated with chronic immune activation. While over 25 percent of females are infected at ages 19-25, less than 5 percent remain infected over 35 years of age, suggesting that in a small but significant proportion of cases, the HPV infection persists. Whilst differences in methodology and sampling error may have explained these observations, a recent longitudinal study of HPV-infected patients, in which the virus was detected using the hybrid capture II assay, demonstrated that a proportion of patients found to have persistent infection after 2 to 3 assessments developed CIN. In contrast, those individuals found to have cleared the infection did not develop any CIN lesions (Clavel *et al.*, 2000). Failure to clear the viral infection results in persistent inflammation with chronic cervicitis and an increased cervical cancer risk (White *et al.*, 1992; Cerqueira *et al.*, 1998; Hsieh *et al.*, 1999). Increased levels of circulating IL-2 soluble receptor, a non-specific marker of inflammation, are seen in a proportion of otherwise normal infected individuals which rise significantly with the development of CIN and, subsequently, invasive cervical cancer (Hildesheim *et al.*, 1997; Ung *et al.*, 1999).

Resolution of HPV infection with clearance of the virus is associated with the development of a CMI response including an IgA antibody response

(Bontkes *et al.*, 1999). In addition, upregulation of IFN-γ in exfoliated cervical cells (Scott *et al.*, 1999), IL-2 Th-1 responses to the C-terminal domain of the HPV16 E2 protein and a hypersensitivity reaction to the HPV16 oncoprotein E7 is also seen. This hypersensitivity reaction is itself associated with the subsequent regression of CIN lesions (Hopfl *et al.*, 2000). In contrast, active CIN is associated with predominant Th-2 immune responses with an increased IL-10/IL-12 ratio seen in whole blood supernatants (Jacobs *et al.*, 1998). Furthermore, the density of IL-2 secreting cells is lower and that of IL-4 positive cells higher in high grade squamous epithelial lesions (CIN III) than in the transformation zone of healthy women with biopsies showing squamous metaplasia (al-Saleh *et al.*, 1998). Although cytotoxic T lymphocyte (CTL) responses have been difficult to detect in HPV-infected patients, CTL responses to E6/E7 proteins are more commonly seen in women with cervical HPV-16 infection without evidence of CIN than in HPV16 positive women with CIN (Sonnex, 1998). These results are supported by studies in women with cervical dysplasia, which have shown reduced lymphocyte Th1 immune responses to HPV16 L1 antigen and E6 and E7 peptides as compared to healthy adults (Luxton *et al.*, 1997). As CIN progresses to carcinoma-in-situ, the levels of $CD4^+$ and $CD3^+$ $DR^+$ antigen peripheral blood T-cells have been shown to decrease while the level of the $CD8^+$ cells increase (Spivak *et al.*, 1999).

More recently, microarray analysis has indicated that infection with HPV16 and 31 may result in downregulation of the response of IFN-inducible genes to IFN (Chang and Laimins, 2000; Nees *et al.*, 2001). In the case of HPV16 infection, the expression of multiple genes known to be inducible by NF-κB and AP-1 was seen. E6 protein increased the secretion of a number of factors including IL-8 and MIP-1α which themselves are capable of suppressing CMI responses, inducing angiogenesis and inhibiting apoptosis (Nees *et al.*, 2001).

Co-infection with chlamydiae may exacerbate the situation, the presence of both organisms being associated with increased proliferation and reduced apoptosis of the ectocervical epithelium (Vaganova, 2000; Antilla *et al.*, 2001). Furthermore, CIN develops in approximately 40 percent of women with HIV infection. A shift towards a Th2 T-cell cytokine profile is seen in biopsy specimens of normal cervix from HIV-positive women as compared to normal healthy controls consistent with the overall bias towards Th-2 responses in HIV-infected individuals (Olaitan *et al.*, 1998).

EBV is implicated in the pathogenesis of lymphomas and solid tumours. In Africa, EBV infection induced Burkitt's lymphoma (BL) arises in children whose immune system is chronically activated by malaria (de The, 1993). In keeping with this, EBV-associated nasopharyngeal cancer (NPC) occurs in China amongst people who are exposed to fish treated by a salt curing process, which may also cause local inflammation (Zheng *et al.*, 1994). Although the majority of the Western population is infected with EBV, only a minority develop associated malignancies, in particular, lymphomas (Yamamoto *et al.*, 1999; Mauray *et al.*, 2000). Other EBV-associated malignancies include squamous oesophageal (Wang *et al.*, 1999), gastric (Takada, 2000), and breast cancer where viral DNA is detected in up to 50 percent of cases studied as compared to normal breast tissue (Bonnet *et al.*, 1999). Although pre-existing chronic immune activation may not be readily apparent prior to the onset of these conditions, nonetheless, EBV gene products may provide the prerequisite environment earlier through the suppression of CMI, induction of angiogenesis, and inhibition of apoptosis. The factors produced by EBV viral DNA and detected in EBV-associated malignancies include the transforming gene product BARF1 (zur Hausen *et al.*, 2000), BHRF1 (Liu *et al.*, 2000), a homologue of the anti-apoptotic factor Bcl-2, EBV-encoded poly(A)(-) RNA which induces IL-10 (Kitagawa, et al. 2000) and EBV-encoded latent membrane protein 1 (LMP1), which activates the p38 mitogen-activated protein kinase pathway and has been demonstrated to coregulate IL-6 and IL-8 production (Eliopoulos *et al.*, 1999; Mauray *et al.*, 2000). EBV LMP1 protein expression has been demonstrated to correlate with the expression of the gelatinase MMP-9, and the presence of metastases in nasopharyngeal cancer (Horikawa *et al.*, 2000). Compared to control tissues, increased IL-1$\alpha$ and IL-1$\beta$ expression is seen in nasopharyngeal cancer which correlates with EBV-encoded viral IL-10 transcript (Huang *et al.*, 1999). This observation is in keeping with the crucial role induction of pro-inflammatory cytokines is postulated to play in carcinogenesis and the progression of malignant disease.

Simian virus-40 (SV-40) has been implicated in playing an important role in the pathogenesis of a number of malignancies including ependymomas, choroid plexus tumours, bone tumours, sarcomas and, in particular, mesothelioma. SV-40 oncoprotein large T antigen binds each of the retinoblastoma family proteins pRb, p107, and pRb2/p130 as well as p53 (Carbone *et al.*, 1999; De Luca *et al.*, 1997). Through these effects, the oncoprotein would facilitate angiogenesis, reduce Th1 cytokine-mediated cytotoxicity and inhibit apoptosis thereby predisposing the infected individual to the development of malignant tumours in infected tissues.

HBV and HCV do not cause cancer unless chronic inflammation occurs and then only after many years have passed (IIHCSG, 1998). Acute HBV and HCV infections require an effective CMI response in order to resolve. In contrast chronic, infection is associated with weak or undetectable CMI responses and/or a predominant Th2 response. The precore antigen (HBeAg), secreted in chronic hepatitis B, has been shown to deplete antihepatitis B-specific Th-1 cells, which are necessary for viral clearance, while enhancing Th-2 cytokine producing cells (Milich *et al.*, 1998). In hepatitis C, the activation of Th-2 responses plays a role in the development of chronicity (Tsai *et al.*, 1997). This shift to a Th-2 phenotype has been confirmed *in vitro* in cultured monocytes from patients with chronic HCV. When compared to normal controls, these monocytes respond to antigen stimulation by increasing the synthesis of the Th-2 cytokine IL-10, but not the Th-1 cytokine IL-12 (Kakumu *et al.*, 1997). Angiogenesis occurs in chronic hepatitis and cirrhosis of the liver induced by hepatitis B and C (Mazzanti *et al.*, 1997; El-Assal *et al.*, 1998). In keeping with this observation, plasma VEGF levels are elevated in chronic hepatitis and cirrhotic liver disease (Jinno *et al.*, 1998) and serum VEGF levels in patients with acute hepatitis as compared to healthy individuals (Akiyoshi *et al.*, 1998). Treatment of chronic HBV and HCV with the therapeutic Th-1 cytokines interferon-α and IL-12 results in varying degrees of clearance of viral particles from the liver and clinical remission (Cacciarelli *et al.*, 1996; Carreno and Quiroga, 1997). When successful, viral clearance is associated with a reduction in circulating IL-4, IL-6 and IL-10 Th-2 cytokine levels (Cacciarelli *et al.*, 1996; Malaguarnera *et al.*, 1997).

In conclusion, failure to clear human oncogenic viruses predisposes to the development of malignant disease through the creation of a HI-predominant, proangiogenic, anti-apoptotic environment which would favour the survival of transformed cells and be conducive to the development of malignant disease. This applies to those infectious states where chronic immune activation is not readily detectable in which non-viral oncogenes lead to transformation in a similar environment. The same may also be true for cancers associated with non-infectious carcinogenic insults, including cigarette smoking and asbestos exposure, which themselves often cause inflammation.

## 7.1 Features of tumours lacking an obvious pre-malignant inflammatory process

Although initially felt to be relevant to only a minority of cancers, our increased understanding of the environment induced by chronic infective or inflammatory conditions indicates that virtually all tumours, including those of the lung, oesophagus, colon and rectum may fit this model. A similar pattern of suppressed CMI, angiogenesis and inhibition of apoptosis is seen even in those tumours, such as melanoma and renal cell cancer, which initially do not appear to readily fit. For example, in melanoma, not only is there a clear genetic susceptibility to the disease (individuals with fair skin, freckles, ginger hair and a tendency to mole formation), but also a history of recurrent sunburn. Sunburn is associated with activation of the EGFR and PI3K pathway (Peus *et al.*, 2000), induction of COX-2 expression (Buckman *et al.*, 1998), angiogenesis in the affected tissue, and local and systemic suppression of the Th-1 immune response (Pamphilon *et al.*, 1991; Luca *et al.*, 1997). The development of renal cell cancer is associated, in the majority of cases, with mutations in the Von Hippel Landau tumour suppressor gene. These mutations are associated with upregulation of the angiogenic growth factor VEGF (Fleming, 1999). Experimental studies clearly demonstrate that VEGF, as well as inducing new microvessel formation, suppresses dendritic cell function, an important mediator of CMI (Gabrilovich *et al.*, 1999). More recently, kidney insults such as dehydration have been shown to be associated with the induction of COX-2. This may give rise to a HI predominant, CMI depressed, pro-angiogenic, anti-apoptotic local environment (Yang *et al.*, 1999).

Likewise, chronic immune activation has not been considered a cause for germ cell, breast and prostate tumours. Testicular cancer, a disease very sensitive to treatment with cytotoxic chemotherapeutic agents, with the majority of cases treated being cured, is increasing rapidly in incidence. The chemosensitivity appears to be related to the low incidence of p53 mutations. Although a specific carcinogen has not yet been identified, these germ cell tumours arise in an immunologically privileged site in which immune responses are suppressed (Guillou *et al.*, 1996).

The inflammatory components in endocrine tumours, such as breast and prostate cancer, may be more subtle than in non-endocrine tumours. This is because the endocrine system interacts directly with the immune response with Th-1 and DHEA steroids counter-regulating Th-2 and cortisol steroid pathways (Rook *et al.*, 1994). Nonetheless, epidemiological evidence exists that both breast and prostate cancer occur more frequently in the presence of chronic mastitis and prostatitis, respectively (Prince and Hildreth, 1986; Nakata *et al.*, 1993; Monson *et al.*, 1976). The role of inflammation in the pathogenesis of prostate cancer is supported by the observation that there is an increased risk of marker relapse in patients whose disease is found to have high grade inflammation surrounding malignant glands in the resected tumour following prostatectomy (Irani *et al.*, 1999). Therefore, it is somewhat surprising that a possible connection between prostatitis and prostate cancer has only rarely been discussed (De Marzo *et al.*, 1999). C-reactive protein is now recognised as being significantly associated with PSA and metastatic disease in prostate cancer (Lehrer *et al.*, 2005; Nelson *et al.*, 2004).

If the biological changes associated with chronic immune activation are essential for carcinogenesis (and these changes do seem to occur in non-inflammatory states which predispose to the subsequent development of malignant disease), it is logical to suppose that the majority of cancers may be amenable to modulation with combination therapies including CMI/Th-1-enhancing, anti-angiogenic, anti-inflammatory agents. In particular, this approach may be of particular benefit in cancer prevention and have a greater impact on cancer mortality than any other measure other than smoking cessation.

## 8. ENVIRONMENT CREATED BY NON-INFLAMMATORY FACTORS WHICH PREDISPOSE TO MALIGNANT DISEASE

Insulin-like growth factors (IGF) appear to have an important role in the initiation of malignant disease. High normal IGF-I levels are associated with the development of prostate and colorectal cancer, and with the development of breast cancer in pre-menopausal women (Hankinson *et al.*, 1998; Chan *et al.*, 1998; Ma *et al.*, 1999). Furthermore, there is evidence that the combined effects of IGF-I and mutagen sensitivity contribute significantly to lung cancer risk (Wu *et al.*, 2000). Recently, both IGF-I and IGF-II have been shown to play a role in the induction of COX-2 and $PGE_2$ in non-malignant and malignant cells (Di Popolo *et al.*, 2000). In keeping with this is the observation that IGF-mediated muscle cell survival is associated with the activation of Akt (Lawlor and Rotwein, 2000) and that IGF-I has been shown to be a pro-angiogenic factor stimulating endothelial cell proliferation and inducing the synthesis of VEGF (Akagi *et al.*, 1998; Dunn, 2000). In adrenocortical tumours, IGF-II has been shown to correlate with VEGF expression and to be inversely associated with the expression of the anti-angiogenic factor thrombospondin-1 (de Fraipont *et al.*, 2000). Moreover, there is increasing evidence to indicate that the IGF-I/IGF-IR system is upregulated by other angiogenic growth factors such as IL-6 and PDGF (Rubini *et al.*, 1994; Franchimont *et al.*, 1997).

Although IGF-I is a proliferative factor for inflammatory cells and plays an important role in maintaining normal immune function, under appropriate circumstances, the growth factor may act as an anti-inflammatory agent suppressing CMI responses to antigens and injury. For example, following experimental renal ischaemic injury, IGF-I therapy inhibits TNF and MHC expression as well as mild interstitial infiltrate normally seen in the affected kidney. IGF-I has also been shown to downregulate TNF serum levels in an *in vivo* sepsis model while overexpression of the IGF-IR protects cells against TNF-induced apoptosis (Wu *et al.*, 1996; Balteskard *et al.*, 1998).

Under normal conditions, IGF-I has been shown to upregulate p53 expression (Wang *et al.*, 1998). In situations where p53 is upregulated, the pro-apoptotic protein represses the transcription of IGF-IR thereby damping down the growth-promoting effects of IGF peptides (Webster *et al.*, 1996). p53 also induces the expression of IGF-binding protein (IGFBP)-3. IGFBP-3 not only antagonises IGF-I activity but is also capable of inducing apoptosis by modulating the expression of Bax and Bcl-2 and potentiating p53-independent radiation-induced apoptosis in human breast cancer cells (Butt *et al.*, 2000). However, in stress inducing conditions, there is evidence that IGF-I may induce the expression of Mdm2 and downregulate p53 thereby inhibiting apoptosis (Leri *et al.*, 1999). Furthermore, some mutations in the p53 protein appear to have the capacity to derepress the IGF-IR promoter leading to growth enhancement by locally produced or systemic IGF-I (Werner *et al.*, 1996).

In keeping with these observations, antisense IGF-I/IGF-IR therapies result in reduced tumour cell growth *in vitro*. They inhibit tumourigenicity and the induction of tumour regression *in vivo*, and result in an increased expression of MHC class I antigen and a tumour-specific immune response (Pass *et al.*, 1996; Lafarge-Frayssinet *et al.*, 1997; Ellouk-Achard *et al.*, 1998).

Obesity is associated with the development of malignant diseases, including breast, colon and prostate cancer (Moller *et al.*, 1994), and has been demonstrated to suppress lymphocyte function, mitogenesis and natural killer cell activity. T-lymphocyte responses to concanavalin A and B-lymphocyte responses to pokeweed mitogen are reduced (Moriguchi *et al.*, 1994). In rats receiving a high fat diet, the cigarette smoke carcinogen NNK induces increasingly high levels of COX-2 expression through progressive stages of lung tumourigenesis (El-Bayoumy *et al.*, 1999). Experiments in obese Zucker rats have shown that exercise restores natural killer cell activity and concanavalin A-induced splenic lymphocyte responses reversing the CMI suppression (Moriguchi *et al.*, 1998).

Long-term treatment with immunosuppressive therapy, using agents such as cyclosporine A following organ transplantation, is associated with an increased incidence of both virally and non-virally induced tumours (Penn, 1988; Nabel, 1999). Cyclosporin-A has recently been demonstrated to induce malignant cell proliferation, invasion and metastasis *in vitro* and/or *in vivo*. Evidence suggests the immunosuppressive agent acts by inducing the expression of functional TGF-β. TGF-β antibodies block the observed effects of cyclosporine-A on the cell lines tested (Hojo *et al.*, 1999). This is interesting as TGF-β may also induce apoptosis. Recent evidence indicates that COX-2 expression converts the apoptotic signalling normally induced by TGF-β to cell proliferation (Saha *et al.*, 1999; Roman *et al.*, 2001). TGF-β is also a potent inhibitor of CMI (Qin *et al.*, 1996; Meert *et al.*, 1996) inducing T-cell anergy (Jarnicki *et al.*, 1996) and directing the immune response towards a Th-2/HI phenotype (D'Orazio *et al.*, 1998). Depending on the environment, TGF-β has also been found to be pro-angiogenic and has been shown to induce the synthesis of VEGF by malignant cells (Pepper *et al.*, 1993). As discussed earlier, tumour-associated macrophages may play a role in tumour angiogenesis. TGF-β is a chemotactic for macrophages, and induces them to produce growth factors and proteases such as IL-6 and urokinase, respectively. These factors induce endothelial cell proliferation and breakdown of the extracellular matrix, respectively, thus facilitating new blood vessel formation (Wahl *et al.*, 1987; Bielefeldt-Ohmann *et al.*, 1996; Hildenbrand *et al.*, 1998). As such, cyclosporine A-induced TGF-β expression may result in the expression of all the essential environmental factors that we hypothesise are necessary for carcinogenesis and tumour development.

## 9. FRACTAL MATHEMATICS, CARCINOGENESIS AND THE PROGRESSION OF MALIGNANT DISEASE

The immune response and cellular control pathways are a complex system of interacting factors. As such, the factors involved in the development of cancer represent non-linear or chaotic processes, and are associated both with unpredictability, because there are too many forces acting on the system, as well as order, in that major attractors are present which are attempting to maintain the system (Coffey, 1998). The simplified concept of CMI and HI immune responses represent two attractors which are both self-regulatory with feedback pathways and are affected by certain outside forces such as chronic infections and non-infectious factors (Dalgleish, 1999).

The major regulatory pathway factors, including p53, p73, Rb and the Bcl-2 family, themselves major cellular policemen in their own right, may also be affected. Once significantly perturbed, further stochastic oncogenic effects can progress. The relevance of this concept is that treatments that return the attractors to normal may be able to have significant indirect anti-cancer activity if applied before the cancer has progressed too far. Therapeutic agents aimed at inducing a pre-dominant CMI response and inhibiting angiogenesis may move the disorder in the system away from tumour cell growth and progression towards inhibition of proliferation and, in some patients, tumour regression. Successful induction of a CMI, anti-angiogenic environment may be responsible for the tumour regressions seen in those patients with renal cell cancer and melanoma following non-specific vaccination with BCG and cytokine therapy using IL-2 and IFN-α (Dalgleish, 1999; Browning and Dalgleish, 1996; Vile *et al.*, 1996).

## 9.1     Implications for chemoprevention and future treatment of malignant disease

Non-steroidal anti-inflammatory drugs (NSAIDs) and specific COX-2 inhibitors inhibit solid malignant cell proliferation *in vitro*. Provided the disease overexpresses COX-2, these agents prevent haematogenous spread of malignancy, suppress angiogenesis and inhibit growth of tumour xenografts (Tsuji *et al.*, 1996; Hida *et al.*, 1998; Sawaoka *et al.*, 1998a; Sawaoka *et al.*, 1998b; Sawaoka *et al.*, 1999; Molina *et al.*, 1999; Tomozawa *et al.*, 1999). However, of greater relevance to the hypothesis that chronic immune activation plays a central role in carcinogenesis is the observation that inhibition of COX-2 activity inhibits carcinogenesis in animal models. Both non-specific COX inhibitors, such as indomethacin, and specific COX-2 inhibitors, such as celocoxib, may inhibit malignant transformation in a variety of experimental *in vivo* models including those for breast, colorectal, lung and skin cancer (Lala *et al.*, 1997; Taketo, 1998; Fischer *et al.*, 1999; Mestre *et al.*, 1999; Yao *et al.*, 2000).

There is already considerable evidence in the literature that long term exposure to aspirin and other NSAIDs reduces the incidence of oesophageal, gastric, colorectal, bladder and lung cancer (Thun and Namboodin, 1991; Giovannucci *et al.*, 1995; Study, 1992; Paganini-Hill, 1994; Giovannucci *et al.*, 1994; Funkhouser and Sharp, 1995; Schreinemachers and Everson, 1994; Castelao *et al.*, 2000; Langman *et al.*, 2000). The effect of aspirin on the inhibition of the COX enzymes and the resultant prostaglandin synthesis may be responsible for the chemoprevention. Inhibition of COX enzymes would prevent susceptible, transformed and/or dysplastic cells from inducing suppression of CMI, inducing angiogenesis and inhibiting apoptosis (Tsujii *et al.*, 1998; Taketo, 1998; Vane *et al.*, 1998; Subbaramaiah *et al.*, 1997; Grinwich and Plescia, 1977). Randomised placebo-controlled studies in thousands of people conducted over several years would be required to prove the efficacy of NSAIDs and selective COX-2 inhibitors in chemoprevention. Recent studies continue to support the hypothesis with randomised trials showing efficacy in reducing colon adenomas for aspirin (Baron *et al.*, 2003).

There is a need to identify individuals at high risk of developing malignant disease and reduce the 'promoter' exposure. Following the success of the Tamoxifen trials in reducing the incidence of breast cancer in an at-risk population, this approach should become a high priority in chemoprevention (reviewed in Savanthanan and O'Byrne, 2001). In the not-too-distant future, an increased understanding of the molecular pathogenesis of malignancies such as lung cancer may make it possible to identify those individuals at risk of developing the disease. In the absence of obvious factors, such as cigarettes, the reduction of inflammation, inhibition of angiogenesis, restoration of CMI and induction of an appropriate pro-apoptotic state should be primary goals. If successful, chemoprevention should decrease the number of patients requiring one-to-one treatment for malignant disease at a later time. Trials could test the relevant contribution of anti-inflammatory, anti-angiogenic and CMI immune stimulatory agents alone and in combination as chemopreventive and adjuvant therapies, and in the management of established inoperable/metastatic malignant disease.

## 9.2    Future Directions

It is only a few years ago that most researchers thought that the link between inflammation and cancer would only be relevant to colitis and colon cancer. It is now clear that many of the solid tumours are clearly linked to inflammation as a precursor. Recent data reports a strong link with B cell lymphomas (Elahi *et al.*, 2005) and even cancer of the pancreas is associated with a poor outcome if there is a systemic inflammatory response (Jamieson, 2005). Moreover, both breast and prostate cancers have been shown to be reduced with regular aspirin or NSAID medication (Swede *et al.*, 2005; Mahmud *et al.*, 2004). Whereas some studies cast doubt on the significance of anti-inflammation precaution in breast and prostate cancer, the majority support the association.

It would appear that multiple myeloma (MM) may emerge as one of the best examples of a chronic inflammatory malignancy. Not only is COX-2 frequently overexpressed in MM but it is an independent predictor of poor outcome (Ladetto *et al.*, 2005). The relevance of this has been recently highlighted by the highly significant effect of the Thalidomide analogue, Revelimid, in controlling metastatic myeloma, recently reported at ASCO 2005 (www.ASCO.com). Revelimid is a COX-2 inhibitor, an anti-angiogenic agent and a Th-1 immunostimulator, thus being one of the first new agents that impact on all three negative features of chronic inflammation (Bartlett *et al.*, 2004).

In addition to chemoprevention in high risk individuals, anti-inflammatory agents are now being used as the major anticancer therapy in some malignancies, such as MM, and are being added to standard chemotherapies/treatments in an attempt to improve the response and long-term outcome.

## 10.  ACKNOWLEDGEMENTS

Professor A. G. Dalgleish is supported by the Cancer Vaccine Institute, The Fischer Family Trust and Celgene, and Dr. Kenneth O'Byrne, by the Institute of Cancer Studies.

# 11. REFERENCES

Akagi Y. *et al.* (1998). Regulation of vascular endothelial growth factor expression in human colon cancer by insulin-like growth factor-I. *Cancer Res.* **58**: 4008-4014.

Akiyoshi, F. *et al.* (1998). Serum vascular endothelial growth factor levels in various liver diseases. *Dig. Dis. Sci.*: **43**: 41-45.

al-Saleh, W. *et al.* (1998). Correlation of T-helper secretory differentiation and types of antigen- presenting cells in squamous intraepithelial lesions of the uterine cervix. *J. Pathol.*: **184**: 283-290.

Anttila, T. *et al.* (2001). Serotypes of Chlamydia trachomatis and risk for development of cervical squamous cell carcinoma. *JAMA* **285**: 47-51.

Asselin-Paturel, C. *et al.* (1998). Quantative analysis of Th1, Th2 and TGF-beta 1 cytokine expression in tumour, TIL and PBL of non-small cell lung cancer patients. *Int. J. Cancer* **77**: 7-12.

Aziz, M. *et al.* (1998). Evaluation of cell-mediated immunity and circulating immune complexes as prognostic indicators in cancer patients. *Cancer Detect. Prev.* **22**: 87-99.

Baron, J.A. *et al.* (2003). A randomized trial of aspirin to prevent colorectal adenomas. *N. Engl. J. Med.* **348**: 891-899.

Bartlett, J.B. *et al.* (2004). The evolution of thalidomide and its IMiD derivatives as anticancer agents. *Nat. Rev. Cancer* **4**: 314-322.

Beraud, C. *et al.* (1999). Involvement of regulatory and catalytic subunits of phosphoinositide 3-kinase in NF-κB activation. *Proc. Natl Acad. Sci. U.S.A.* **96**: 429-434.

Bielefeldt-Ohmann, H. *et al.* (1996). Molecular pathobiology and immunology of malignant mesothelioma. *J. Pathol.* **178**: 369-378.

Bonnet, M. *et al.* (1999). Detection of Epstein-Barr virus in invasive breast cancers. *J. Natl Cancer Inst.* **91**: 1376-1381.

Bontkes, H.J. *et al.* (1999). Human papillomavirus type 16 E2-specific T-helper lymphocyte responses in patients with cervical intraepithelial neoplasia. *J. Gen. Virol.*: **80**: 2453-2459.

Brooks, L.A. *et al.* (1997). Kaposi's sarcoma-associated herpesvirus (KSHV)/human herpesvirus 8 (HHV8) - a new human tumour virus. *J. Pathol.* **182**: 262-265.

Browning, M.J. and Bodmer, W.F. (1992). MHC antigens and cancer: implications for T-cell surveillance. *Curr. Opin. Immunol.* **4**: 613-618.

Browning, M. and Dalgleish, A.G. (1996). 'Introduction and historical perspective' in *Tumour Immunology*, Sikora, K., Dalgleish, A.G. and Browning, M. (eds). Cambridge University Press, London.

Buckman, S.Y. *et al.* (1998). COX-2 expression is induced by UVB exposure in human skin: implications for the development of skin cancer. *Carcinogenesis* **19**: 723-729.

Butt, AJ. *et al.* (2000). Insulin-like growth factor-binding protein-3 modulates expression of Bax and Bcl-2 and potentiates p53-independent radiation-induced apoptosis in human breast cancer cells. *J. Biol. Chem.* **275**: 39174-39181.

Cacciarelli, T.V. *et al.* (1996). Immunoregulatory cytokines in chronic hepatitis C virus infection: pre- and posttreatment with interferon alpha. *Hepatology* **24**: 6-9.

Cainzos, M. (1989). Anergy in patients with gastric cancer. *Hepatogastroenterol.* **36**: 36-39.

Carbone, M. (1999). Simian virus 40 and human tumors: It is time to study mechanisms. *J. Cell. Biochem.* **76**: 189-193.

Cardone, M.H. *et al.* (1998). Regulation of cell death protease caspase-9 by phosphorylation. *Science* **282**: 1318-1321.

Carreno, V. and Quiroga, J.A. (1997). Biological properties of interleukin-12 and its therapeutic use in persistent hepatitis B virus and hepatitis C virus infection. *J. Viral. Hepatitis* **4** (Suppl. 2): 83-86.

Casaco, A. *et al.* (2004). Effect of an EGF-cancer vaccine on wound healing and inflammation models. *J. Surg. Res.* **122**:130-134.

Castelao, J.E. *et al.* (2000). Non-steroidal anti-inflammatory drugs and bladder cancer prevention. *Br. J. Cancer* **82**: 1364-1369.

Cerqueira, E.M. *et al.* (1998). Genetic damage in exfoliated cells of the uterine cervix. Association and interaction between cigarette smoking and progression to malignant transformation? *Acta Cytol.* **42**: 639-649.

Chan, J.M. *et al.* (1998). Plasma insulin-like growth factor-I and prostate cancer risk: a prospective study. *Science* **279**: 563-566.

Chang, Y.E. and Laimins, L.A. (2000). Microarray analysis identifies interferon-inducible genes and Stat-1 as major transcriptional targets of human papillomavirus type 31. *J Virol.* **74**: 4174-4182.

Chen, E.K. *et al.* (1998). Not just another meeting: the coming of age of JAKs and STATs. *Immunol. Today*, **19**: 338-341.

Chen, Y.M. *et al.* (1997). Cross regulation by IL-10 and IL-2/IL-12 of the helper T cells and the cytolytic activity of lymphocytes from malignant effusions of lung cancer patients. *Chest* **112**: 960-966.

Clavel, C. *et al.* (2000). Human papillomavirus detection by the hybrid capture II assay: a reliable test to select women with normal cervical smears at risk for developing cervical lesions. *Diagn. Mol. Pathol.* **9**: 145-150.

Coffey, D.S. (1998). Self-organization, complexity and chaos: the new biology for medicine. *Nat. Med.* **4**: 882-885.

Coffey, R.J. *et al.* (1997). Epidermal growth factor receptor activation induces nuclear targeting of cyclooxygenase-2, basolateral release of prostaglandins, and mitogenesis in polarizing colon cancer cells. *Proc. Natl Acad. Sci. U.S.A.* **94**: 657-662.

Cordon-Cardo, C. and Prives, C. (1999). At the crossroads of inflammation and tumorigenesis. *J. Exp. Med.* **190**: 1367-1370.

Dalgleish, A. (1999). The relevance of non-linear mathematics (chaos theory) to the treatment of cancer, the role of the immune response and the potential for vaccines. *QJM* **92**: 347-359.

Dalgleish, A.G. (1991). Viruses and cancer. *Br. Med. Bull.* **47**: 21-46.

Dameron, K.M. *et al.* (1994). The p53 tumor suppressor gene inhibits angiogenesis by stimulating the production of thrombospondin. *Cold Spring Harb. Symp. Quant. Biol.* **59**: 483-489.

Das, T. *et al.* (1999). Induction of cell proliferation and apoptosis: dependence on the dose of the inducer. *Biochem. Biophys. Res. Commun.* **260**: 105-110.

de Fraipont, F. *et al.* (2000). Expression of the angiogenesis markers vascular endothelial growth factor-A, thrombospondin-1, and platelet-derived endothelial cell growth factor in human sporadic adrenocortical tumors: correlation with genotypic alterations. *J. Clin. Endocrinol. Metab.* **85**: 4734-4741.

De Luca, A. *et al.* (1997). The retinoblastoma gene family pRb/p105, p107, pRb2/p130 and simian virus-40 large T-antigen in human mesotheliomas. *Nat. Med.* **3**: 913-916.

De Marzo, A.M. *et al.* (1999). New concepts in tissue specificity for prostate cancer and benign prostatic hyperplasia. *Urology* **53**: 29-39; discussion 39-42.

De The, G. (1993) The etiology of Burkitt's lymphoma and the history of shaken dogmas. *Blood Cells* **19**: 667-675.

de Visser, K.E. and Coussens, L.M. (2005). The interplay between innate and adaptive immunity regulates cancer development. *Cancer Immunol. Immunother.* in press.

de Visser, K,E. *et al.* (2005). De novo carcinogenesis promoted by chronic inflammation is B lymphocyte dependent. *Cancer Cell* **7**: 411-423.

del Peso, L. *et al.* (1997). Interleukin-3-induced phosphorylation of BAD through the protein kinase Akt. *Science* **278**: 687-689.

Della Bella, S. *et al.* (1997). Differential effects of cyclo-oxygenase pathway metabolites on cytokine production by T lymphocytes. *Prostaglandins Leukot. Essent. Fatty Acids* **56**: 177-184.

Di Popolo, A. *et al.* (2000). IGF-II/IGF-I receptor pathway up-regulates COX-2 mRNA expression and PGE2 synthesis in Caco-2 human colon carcinoma cells. *Oncogene* **19**: 5517-5524.

Doherty, P.C. *et al.* (1994). Evasion of host immune responses by tumours and viruses. *Ciba Found. Symp.* **187**: 245-256.

D'Orazio, T.J. and Niederkorn, J.Y. (1998). A novel role for TGF-beta and IL-10 in the induction of immune privilege. *J. Immunol.* **160**: 2089-2098.

Dunn, S.E. (2000). Insulin-like growth factor I stimulates angiogenesis and the production of vascular endothelial growth factor. *Growth Horm. IGF Res.* **10** Suppl A: S41-S42.

Dvorak, H.F. (1986).Tumors: wounds that do not heal. Similarities between tumor stroma generation and wound healing. *N. Engl. J. Med.* **315**:1650-1659.

Elahi, M.M. *et al.* (2005). The systemic inflammatory response predicts overall and cancer specific survival in patients with malignant lymphoma. *Med. Sci. Monit.* **11**: CR75-CR78.

Eliopoulos, A.G. *et al.* (1999). Activation of the p38 mitogen-activated protein kinase pathway by Epstein-Barr virus-encoded latent membrane protein 1 coregulates interleukin-6 and interleukin-8 production. *J. Biol. Chem.* **274**: 16085-16096.

Ellouk-Achard, S. *et al.* (1998) Induction of apoptosis in rat hepatocarcinoma cells by expression of IGF-I antisense c-DNA. *J. Hepatol.* **29**: 807-818.

El-Assal, O.N. *et al.* (1998). Clinical significance of microvessel density and vascular endothelial growth factor expression in hepatocellular carcinoma and surrounding liver: possible involvement of vascular endothelial growth factor in the angiogenesis of cirrhotic liver. *Hepatology* **27**: 1554-1562.

El-Bayoumy, K. *et al.* (1999). Increased expression of cyclooxygenase-2 in rat lung tumors induced by the tobacco-specific nitrosamine 4-(methylnitrosamino)-4-(3-pyridyl)-1-butanone: the impact of a high-fat diet. *Cancer Res.* **59**: 1400-1403.

Faux, S.P. *et al.* (2000). Increased expression of epidermal growth factor receptor in rat pleural mesothelial cells correlates with carcinogenicity of mineral fibres. *Carcinogenesis* **21**: 2275-2280.

Faux, S.P. *et al.* (2001). EGFR induced activation of NF-κB in mesothelial cells by asbestos is important in cell survival. *Proc. Am. Assoc. Cancer Res.* abstract 1315.

Ferre, F. *et al.* (1995). Viral load in peripheral blood mononuclear cells as surrogate for clinical progression. *J. Acquir. Immune Defic. Syndr. Hum. Retrovirol.* **10**: S51-S56.

Fischer, S.M. *et al.* (1999). Chemopreventive activity of celecoxib, a specific cyclooxygenase-2 inhibitor, and indomethacin against ultraviolet light-induced skin carcinogenesis. *Mol. Carcinog.* **25**: 231-240.

Fisseler-Eckhoff, A. *et al.* (1996). Neovascularisation in hyperplastic, metaplastic and potentially preneoplastic lesions of the bronchial mucosa. *Virchows Arch.* **429**: 95-100.

Fontanini, G. *et al.* (1996). Neoangiogenesis: a putative marker of malignancy in non-small cell lung cancer (NSCLC) development. *Int. J. Cancer* **67**: 615-619.

Fleming, S. (1999). Renal cancer genetics: von Hippel Lindau and other syndromes. *Int. J. Dev. Biol.* **43**: 469-471.

Folkman, J. (1995). Seminars in Medicine of the Beth Israel Hospital, Boston. Clinical applications of research on angiogenesis. *N. Engl. J. Med.* **333**: 1757-1763.

Forni, G. and Foa, R. (1996). 'The role of cytokines in tumor rejection' in Tumour Immunology: Immunotherapy and Cancer Vaccines. Dalgleish A.G. and Browning M (eds) Cambridge University Press: 199-218.

Franchimont, N. *et al.* (1997). Interleukin-6 with its soluble receptor enhances the expression of insulin-like growth factor-I in osteoblasts. *Endocrinology* **138**: 5248-5255.

Funkhouser, E.M. and Sharp, G.B. (1995). Aspirin and reduced risk of esophageal carcinoma. *Cancer*, **76**: 1116-1119.

Gabrilovich, D.I. *et al.* (1999). Antibodies to vascular endothelial growth factor enhance the efficacy of cancer immunotherapy by improving endogenous dendritic cell function. *Clin. Cancer Res.* **5**: 2963-2970.

Gallucci, R.M. *et al.* (2000). Impaired cutaneous wound healing in interleukin-6-deficient and immunosuppressed mice. *FASEB J.* **14**: 2525-2531.

Ganss, R. and Hanahan, D. (1998). Tumor microenvironment can restrict the effectiveness of activated antitumor lymphocytes. *Cancer Res.* **58**: 4673-4681.

Garrido, F. *et al.* (1993). Natural history of HLA expression during tumour development. *Immunol. Today* **14**: 491-499.

Giovannucci, E. *et al.* (1995). Aspirin and the risk of colorectal cancer in women. *N. Engl. J. Med.* **333**: 609-614.

Giovannucci, E. *et al.* (1994). Aspirin use and the risk for colorectal cancer and adenoma in male health professionals. *Ann. Intern. Med.* **121**: 241-246.

Gjertsen, M.K. *et al.* (1997). Cytotoxic CD4[+] and CD8[+] T lymphocytes, generated by mutant p21-ras (12Val) peptide vaccination of a patient, recognize 12Val-dependent nested epitopes present within the vaccine peptide and kill autologous tumour cells carrying this mutation. *Int. J. Cancer* **72**: 784-790.

Glinghammar, B. and Rafter, J. (2001). Colonic luminal contents induce cyclooxygenase 2 transcription in human colon carcinoma cells. *Gastroenterology* **120**: 401-410.

Gorter, A. and Meri, S. (1999). Immune evasion of tumor cells using membrane-bound complement regulatory proteins. *Immunol. Today* **20**: 576-582.

Grange, J.M. *et al.* (1995). Tuberculosis and cancer: parallels in host responses and therapeutic approaches? *Lancet* **345**: 1350-1352.

Greenberg, P.D. (1991). Adoptive T cell therapy of tumors: mechanisms operative in the recognition and elimination of tumor cells. *Adv. Immunol.* **49**: 281-355.

Grinwich, K.D. and Plescia, O.J. (1977). Tumor-mediated immunosuppression: prevention by inhibitors of prostaglandin synthesis. *Prostaglandins* **14**: 1175-1182.

Guillou, L. *et al.* (1996). Germ cell tumors of the testis overexpress wild-type p53. *Am. J. Pathol.* **149**: 1221-1228.

Hankinson, S.E. *et al.* (1998) Circulating concentrations of insulin-like growth factor-I and risk of breast cancer. *Lancet* **351**: 1393-1396.

Harris, R.E. *et al.* (2005). Aspirin, ibuprofen, and other non-steroidal anti-inflammatory drugs in cancer prevention: a critical review of non-selective COX-2 blockade. *Oncol. Rep.* **13**: 559-583.

Heeschen, C. *et al.* (2001). Nicotine stimulates angiogenesis and promotes tumor growth and atherosclerosis. *Nat. Med.* **7**: 775-777.

Heriot, A.G. *et al.* (2000). Reduction in cytokine production in colorectal cancer patients: association with stage and reversal by resection. *Br. J. Cancer* **82**: 1009-1012.

Hida, T. *et al.* (1998). Non-small cell lung cancer cycloxygenase activity and proliferation are inhibited by non-steroidal antiinflammatory drugs. *Anticancer Res.* **18**: 775-782.

Hildenbrand, R. *et al.* (1998). Transforming growth factor-beta stimulates urokinase expression in tumor-associated macrophages of the breast. *Lab Invest.* **78**: 59-71.

Hildesheim, A. *et al.* (1997). Immune activation in cervical neoplasia: cross-sectional association between plasma soluble interleukin 2 receptor levels and disease. *Cancer Epidemiol. Biomarkers Prevention* **6**: 807-813.

Hojo, M. *et al.* (1999). Cyclosporine induces cancer progression by a cell-autonomous mechanism. *Nature* **397**: 530-534.

Hong, S.H. *et al.* (2000). Cyclooxygenase regulates human oropharyngeal carcinomas via the proinflammatory cytokine IL-6: a general role for inflammation? *FASEB J.*, **14**: 1499-1507.

Hopfl, R. *et al.* (2000). Spontaneous regression of CIN and delayed-type hypersensitivity to HPV-16 oncoprotein E7. *Lancet* **356**: 1985-1986.

Horikawa, T. *et al.* (2000). Association of latent membrane protein 1 and matrix metalloproteinase 9 with metastasis in nasopharyngeal carcinoma. *Cancer* **89**: 715-723.

Hrouda, D. *et al.* (1998). Immunotherapy of advanced prostate cancer: a phase I/II trial using mycobacterium vaccae. *Br. J. Urol.* **82**: 568-573.

Hsieh, C.Y., You, S.L., Kao, C.L. and Chen, C.J. (1999). Reproductive and infectious risk factors for invasive cervical cancer in Taiwan. *Anticancer Res.* **19**: 4495-4500.

Hu, H.M. *et al.* (1998). Gene-modified tumor vaccine with therapeutic potential shifts tumor-specific T cell response from a type 2 to a type 1 cytokine profile. *J. Immunol.* **16**: 3033-3041.

Huang, M. *et al.* (1998). Non-small cell lung cancer cyclooxygenase-2-dependent regulation of cytokine balance in lymphocytes and macrophages: up-regulation of interleukin 10 and down-regulation of interleukin 12 production. *Cancer Res.* **58**: 1208-1216.

Huang, R.P. *et al.* (1996) UV activates growth factor receptors via reactive oxygen intermediates. *J. Cell Biol.* **133**: 211-220.

Huang, Y.T. *et al.* (1999). Profile of cytokine expression in nasopharyngeal carcinomas: a distinct expression of interleukin 1 in tumor and CD4$^+$ T cells. *Cancer Res.* **59**: 1599-1605.

Hudson, J.D. *et al.* (1999). A proinflammatory cytokine inhibits p53 tumor suppressor activity. *J. Exp. Med.* **190**: 1375-1382.

Igney, F.H. and Krammer, P.H. (2005). Tumor counterattack: fact or fiction? *Cancer Immunol. Immunother.* in press.

Irani, J. *et al.* (1999). High-grade inflammation in prostate cancer as a prognostic factor for biochemical recurrence after radical prostatectomy. Pathologist Multi Center Study Group. *Urology* **54**: 467-472.

Jacobs, N. *et al.* (1998). Inverse modulation of IL-10 and IL-12 in the blood of women with preneoplastic lesions of the uterine cervix. *Clin. Exp. Immunol.* **111**: 219-224.

Jamieson, N.B. *et al.* (2005). Systemic inflammatory response predicts outcome in patients undergoing resection for ductal adenocarcinoma head of pancreas. *Br. J. Cancer* **92**: 21-23.

Janssen, Y.M. *et al.* (2000). Asbestos causes translocation of p65 protein and increases NF-kappaB DNA binding activity in rat lung epithelial and pleural mesothelial cells. *Am. J. Pathol.* **151**: 389-401.

Jarnicki, A.G. *et al.* (1996). Altered CD3 chain and cytokine gene expression in tumor infiltrating T lymphocytes during the development of mesothelioma. *Cancer Lett.* **15**: 1-9.

Jinno, K. *et al.* (1998). Circulating vascular endothelial growth factor (VEGF) is a possible tumor marker for metastasis in human hepatocellular carcinoma. *J. Gastroenterol.* **33**: 376-382.

Johnston-Early, A. *et al.* (1983). Delayed hypersensitivity skin testing as a prognostic indicator in patients with small cell lung cancer. *Cancer* **52**: 1395-1400.

Jost, M. *et al.* (2001). Epidermal growth factor receptor-dependent control of keratinocyte survival and Bcl-xL expression through a MEK-dependent pathway. *J. Biol. Chem.* **276**: 6320-6326.

Kakumu, S. *et al.* (1997). Production of interleukins 10 and 12 by peripheral blood mononuclear cells (PBMC) in chronic hepatitis C virus (HCV) infection. *Clin. Exp. Immunol.* **108**: 138-143.

Kano, A. *et al.* (1999). IRF-1 is an essential mediator in IFN-gamma-induced cell cycle arrest and apoptosis of primary cultured hepatocytes. *Biochem. Biophys. Res. Commun.* **257**: 672-677.

Kaplan, M.H. *et al.* (1998). A signal transducer and activator of transcription (Stat)4-independent pathway for the development of T helper type 1 cells. *J. Exp. Med.* **188**: 1191-1196.

Keith, R.L. *et al.* (2000). Angiogenic squamous dysplasia in bronchi of individuals at high risk for lung cancer. *Clin. Cancer Res.* **6**: 1616-1625.

Kieser, A. *et al.* (1994). Mutant p53 potentiates protein kinase C induction of vascular endothelial growth factor expression. *Oncogene* **9**: 963-969.

Kiessling, R. *et al.* (2000). Have tumor cells learnt from microorganisms how to fool the immune system? Escape from immune surveillance of tumors and microorganisms: emerging mechanisms and shared strategies. *Mol. Med. Today* **6**: 344-346.

Kirk, G.R. and Clements, W.D. (1999). Crohn's disease and colorectal malignancy. *Int. J. Clin. Pract.* **53**: 314-315.

Kitagawa, N. *et al.* (2000). Epstein-Barr virus-encoded poly(A)(-) RNA supports Burkitt's lymphoma growth through interleukin-10 induction. *EMBO J.* **19**: 6742-50.

Kodelja, V. *et al.* (1997). Differences in angiogenic potential of classically vs alternatively activated macrophages. *Immunobiology* **197**: 478-493.

Konturek, S.J. *et al.*(2000). *Helicobacter pylori* infection delays healing of ischaemia-reperfusion induced gastric ulcerations: new animal model for studying pathogenesis and therapy of *H. pylori* infection. *Eur. J. Gastroenterol. Hepatol.* **12**: 1299-313.

Koshiba, T. *et al.* (1999). Immunohistochemical analysis of cyclooxygenase-2 expression in pancreatic tumors. *Int. J. Pancreatol.* **26**: 69-76.

Ladetto, M. *et al.* (2005). Cyclooxygenase-2 (COX-2) is frequently expressed in multiple myeloma and is an independent predictor of poor outcome. *Blood* **105**: 4784-91.

Lafarge-Frayssinet, C. *et al.* (1997). Antisense insulin-like growth factor I transferred into a rat hepatoma cell line inhibits tumorigenesis by modulating major histocompatibility complex I cell surface expression". *Cancer Gene Ther.* **4**: 276-285.

Lala, P.K. *et al.* (1997). Effects of chronic indomethacin therapy on the development and progression of spontaneous mammary tumors in C3H/HEJ mice. *Int. J. Cancer* **73**: 371-380.

Lang, J.M. *et al.* (1980). Delayed cutaneous hypersensitivity testing in untreated Hodgkin's disease using a standardised new device. *Biomedicine* **33**: 62-64.

Langman, M.J. *et al.* (2000). Effect of anti-inflammatory drugs on overall risk of common cancer: case-control study in general practice research database. *Br. Med. J.* **320**: 1642-1646.

Lawlor MA and Rotwein P. (2000). Insulin-like growth factor-mediated muscle cell survival: central roles for Akt and cyclin-dependent kinase inhibitor p21. *Mol. Cell Biol.* **20**: 8983-8995.

Lee, J. *et al.* (1998). Interleukin 2 expression by tumor cells alters both the immune response and the tumor microenvironment. *Cancer Res.* **58**: 1478-1485.

Lee, P.P. *et al.* (1997). T helper 2-dominant antilymphoma immune response is associated with fatal outcome. *Blood* **90**: 1611-1617.

Lehrer, S. *et al.* (2005). C-reactive protein is significantly associated with prostate-specific antigen and metastatic disease in prostate cancer. *BJU Int.* **95**: 961-962.

Leri, A. *et al.* (1999) "Insulin-like growth factor-1 induces Mdm2 and down-regulates p53, attenuating the myocyte renin-angiotensin system and stretch-mediated apoptosis. *Am. J. Pathol.* **154**: 567-580.

Liu, M.Y. *et al.* (2000). Expression of the Epstein-Barr virus BHRF1 gene, a homologue of Bcl-2, in nasopharyngeal carcinoma tissue. *J. Med. Virol.* **61**: 241-250.

Luca, M. *et al.* (1997). Expression of interleukin-8 by human melanoma cells up-regulates MMP-2 activity and increases tumor growth and metastasis. *Am. J. Pathol.* **151**: 1105-1113.

Luxton, J.C. *et al.* (1997). Serological and T-helper cell responses to human papillomavirus type 16 L1 in women with cervical dysplasia or cervical carcinoma and in healthy controls. *J. Gen. Virol.* **78**: 917-923.

Ma, J. *et al.* (1999). Prospective study of colorectal cancer risk in men and plasma levels of insulin-like growth factor (IGF)-I and IGF-binding protein-3. *J. Natl Cancer Inst.* **91**: 620-625.

Madrid, L.V. *et al.* (2001). Akt stimulates the transactivation potential of the RelA/p65 subunit of NF-{kappa}B through utilization of the IκB kinase and activation of the mitogen activated protein kinase p38. *J. Biol. Chem.* **276**: 18934-18940.

Mahmud, S. *et al.* (2004). Prostate cancer and use of nonsteroidal anti-inflammatory drugs: systematic review and meta-analysis. *Br. J. Cancer* **90**: 93-99.

Malaguarnera, M. *et al.* (1997). Serum interleukin 6 concentrations in chronic hepatitis C patients before and after interferon-alpha treatment. *Int. J. Clin. Pharmacol. Ther.* **35**: 385-388.

Maraveyas, A. *et al.* (1999). Possible improved survival of patients with stage IV AJCC melanoma receiving SRL 172 immunotherapy: correlation with induction of increased levels of intracellular interleukin-2 in peripheral blood lymphocytes. *Ann. Oncol.* **10**: 817-824.

Markham, A.F. (1996). Carcinoma of the lung: warts and all. *Thorax* **51**: 878-879.

Mauray, S. *et al.* (2000). Epstein-Barr virus-dependent lymphoproliferative disease: critical role of IL-6. *Eur. J. Immunol.* **30**: 2065-2073.

Mayne, S.T. *et al.* (1999). Previous lung disease and risk of lung cancer among men and women nonsmokers. *Am. J. Epidemiol.* **149**: 13-20.

Mazzanti, R. *et al.* (1997). Chronic viral hepatitis induced by hepatitis C but not hepatitis B virus infection correlates with increased liver angiogenesis *Hepatology* **25**: 229-234.

McGinty, A. *et al.* (2000). Cyclooxygenase-2 expression inhibits trophic withdrawal apoptosis in nerve growth factor-differentiated PC12 cells. *J. Biol. Chem.* **275**: 12095-12101.

Meert, K.L. *et al.* (1996). Elevated transforming growth factor-beta concentration correlates with post-trauma immunosuppression. *J. Trauma* **40**: 901-906.

Melief, C.J. and Kast, W.M. (1991). Cytotoxic T lymphocyte therapy of cancer and tumor escape mechanisms. *Semin. Cancer Biol.* **2**: 347-354.

Mestre, J.R. *et al.* (1999). Inhibition of cyclooxygenase-2 expression. An approach to preventing head and neck cancer. *Ann. N.Y. Acad. Sci.* **889**: 62-71.

Milich, D.R. *et al.* (1998). The secreted hepatitis B precore antigen can modulate the immune response to the nucleocapsid: a mechanism for persistence. *J. Immunol.* **160**: 2013-2021.

Mizoguchi, H. *et al.* (1992). Alterations in signal transduction molecules in T lymphocytes from tumor-bearing mice. *Science* **258**: 1795-1798.

Molina, M.A. *et al.* (1999). Increased cyclooxygenase-2 expression in human pancreatic carcinomas and cell lines: growth inhibition by nonsteroidal anti-inflammatory drugs. *Cancer Res.* **59**: 4356-4362.

Moller, H. *et al.* (1994). Obesity and cancer risk: a Danish record-linkage study. *Eur. J. Cancer* **30A**: 344-350.

Monson, R.R. *et al.* (1976). Chronic mastitis and carcinoma of the breast. *Lancet* **2**: 224-226.

Moore, R.J. *et al.* (1999). Mice deficient in tumor necrosis factor-alpha are resistant to skin carcinogenesis. *Nat. Med.* **5**: 828-831.

Moriguchi, S. *et al.* (1998). Exercise training restores decreased cellular immune functions in obese Zucker rats. *J. Appl. Physiol.* **84**: 311-317.

Mosmann, T.R. and Coffman, R.L. (1989). TH1 and TH2 cells: different patterns of lymphokine secretion lead to different functional properties. *Annu. Rev. Immunol.* **7**: 145-173.

Murata, H. *et al.* (1999). Cyclooxygenase-2 overexpression enhances lymphatic invasion and metastasis in human gastric carcinoma. *Am. J. Gastroenterol.* **94**: 451-455.

Nabel, G.J. (1999). A transformed view of cyclosporine. *Nature* **397**: 471-472.

Nakata, S. *et al.* (1993). Study of risk factors for prostatic cancer. *Hinyokika Kiyo* **39**: 1017-1024. Discussion: 1024-1025.

Nees, M. *et al.* (2001). Papillomavirus type 16 oncogenes downregulate expression of interferon-responsive genes and upregulate proliferation-associated and NF-kappaB-responsive genes in cervical keratinocytes. *J. Virol.* **75**: 4283-4296.

Nelson, W.G. *et al.* (2004). The role of inflammation in the pathogenesis of prostate cancer. *J. Urol.* **172**: S6-S11. Discussion: S11-S12.

O'Byrne, K.J. *et al.* (2000a). The relationship between angiogenesis and the immune response in carcinogenesis and the progression of malignant disease. *Eur. J. Cancer.* **36**: 151-169.

O'Byrne, K.J. *et al.* (2000b). Vascular endothelial growth factor, platelet-derived endothelial cell growth factor and angiogenesis in non-small cell lung cancer. *Br. J. Cancer* **82**: 1427-1432.

O'Hara, R.J. *et al.* (1998). Advanced colorectal cancer is associated with impaired interleukin 12 and enhanced interleukin 10 production. *Clin. Cancer Res.* **4**: 1943-1948.

O'Sullivan, G.C. *et al.* (1996). Regional immunosuppression in esophageal squamous cancer: evidence from functional studies with matched lymph nodes. *J. Immunol.* **157**: 4717-4720.

Oka, M. *et al.* (1992). Immunosuppression in patients with Barrett's esophagus. *Surgery* **112**: 11-17.

Olaitan, A. *et al.* (1998). Changes to the cytokine microenvironment in the genital tract mucosa of HIV⁺ women. *Clin. Exp. Immunol.* **112**: 100-104.

Paganini-Hill, A. (1994). Aspirin and the prevention of colorectal cancer: a review of the evidence. *Semin. Surg. Oncol.* **10**: 158-164.

Pamphilon, D.H. *et al.* (1991). Immunomodulation by ultraviolet light: clinical studies and biological effects. *Immunol. Today* **12**: 119-123.

Papadopoulos, E.B. *et al.* (1994). Infusions of donor leukocytes to treat Epstein-Barr virus-associated lymphoproliferative disorders after allogeneic bone marrow transplantation. *New Engl. J. Med.* **330**: 1185-1191.

Pass, H.I. *et al.* (1996). Inhibition of hamster mesothelioma tumorigenesis by an antisense expression plasmid to the insulin-like growth factor-I receptor. *Cancer Res.* **56**: 4044-4048.

Penn, I. (1988). Tumors of the immunocompromised patient. *Annu. Rev. Med.* **39**: 63-73.

Pepper, M.S. *et al.* (1993). Biphasic effect of transforming growth factor factor-beta 1 on in vitro angiogenesis. *Exp. Cell Res.* **204**: 356-363.

Pettit, S.J. *et al.* (2000). Immune selection in neoplasia: towards a microevolutionary model of cancer development. *Br. J. Cancer* **82**: 1900-1906.

Peus, D. *et al.* (2000). UVB-induced epidermal growth factor receptor phosphorylation is critical for downstream signaling and keratinocyte survival. *Photochem. Photobiol.* **72**: 135-140.

Pianetti, S. *et al.* (2001). Her-2/neu overexpression induces NF-kappaB via a PI3-kinase/Akt pathway involving calpein-mediated degradation of IkappaB-alpha that can be inhibited by the tumour suppressor PTEN. *Oncogene* **20**: 1287-1299.

Piccinni, M.P. *et al.* (1998). Defective production of both leukemia inhibitory factor and type 2 T-helper cytokines by decidual T cells in unexplained recurrent abortions. *Nat. Med.* **4**: 1020-1024.

Prince, M.M. and Hildreth, N.G. (1986). The influence of potential biases on the risk of breast tumors among women who received radiotherapy for acute postpartum mastitis. *J. Chronic. Dis.* **39**: 553-560.

Qin, L. *et al.* (1996). Gene transfer of transforming growth factor-beta 1 prolongs murine cardiac allograft survival by inhibiting cell mediated immunity. *Human. Gene Ther.* **7**: 1981-1988.

Richards, J.S. *et al.* (1995). Ovarian cell differentiation: a cascade of multiple hormones, cellular signals, and regulated genes. *Recent Prog. Horm. Res.* 50: 223-254.

Richtsmeier W.J. and Eisele, D. (1986). *In vivo* anergy reversal with cimetidine in patients with cancer. *Arch. Otolaryngol. Head and Neck Surg.* **112**: 1074-1077.

Roman, C. *et al.* (2001) TGF-beta and colorectal carcinogenesis. *Microsc. Res. Tech.* **52**: 450-457.

Rook, G.A. *et al.* (1994). Hormones, peripherally activated prohormones and regulation of the Th1/Th2 balance. *Immunol. Today* **15**: 301-303.

Rooney, C.M. *et al.* (1995). Use of gene-modified virus-specific T lymphocytes to control Epstein-Barr-virus-related lymphoproliferation. *Lancet* **345**: 9-13.

Rosenberg, S.A. *et al.* (1986). A new approach to the adoptive immunotherapy of cancer with tumor-infiltrating lymphocytes. *Science* **233**: 1318-1321.

Roses, D.F. *et al.* (1979). Malignant melanoma. Delayed hypersensitivity skin testing. *Arch. Surg.* **114**: 35-38.

Rubini, M. *et al.* (1994). Platelet-derived growth factor increases the activity of the promoter of the insulin-like growth factor-I (IGF-I) receptor gene. *Exp. Cell Res.* **211**: 374-379.

Saareks, V. *et al.* (1998). Nicotine stereoisomers and cotinine stimulate prostaglandin E2 but inhibit thromboxane B2 and leukotriene E4 synthesis in whole blood. *Eur. J. Pharmacol.* **353**: 87-92.

Saha, D. *et al.* (1999). Synergistic induction of cyclooxygenase-2 by transforming growth factor-beta1 and epidermal growth factor inhibits apoptosis in epithelial cells. *Neoplasia* **1**: 508-517.

Sairam, M. *et al.* (1998). Effect of hypobaric hypoxia on immune function in albino rats. *Int. J. Biometeorol.* **42**: 55-59.

Salgado, R. *et al.* (1999). Platelet number and interleukin-6 correlate with VEGF but not with bFGF serum levels of advanced cancer patients. *Br. J. Cancer* **80**: 892-897.

Salvadori, S. *et al.* (1994). Abnormal signal transduction by T cells of mice with parental tumors is not seen in mice bearing IL-2 secreting tumors. *J. Immunol.* **153**: 5176-5182.

Savanthanan, S. and O'Byrne, K.J. (2001). Antiestrogens. *J. Br. Meno. Soc.* **7**: 21-26.

Sawaoka, H. *et al.* (1998a). Helicobacter pylori infection induces cyclooxygenase-2 expression in human gastric mucosa. *Prostaglandins Leukot. Essent. Fatty Acids* **59**: 313-316.

Sawaoka, H. *et al.* (1998b). Cyclooxygenase-2 inhibitors suppress the growth of gastric cancer xenografts via induction of apoptosis in nude mice. *Am. J. Physiol.* **274**: G1061-G1067.

Sawaoka, H. *et al.* (1999). Cyclooxygenase inhibitors suppress angiogenesis and reduce tumor growth *in vivo*. *Lab. Invest.* **79**: 1469-1477.

Schaffer, M. and Barbul, A. (1998). Lymphocyte function in wound healing and following injury. *Br. J. Surg.* **85**: 444-460.

Schreinemachers, D.M. and Everson, R.B. (1994). Aspirin use and lung, colon, and breast cancer incidence in a prospective study. *Epidemiology* **5**: 138-146.

Schror, K. *et al.* (1998). Augmented myocardial ischaemia by nicotine - mechanisms and their possible significance. *Br. J. Pharmacol.* **125**: 79-86.

Singer, A.J. and Clark, R.A. (1999). Cutaneous wound healing. *N. Engl. J. Med.* **341**: 738-746.

Sonnex, C. (1998). Human papillomavirus infection with particular reference to genital disease. *J. Clin. Pathol.* **51**: 643-648.

Sparmann A. and Bar-Sagi D. (2005). Ras oncogene and inflammation: partners in crime. *Cell Cycle* **4** in press.

Spivak, M. *et al.* (1999). Interrelation of lymphocyte subpopulations in peripheral blood under cervical papillomavirus infection. *Folia Microbiol.* **44**: 721-725.

Strand, S. and Galle, P.R. (1998). Immune evasion by tumours: involvement of the CD95 (APO-1/Fas) system and its clinical implications. *Mol. Med. Today* **4**: 63-68.

Sredni, B. *et al.* (1996). Predominance of TH1 response in tumor-bearing mice and cancer patients treated with AS101. *J. Natl. Cancer Inst.* **88**: 1276-1284.

Study, C.P. (1992). The American Cancer Society Prospective Study. *Stat. Bull. Metrop. Insur. Co.* **73**: 21-29.

Subbaramaiah, K. *et al.* (1997). Inhibition of cyclooxygenase: a novel approach to cancer prevention. *Proc. Soc. Exp. Biol. Med.* **216**: 201-210.

Swede, H. *et al.* (2005). Association of regular aspirin use and breast cancer risk. *Oncology* **68**: 40-47.

Takagi, A. *et al.* (2000). The effect of Helicobacter pylori on cell proliferation and apoptosis in gastric epithelial cell lines. *Aliment. Pharmacol. Ther.* **14**: 188-192.

Takada, K. (2000). Epstein-Barr virus and gastric carcinoma. *Mol. Pathol.* **53**: 255-261.

Takahashi, Y. *et al.* (1999). Activation of matrix metalloproteinase-2 in human breast cancer cells overexpressing cyclooxygenase-1 or -2. *FEBS Lett.* **460**: 145-148.

Taketo, M.M. (1998). Cyclooxygenase-2 inhibitors in tumorigenesis (Part II). *J. Natl Cancer Inst.* **90**: 1609-1620.

Thanos, D. and Maniatis, T. (2000). NF-κB: a lesson in family values. *Cell* **80**: 529-532.

Thun, M.J. and Namboodin, M.M. (1991). Aspirin use and reduced risk of fatal colon cancer. *N. Eng. J. Med.* **325**: 1593-1596.

Tomozawa, S. *et al.* (1999). Inhibition of haematogenous metastasis of colon cancer in mice by a selective COX-2 inhibitor, JTE-522. *Br. J. Cancer.* **81**: 1274-1279.

Tsai, S.L. *et al.* (1997). Detection of type-2-like T-helper cells in hepatitis C virus infection: implications for hepatitis C virus chronicity. *Hepatology* **25**: 449 -458.

Tsuji, S. *et al.* (1996). Evidences for involvement of cyclooxygenase-2 in proliferation of two gastrointestinal cancer cell lines. *Prostaglandins Leukot. Essent. Fatty Acids* **55**: 179-183.

Tsujii, M. and DuBois, R.N. (1995). Alterations in cellular adhesion and apoptosis in epithelial cells overexpressing prostaglandin endoperoxide synthase 2. *Cell* **83**: 493-501.

Tsujii, M. *et al.* (1997). Cyclooxygenase-2 expression in human colon cancer cells increases metastatic potential. *Proc. Natl Acad. Sci. U.S.A.* **94**: 3336-3340.

Tsujii, M. *et al.* (1998). Cyclooxygenase regulates angiogenesis induced by colon cancer cells". *Cell*, **93**: 705-716.

Ung, A. *et al.* (1999). Soluble interleukin 2 receptor levels and cervical neoplasia: results from a population-based case-control study in Costa Rica. *Cancer Epidemiol. Biomarkers Prev.* **8**: 249-253.

Uotila, P. (1996). The role of cyclic AMP and oxygen intermediates in the inhibition of cellular immunity in cancer. *Cancer Immunol. Immunother.* **43**: 1-9.

Um, S.J. *et al.* (2000). Antiproliferative effects of retinoic acid/interferon in cervical carcinoma cell lines: cooperative growth suppression of IRF-1 and p53. *Int. J. Cancer* **85**: 416-423.

Vaganova, I.G. (2000). Apoptosis and proliferation of epithelial cells in papillomaviral and chlamydial cervicitis. *Vopr. Onkol.* **46**: 578-582.

Vainio, H. and Morgan, G. (1998). Cyclo-oxygenase 2 and breast cancer prevention. Non-steroidal anti-inflammatory agents are worth testing in breast cancer. *Br. Med. J.* **317**: 828.

Vane, J.R. *et al.* (1998). Cyclooxygenases 1 and 2. *Annu. Rev. Pharmacol. Toxicol.* **38**: 97-120.

Vile, R. *et al.* (1996). 'Tumour Vaccines' in *Immunotherapy in Cancer*. Gore, M. and Riches, P. (eds). Wiley, Chichester.

White, R. *et al.* (1988). Genetic alterations during colorectal-tumor development. *N. Engl. J. Med.* **319**: 525-32.

Volpert, O.V. *et al.* (1997). Sequential development of an angiogenic phenotype by human fibroblasts progressing to tumorigenicity. *Oncogene* **14**: 1495-1502.

Wahl, S.M. *et al.* (1987). Transforming growth factor type β induces monocyte chemotaxis and growth factor production. *Proc. Natl Acad. Sci. U.S.A.* **84**: 5788-5792.

Wallenius, V. *et al.* (2000). Normal pharmacologically-induced, but decreased regenerative liver growth in interleukin-6-deficient (IL-6(-/-) mice. *J. Hepatol.* **33**: 967-974.

Wang, L.S. *et al.* (1999). Detection of Epstein-Barr virus in esophageal squamous cell carcinoma in Taiwan. *Am. J. Gastroenterol.* **94**: 2834-2839.

Wang, P.H. *et al.* (1998). IGF-I induction of p53 requires activation of MAP kinase in cardiac muscle cells. *Biochem. Biophys. Res. Commun.* **245**: 912-917.

Wang, X. *et al.* (2000). Epidermal growth factor receptor-dependent Akt activation by oxidative stress enhances cell survival. *J. Biol. Chem.* **275**: 14624-14631.

Watanabe, M. *et al.* (1997). Regulation of local host-mediated anti-tumor mechanisms by cytokines: direct and indirect effects on leukocyte recruitment and angiogenesis. *Am. J. Pathol.* **150**: 1869-1880.

Webster, N.J. *et al.* (1996). Repression of the insulin receptor promoter by the tumor suppressor gene product p53: a possible mechanism for receptor overexpression in breast cancer. *Cancer Res.* **56**: 2781-2788.

Werner, H. *et al.* (1996). Wild-type and mutant p53 differentially regulate transcription of the insulin-like growth factor I receptor gene. *Proc. Natl Acad. Sci. U.S.A.* **93**: 8318-8323.

White, C.D. *et al.* (1992). Inflammatory cell infiltrate in the cervix as a predictor of residual cervical intraepithelial neoplasia after conization. *J. Reprod. Med.* **37**: 799-802.

Williams, M.P. and Pounder, R.E. (1999). *Helicobacter pylori*: from the benign to the malignant. *Am. J. Gastroenterol.* **94**: S11-S16.

Wolff, H. *et al.* (1998). Expression of cyclooxygenase-2 in human lung carcinoma. *Cancer Res.* **58**: 4997-5001.

Wu, X. *et al.* (2000). Joint effect of insulin-like growth factors and mutagen sensitivity in lung cancer risk. *J. Natl Cancer Inst.* **92**: 737-743.

Wu, Y. *et al.* (1996). Activation of the insulin-like growth factor-I receptor inhibits tumor necrosis factor-induced cell death. *J. Cell Physiol.* **168**: 499-509.

Yamamoto, T. *et al.* (1999). Epstein-Barr virus (EBV)-infected cells were frequently but dispersely detected in T-cell lymphomas of various types by in situ hybridization with an RNA probe specific to EBV-specific nuclear antigen 1. *Virus Res.* **65**: 43-55.

Yang, C.H. *et al.* (2001). IFNalpha/beta promotes cell survival by activating NF-kappaB through phosphatidyl inositol-3 kinase and Akt. *J. Biol. Chem.* **276**: 13756-13761.

Yang, T. *et al.* (1999). Regulation of cyclooxygenase-2 expression in renal medulla by tonicity in vivo and *in vitro. Am. J. Physiol.* **277**: F1-F9.

Yao, R. *et al.* (2000). Inhibition of COX-2 and induction of apoptosis: two determinants of nonsteroidal anti-inflammatory drugs' chemopreventive efficacies in mouse lung tumorigenesis. *Exp. Lung Res.* **26**: 731-742

Yeung, M.C. and Lau, A.S. (1998). Tumor suppressor p53 as a component of the tumor necrosis factor-induced, protein kinase PKR-mediated apoptotic pathway in human promonocytic U937 cells. *J. Biol. Chem.* **273**: 25198-25202.

Zea, A.H. *et al.* (1995). Alterations in T cell receptor and signal transduction molecules in melanoma patients. *Clin. Cancer Res.* **1**: 1327-1335.

Zhang, F. *et al.* (1999). Curcumin inhibits cyclooxygenase-2 transcription in bile acid- and phorbol ester-treated human gastrointestinal epithelial cells. *Carcinogenesis* **20**: 445-451.

Zheng, X. *et al.* (1994). Epstein-Barr virus infection, salted fish and nasopharyngeal carcinoma. A case control study in Southern China. *Acta Oncol.* **33**: 867-872.

Zhou, B.P. *et al.* (2000). HER-2/neu blocks tumour necrosis factor-induced apoptosis via the Akt/NF-κB pathway. *J. Biol. Chem.* **275**: 8027-8031.

Zhu, K. *et al.* (1999). p53 induces TAP1 and enhances the transport of MHC class I peptides. *Oncogene* **18**: 7740-7747.

zur Hausen, A. *et al.*(2000). Unique transcription pattern of Epstein-Barr virus (EBV) in EBV-carrying gastric adenocarcinomas: expression of the transforming BARF1 gene. *Cancer Res.* **60**: 2745-2748.

Chapter 2

# CHRONIC INFLAMMATION AND PATHOGENESIS OF GI AND PANCREATIC CANCERS

Lindsey Jackson[1] and B. Mark Evers[1, 2]
*[1]Department of Surgery and [2]The Sealy Center for Cancer Cell Biology*
*The University of Texas Medical Branch Galveston, Texas*

Abstract:    The pathogenesis of cancer represents a complex and multifactorial process requiring a number of acquired and genetic defects. It is becoming increasingly apparent that many cancers originate from a chronic inflammatory process. The topic of this review is the inflammatory response and development of gastrointestinal (GI) and pancreatic cancers. Here, we describe the development of various gastric colorectal and pancreatic cancers through an inflammatory process. The tumor microenvironment which predisposes to tissue destruction, subsequent attempts at healing and accumulation of cellular damage with loss of cell cycle control mechanisms is discussed. Components of the tumor microenvironment that are important in the final common pathway leading to cancer include the tumor stroma, tumor-associated macrophages, cytokines and chemokines and reactive oxygen and nitrogen species. Common signaling pathways that link inflammation with cancer are described and include the COX-2, NF-κB and phosphatidyl inositol 3-kinase (PI3K) pathways. Finally, therapies that can be directed to the inflammatory process as either treatment or prevention of these cancers will be discussed including novel inhibitors of signaling pathways which are currently in development.

Keywords:    inflammation; carcinogenesis; GI; pancreatitis; inflammatory bowel disease; reactive oxygen species; cytokines; COX-2; NF-κB; PI3K; Akt; PTEN

# 1.    INTRODUCTION

The link between chronic inflammation and cancer was first reported by the French surgeon Jean Nicholas Marjolin who, in 1828, described the occurrence of squamous cell carcinoma in a post-traumatic, chronically inflamed wound (Balkwill and Mantovani, 2001). In 1863, Rudolf Virchow identified leukocytes in tumor stroma and suggested that malignancy originated at sites of chronic inflammation, challenging the popular opinion that lymphoreticular infiltrate was simply a reaction to the neoplastic process (Balkwill and Mantovani, 2001). The clinical entity of a cancer arising from a chronic wound is now commonly referred to as a Marjolin's ulcer and can occur in the setting of burn injury, osteomyelitis, venous stasis ulceration, frost bite injury, chronic decubitus ulcers, gunshot wounds, occult trauma, and colostomy sites (Celik *et al.*, 2003). The time between the inciting inflammatory event and the development of cancer is typically 25-40 years but can occur as early as 14 years, with a latency period that is inversely proportional to the patient's age at the time of injury; thus, the younger the patient at the time of injury, the longer the latency period (Celik *et al.*, 2003). Cancer development can be prevented in this setting by early excision of burn wounds or ulcerations and skin grafting to the area. Although far more complicated than treating visible external wounds, perhaps successful elimination of chronic inflammation in other organ systems would have such a preventive effect.

The occurrence of cancers arising after prolonged inflammation has been described in other organs as well (Table 1). Many of these cancers are attributable to infectious, mechanical, or chemical agents that elicit a chronic immune response. For example, mesothelioma, a relatively uncommon form of lung cancer, is associated with asbestos exposure (mechanical agent), and hepatitis B and C infection has a well-defined relationship with the development of hepatocellular carcinoma. It is estimated that 15% of cancers worldwide (approximately 1.2 million cases) are attributable to infectious agents alone (Stoicov et al., 2004). Injury resulting from infections results in cellular proliferation and regeneration which would normally subside once the offending agent was removed or once the tissue was satisfactorily repaired. If the immune response fails to eliminate the inciting agent, proliferation continues in a microenvironment rich in cytokines, growth factors, and accumulating breakdown products of cellular function in a prolonged attempt to repair, often resulting in an accumulation of genetic errors and further inappropriate proliferation. Recent evidence implicates a role for such an inflammatory response in the development of gastrointestinal (GI) and pancreatic cancer, which is the focus of this review.

*Table 1.* Conditions associated with development of cancer

| Inciting agent | Associated cancer |
| --- | --- |
| Burn injury ⟶ | Marjolin's ulcer |
| Hepatitis B/C infection ⟶ | Hepatocellular carcinoma |
| HHV8 ⟶ | Kaposi's sarcoma |
| Papillomavirus ⟶ | Cervical cancer |
| Schistosomiasis ⟶ | Bladder cancer |
| Epstein-Barr virus ⟶ | Burkitt's lymphoma |
| Asbestosis ⟶ | Mesothelioma |
| Cigarette smoke ⟶ | Lung cancer |
| Hashimoto's thyroiditis ⟶ | Papillary cancer of thyroid |

# 2. INFLAMMATION IN GI AND PANCREATIC CANCER

## 2.1 Gastric cancer

While the overall incidence of gastric cancer in the United States has significantly decreased over the past 50 years, it remains the second most common cancer-related mortality in developing countries (Stoicov *et al.*, 2004). The single most identifiable factor contributing to the development of gastric adenocarcinoma is chronic infection with the bacterium *Helicobacter pylori* (*H. pylori*), which has led to its recent classification as a class I carcinogen by the World Health Organization (WHO) (Stoicov *et al.*, 2004). Case-controlled studies have estimated an approximate 2- to 17-fold increased risk of patients seropositive for *H. pylori* to develop gastric cancer when compared with seronegative patients (Stolte and Meining, 1998). A recent Japanese study demonstrated similar results in a cohort of 1,246 patients with documented *H. pylori* infection for approximately 7 years. Of these, 36 patients (3%) developed cancer; individuals with preexisting gastric ulcer or atrophy were at greatest risk (Uemura *et al.*, 2001).

Over half of the world's population is colonized by *H. pylori*, and yet only a small percentage of these individuals will develop gastric disease (Stoicov *et al.*, 2004; Stolte and Meining, 1998). Overall, 15-20% of patients with *H. pylori* infection will develop gastritis or gastric/peptic ulcer disease, while only approximately 1-3% will develop gastric adenocarcinoma or, rarely, non-Hodgkin (MALT) lymphoma of the stomach (Stoicov *et al.*, 2004; Stolte and Meining, 1998). It is apparent that a combination of factors, which may include bacterial virulence, host genetic, environmental and dietary factors, contributes to the risk of an individual infected with *H. pylori* to develop gastric carcinoma (Stolte and Meining, 1998; Correa, 2003). Such determinants of oncogenic outcome continue to be explored in an effort to identify those individuals at greatest risk for the development of gastric cancer as a result of infection and inflammation. A striking 80% of patients with adenocarcinoma of the stomach are seropositive for *H. pylori* (Stoicov *et al.*, 2004). It is important to distinguish between two histologically distinct forms of noncardia gastric cancer: an intestinal-type and diffuse-type adenocarcinoma. The diffuse type generally affects patients at a younger age and lacks a stepwise progression from premalignant lesion to malignancy. Thought to have a predominantly genetic basis, Parsonnet *et al.* (1991) found that only 32% of patients with this type of adenocarcinoma were *H. pylori* seropositive. The intestinal type generally involves the distal stomach. In contrast to the diffuse type, there is a clear transition from normal mucosa to atrophy, metaplasia, and, eventually, dysplasia, supporting the hypothesis that this form of noncardia gastric cancer arises from a background of chronic inflammation. It is this form most commonly associated with *H. pylori* infection, with approximately 89% seropositivity (Parsonnet *et al.* 1991).

Aggressive treatment of this infection was not initiated until the 1990's, so definitive long-term data on the prevention of gastric cancer by eradication of *H. pylori* is not yet available. However, several studies have shown promising results. Correa *et al.* (2000) performed a nonrandomized chemoprevention trial in a high risk population in Columbia. Individuals received anti-*H. pylori* triple therapy and/or dietary supplementation with ascorbic acid, β-carotene, or placebo; gastric biopsies were performed over a 6-year period. Statistically significant regression of intestinal metaplasia and nonmetaplastic atrophy and prevention of progression was noted in those who underwent triple therapy. Uemura *et al.* (1997) reported that *H. pylori* seropositive patients who underwent early gastric cancer resection with subsequent eradication of the infection demonstrated no recurrence during the 2-year follow-up period, while in a similar group of patients with persistent *H. pylori* infection, almost 9% developed a secondary cancer, further supporting the role of *H. pylori* treatment in gastric cancer prevention. Treatment of *H. pylori* infection is currently reserved only for those with symptomatic dyspepsia or those with confirmed gastritis or peptic ulcer disease, since these individuals are at greatest risk for the development of gastric cancer.

## 2.2       Pancreatic cancer

Pancreatic cancer, the fourth leading cause of cancer death in the US, remains the deadliest of all GI malignancies with an overall five-year survival rate of less than 3% (Farrow *et al.*, 2004; Shi *et al.*, 1999). The propensity for early invasion of local structures and rapid growth contribute to its lethality. Current research and epidemiology indicate a correlation between chronic pancreatitis and the subsequent development of pancreatic cancer, with cancer risk increased 10- to 20-fold in this population (Farrow and Evers, 2002). Hereditary pancreatitis, a rare form of pancreatitis accounting for <1% of all cases, causes wide-spread inflammation and fibrosis affecting the entire organ and is associated with a 53-fold greater risk for cancer development in affected individuals as compared with normal subjects, further supporting such a correlation (Farrow and Evers, 2002).

A large international, multicenter cohort study published in 1993 recruited 1,552 patients from 1946-1989 who fulfilled the diagnostic criteria for chronic pancreatitis and were deemed free of pancreatic cancer for at least 2 years after diagnosis (Lowenfels *et al.*, 1993). Of these subjects, 29 (21 male and 8 female) had evidence of pancreatic cancer two or more years after the diagnosis of pancreatitis was made. The expected number of patients with pancreatic cancer, when adjusted for location, age, and sex was approximately 2, a 17-fold greater incidence in this population with chronic pancreatitis. The effects of several variables on the risk of pancreatic cancer development were compared, including demographic (age, sex, nationality), clinical (comorbidities), and lifestyle variables (smoking, alcohol use), with the only statistically significant predictor proving to be advanced age. This confirmed that the etiology of pancreatic cancer in these individuals was likely the underlying chronic pancreatic inflammation.

## 2.3       Colorectal cancer

Inflammatory bowel disease (IBD), including both ulcerative colitis (UC) and Crohn's disease, has a well established association with the development of colorectal cancer (CRC). In contrast to conditions such as familial adenomatous polyposis (FAP) and hereditary nonpolyposis colorectal cancer (HNPCC), which have a well-defined genetic basis and follow an "adenoma-carcinoma" sequence of development, it appears that chronic inflammation predisposes to the development of CRC in the setting of IBD, following an "inflammation-dysplasia-carcinoma" model (Itzkowitz and Yio, 2004; Lichtenstein, 2002). This is supported by the fact that: 1) anti-inflammatory agents decrease the risk of developing CRC in IBD patients, 2) the risk of

CRC increases with duration of illness, 3) the risk of CRC increases with severity of inflammation, 4) the risk of CRC increases in those patients who demonstrate other inflammatory manifestations of IBD, such as primary sclerosing cholangitis (Itzkowitz and Yio, 2004). Other differences in colorectal cancer development in patients with IBD include a younger age at tumor development, mucinous or signet ring histology, higher incidence of two or more primary tumors, and a more proximal distribution of tumors (Itzkowitz and Yio, 2004).

A large meta-analysis by Eaden *et al.* (2001) identified 116 published studies dating from 1925 that reported incidence of CRC occurring in patients with UC. From these pooled results, they calculated the cumulative probability of a patient with UC to develop cancer by decade of disease, and found incidence rates to be 2% by 10 years, 8% by 20 years, and 18% by 30 years of disease. This approximates the risk cited in a review by Itzkowitz and Yio (Itzkowitz and Yio, 2004), who reported a relative increase in tumor incidence of 0.5-1% per year after seven years of disease. Therefore, patients with UC duration greater than 10 years are at a 20- to 30-fold greater risk of CRC development than the general population (Eaden *et al.*, 2001; Cotran *et al.*, 1999). These estimates likely underestimate true risk as they exclude patients at greatest risk for the development of CRC, since those with the most severe, extensive colitis generally undergo early colectomy.

## 3.     CHRONIC INFLAMMATION AND THE TUMOR MICROENVIRONMENT

The chronic inflammatory response represents a fine balance between active inflammation, repair, and destruction that occurs in response to a persistent stimulus over a prolonged period of time. Activation of leukocytes in response to such an ongoing stimulus leads to the production of chemokines, cytokines, and reactive oxygen species (ROS), resulting in accumulated tissue destruction and subsequent attempts at healing via remodeling, angiogenesis, and connective tissue replacement. Accumulation of cellular damage with loss of cell cycle control mechanisms is thought to be the final common pathway leading to tumor initiation (Balkwill and Mantovani, 2001; Coussens and Werb, 2002).

### 3.1     Chronic inflammation and tumor stroma

Tumor stroma is far more likely to contribute to tumor growth, invasion, and immunosuppression than it is to mount an effective anti-tumor response. Pancreatic, gastric, and colorectal cancer stroma all share the common composition of macrophages, dendritic cells, lymphocytes, fibroblasts, connective tissue, and a fibrin-gel matrix. Farrow *et al.*(2004) compared the inflammatory components of chronic pancreatitis to the tumor stroma associated with pancreatic adenocarcinoma, and subsequently utilized laser-capture microdissection (LCM) to separate stroma from tumor for further analysis. The fibrotic stroma which forms in chronic pancreatitis strongly resembles pancreatic cancer histologically, composed of proliferating fibroblasts, inflammatory cells, and cytokines; only by comparing patterns of gene expression are differences appreciated. Mediators of tumor growth and invasion, such as cyclin E1, the calcium-binding protein S100A4, matrix metalloproteinase 2 (MMP-2), and epidermal growth factor (EGF) were found to be more highly expressed in pancreatic tumor stroma than in chronic pancreatitis. Upon separation of tumor from surrounding stroma, immunohistochemistry demonstrated that while the expression of EGF was higher in the tumor stroma, EGF receptor (EGFR) expression was higher on tumor cells. This suggests a mitogenic relationship between stroma and adjacent tumor, one in which the stroma provides the growing tumor with growth factors and invasion-promoting proteinases. Additionally, NF-κB, a transcription factor whose products regulate oncogenesis, inflammation, and apoptosis, and its activator, IκB kinase, were elevated in both chronic pancreatitis and tumor samples, with staining localized predominantly to either ductal or acinar cells or tumor cells. Upregulation of this protein occurs in response to factors produced by the chronic pancreatitis or tumor stroma, such as IL-8 (9-fold increased expression in chronic pancreatitis as compared to normal tissue) or tumor necrosis factor α (TNF-α), which provides additional evidence for the existence of a mitogenic relationship.

### 3.1.1   Tumor-associated macrophages

Of the stromal elements, the tumor-associated macrophages are the chief effectors of chronic inflammation in the pathogenesis of pancreatic, gastric, and colon cancer, which produce a large array of inflammatory mediators (Table 2). These inflammatory mediators include growth and angiogenic factors (PDGF, TGF-β, EGF), cytokines and chemokines (IL-1, IL-8, and TNF-α), proteolytic enzymes that degrade the extracellular matrix, promoting invasiveness (proteases, elastase, collagenase, hydrolases, phosphatases, matrix metalloproteinase-9 (MMP-9), and lipases), and cytotoxic agents which likely contribute to host cell genomic damage and promote carcinogenesis (ROS, hydrogen peroxide ($H_2O_2$), nitric oxide) (Balkwill and Mantovani, 2001; Coussens and Werb, 2002; Mantovani *et al.*, 1992). Macrophages also produce migration inhibitory factor (MIF), which contributes to mononuclear cell immobilization at the site of active, chronic inflammation; however, MIF also has the dual role of suppressing transcriptional activation of the tumor suppressor gene p53, which may also contribute to carcinogenesis (Balkwill and Mantovani, 2001; Farrow and Evers, 2002; Coussens and Werb, 2002). $H_2O_2$, a byproduct of macrophage activation, has the ability to activate NF-κB by displacing its inhibitor IκB, leading to translocation of the transcription factor to the nucleus, where it drives the expression of genes regulating inflammation and cell survival, as described in the next section (Farrow and Evers, 2002). TNF-α also activates the NF-κB complex, effectively inhibiting apoptosis (Farrow and Evers, 2002).

*Table 2.* Mechanisms by which macrophages contribute to tumorigenesis

| | |
|---|---|
| A. | Direct DNA damage: reactive oxygen species (ROS) |
| B. | Bypassing p53, leading to inappropriate cell survival: macrophage inhibiting factor (MIF) |
| C. | Growth and survival factors: IL-1, IL-6, IL-8, TNF-α |
| D. | Angiogenesis: TNF-α, IL-1, and IL-6 associated with vascular endothelial growth factor (VEGF) production; transforming growth factor-β1 (TGF-β1), nitric oxide (NO) |
| E. | Increased microvascular permeability |
| F. | Invasion and metastasis: proteases, MMP-9 allow direct invasion; TNF-α and IL-1 augment expression of adhesion molecules on endothelial cells |
| G. | Subversion of immunity: IL-10 and TGF-β are immunosuppressive |

### 3.1.2 Cytokines and chemokines

TNF-α, IL-1, and IL-6, produced by activated leukocytes, are major mediators of inflammation and tumorigenesis (Cotran *et al.*, 1999; McCawley and Matrisian, 2001; Dvorak, 1986). Together they induce production of adhesion molecules, growth factors, eicosanoids, nitric oxide, chemotactic and angiogenic factors such as VEGF, and are capable of NF-κB and PI3K pathway activation, thus supporting tumor initiation, growth, and invasion. Receptors are found both on stromal elements and tumor cells, suggesting both autocrine and paracrine local effects (Balkwill and Mantovani, 2001; Farrow *et al.*, 2004). Direct evidence for the vital role of TNF-α in tumor development was recently reported in two independent studies (Suganuma *et al.*, 1999; Moore *et al.*, 1999) which found that TNF-α deficient mice were resistant to skin carcinogenesis. In a mouse model of melanoma, treatment with an IL-1 receptor antagonist significantly decreased tumor growth, and mice deficient in IL-1β were resistant to tumor metastasis (Vidal-Vanaclocha *et al.* 2000). Another study found that IL-6 deficient mice were resistant to chronic inflammation and neoplasia formation in response to intraperitoneal mineral oil injection (Tricot, 2000). The CXC chemokine IL-8 has recently been explored as an important growth and angiogenic factor for pancreatic, gastric, and colorectal tumors. Shi *et al.* (1999) confirmed that inhibition of IL-8 with antisense oligonucleotide *in vivo* suppressed pancreatic tumor growth and metastasis, while increased IL-8 expression increased tumor growth and metastasis.

### 3.1.3     Reactive oxygen and nitrogen species

Neoplasia developing in the setting of chronic inflammation is a multi-hit process, resulting from the accumulation of genetic mutations. These mutations may largely be due to the effects of ROS such as superoxide anions, $H_2O_2$, hydroxyl and hydroperoxyl radicals, and reactive nitrogen species such as NO, peroxynitrite, nitrogen dioxide, and nitrosoperoxy carbonate, collectively known as reactive oxygen and nitrogen species (RONS), that are elaborated by activated inflammatory cells (Stoicov *et al.* 2004; Gasche *et al.* 2001). The toxic effects of RONS include DNA strand breaks, mismatches, mutations, and the formation of adducts with DNA, such as nitrotyrosine (Farrow and Evers, 2002; Hussain *et al.*, 2000). NO is also responsible for the nitrosylation and nitosation of proteins involved in apoptosis, such as caspases-3, -8, and -9, resulting in inactivation and prevention of cell death in response to injury.

To further support the role of RONS in carcinogenesis, Hussain *et al.* (2000) compared the spectrum of p53 mutations in biopsies taken from inflamed and non-inflamed, non-neoplastic colonic mucosa of UC patients to normal, age-matched controls. They noted that greater than half of the inflamed mucosal samples demonstrated p53 mutations that were associated with a concurrent increase in NO synthase-2 (NOS-2) activity, suggesting that oxidative stress was a major contributor. They also noted an increase in post-translational modifications of p53 associated with elevated NOS activity in inflamed samples. Such mutations were not present in non-inflamed mucosal samples. Another study by Gasche *et al* (2001) examining the effects of $H_2O_2$ on *in vitro* colon cancer cell lines demonstrated that $H_2O_2$ was capable of damaging the protein complexes responsible for DNA mismatch repair, resulting in inactivation. With higher concentrations of $H_2O_2$, they also demonstrated the presence of frameshift mutations within previously normal mismatch repair genes.

# 4. CELL SIGNALING PATHWAYS THAT LINK INFLAMMATION WITH CANCER

Many derangements in cell signaling occur during the transformation of a normal cell to a malignant phenotype. It is useful to identify cell signaling pathways which may inhibit apoptosis and promote tumor growth which are similarly upregulated in multiple cancer cell lines. Three prominent pathways include the COX-2, NF-κB, and PI3K pathways.

## 4.1 COX-2

Cyclooxygenase (COX), also known as prostaglandin G/H synthase, is the rate-limiting enzyme catalyzing the conversion of arachidonic acid to a variety of inflammatory and physiological mediators, including prostaglandins and thromboxane (Fig. 1). Two isoforms of this enzyme exist which vary in tissue distribution and expression patterns. COX-1 is constitutively expressed in most tissues, and its products regulate homeostatic processes such as platelet function and gastric cytoprotection (Bing *et al.*, 2001; Sheng *et al.*, 1997). In contrast, COX-2 belongs to a class of genes known as immediate early or early growth response genes inducible by inflammatory cytokines and growth factors, including IL-1 and TNF-α, and its products are predominantly pro-inflammatory prostaglandins and eicosanoids involved in regulation of the immune response (Sheng *et al.*, 1997).

COX-2 is not normally expressed in the human intestine, but its activity is significantly elevated in the majority of human colorectal, pancreatic, gastric and other non-GI cancers. A significant and early COX-2 overexpression is associated with UC, both in inflamed and noninflamed mucosa, and with UC-associated dysplasia and neoplasia (Agoff *et al.*, 2000). Similarly, pancreatitis is associated with increased COX-2 expression, and selective genetic deletion of COX-2 or inhibition of its activity significantly reduces the effect of cerulein in the induction of acute pancreatitis and associated acute lung injury in mouse models (Ethridge *et al.*, 2002a). This has led to interest in defining its specific mechanism of action in chronic inflammation and neoplasia to determine if its inhibition may act as an adjunct to current chemotherapy. Large epidemiologic studies have demonstrated a 30-50% reduction in adenomatous polyp formation, incident disease, and death from colorectal cancer by inhibiting COX-2 activity with nonsteroidal anti-inflammatory medications (NSAIDs) (Thun *et al.*, 2002).

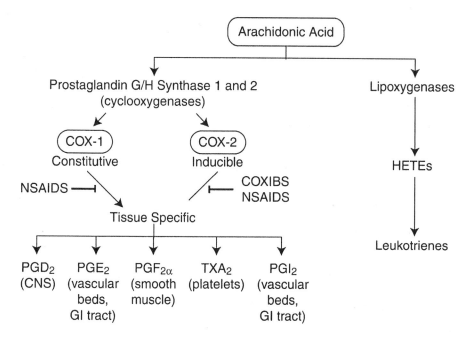

*Figure 1.* Arachidonic acid metabolism and the role of COX-1 and COX-2. Tissues of major prostaglandin expression are indicated in parenthesis. $PGD_2$ = prostaglandin $D_2$; $PGE_2$ = prostaglandin $E_2$; $PGF_{2\alpha}$ = prostaglandin $F2_{2\alpha}$; $TXA_2$ = thromboxane $A_2$; $PGI_2$ = prostaglandin $I_2$, HETE = hydroxyeicosatetraenoic acid

Several mechanisms linking COX-2 overexpression to tumor initiation and progression have been proposed. Two prostaglandin products of COX-2 activity, $PGE_2$ and $PGI_2$, possess angiogenic activity, and are thus believed to support tumor growth and extension. This is supported by the fact that when human or rodent colorectal cancer cells are cocultured with vascular endothelial cells and treated with selective COX-2 inhibitors *in vitro*, migration and tube formation by the endothelial cells can be inhibited (Thun *et al.*, 2002). Agoff *et al.* (2000) suggest two additional mechanisms by which COX-2 activation may promote tumorigenesis - a resultant increase in the derivative malondialdehyde and an up-regulation of the antiapoptotic protein Bcl-2. Malondialdehyde, a genotoxic byproduct of COX-mediated lipid peroxidation and prostaglandin synthesis, has been detected in both sporadic colon cancer and inflammatory bowel disease and is capable of contributing to genomic instability. Bcl-2 inhibits cytochrome c release from the mitochondria and prevents caspase activation, resulting in inhibition of apoptosis. Sun *et al.* (2002) demonstrated that HCT-15 colon cancer cells overexpressing COX-2 underwent upregulation of the antiapoptotic Bcl-2 protein relative to parental cells, leading to inappropriate cell survival. NSAIDs decrease malondialdehyde levels and Bcl-2 expression, perhaps contributing to the decreased incidence of polyp formation in patients treated with these medications.

Sheng et al. (Sheng et al., 1997) observed increased COX-2 mRNA and protein in colonic tumors that developed in rodents exposed to carcinogens. To define the relationship of COX-2 to tumorigenesis, human colon cancer xenografts constitutively expressing COX-2 were implanted into nude mice, and the mice were treated with the highly selective COX-2 inhibitor SC-58125. Mice treated with SC-58125 demonstrated a 90% reduction in tumor development when compared with control mice. Oshima et al. (1996) crossed APC$^{\Delta 716}$ mice, known to develop hundreds of intestinal tumors, with COX-2 null mice, and noted an 80-90% reduction in tumor multiplicity in the homozygous COX-2 null offspring. Moreover, a marked reduction in tumor number and size in APC$^{\Delta 716}$ mice treated with a highly selective COX-2 inhibitor was shown, further supporting the role of COX-2 in the development of colorectal cancer.

## 4.2    NF-κB

NF-κB is a ubiquitously expressed transcription factor that plays a pivotal role in cellular responses to environmental changes, such as stress, inflammation, and infection. NF-κB is activated in response to infectious agents or cytokines, including TNF-$\alpha$, IL-1, platelet activating factor (PAF), ROS, lipopolysaccharide (LPS), and leukotriene B4 (Gustin et al., 2004). Its products include growth factors, cytokines, cell adhesion molecules, immunoreceptors, and cell survival proteins, making it an important and complex regulator of the immune response (Gustin et al., 2004; Schwartz et al., 1999). Constitutive activation of NF-κB has been described in inflammatory conditions such as acute and chronic pancreatitis, gastritis, and inflammatory bowel disease, as well as many solid tumors, including GI cancers. The activation of NF-κB by proinflammatory stimuli and its ability to inhibit apoptosis have led to the assumption that the NF-κB pathway provides a mechanistic link between inflammation and cancer (Greten et al., 2004).

The functional NF-κB protein is a heterodimer, most commonly composed of a p65/RelA and a p50 subunit, although many dimers are known to exist *in vivo* (Fig. 2). In a resting cell, NF-κB is bound by inhibitor of NF-κB (IκB) proteins, masking its nuclear localization signal and sequestering inactive NF-κB in the cytoplasm (Baldwin, Jr., 1996; Ethridge et al., 2002b; May and Ghosh, 1998). Stimulation of a cell by an activator

such as TNF-α results in a cascade of events, beginning with the activation
of the IKK complex, composed of IKKα, IKKβ, and IKKγ. This complex
then phosphorylates IκB, marking it for ubiquitination at specific lysine
residues and targeting it to the 26S proteasome. The 26S proteasome
degrades IκB, unmasking the nuclear localization signal of NF-κB, thus
allowing its translocation to the nucleus where it regulates target gene
transcription (Baldwin, Jr., 1996; Ethridge *et al.*, 2002b; May and Ghosh,
1998).

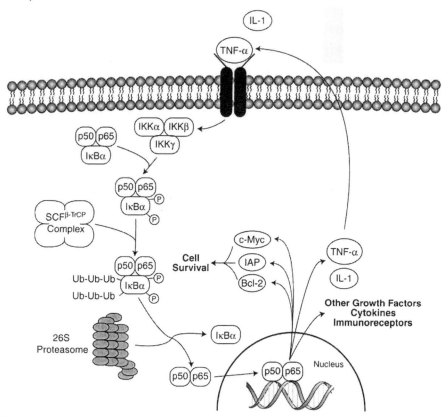

*Figure 2.* The NF-κB pathway. IKKα, β, γ = IκB kinase complex; p50,
p65 = NF-κB heterodimer; IκBα = inhibitor of κB; E3-SCF$^{\beta\text{-TrCP}}$ complex =
ubiquitin ligase complex; Ub = ubiquitination site; P = phosphorylation site;
IAP = inhibitor of apoptosis protein.

TNF-α binding to TNF receptor-1 (TNFR1) leads to signal transduction
resulting in NF-κB activation and subsequent upregulation of proteins
responsible for modulating the immune response and inhibiting apoptosis,

including the c-*myc* proto-oncogene, inhibitor of apoptosis proteins (IAP), and Bcl-2. A positive autoregulatory loop exists whereby some stimulators of NF-κB activation, including TNF-α and IL-1, are upregulated by NF-κB activation, thus potentiating its effect (Kim *et al.*, 2002).

Activated NF-κB has been isolated in macrophages and epithelial cells from biopsy samples and cultured cells of patients with IBD and colorectal cancer, while levels in adjacent normal tissue remain normal. In an effort to further delineate the role of NF-κB specific to the development of colorectal cancer in the setting of chronic inflammation, Greten *et al.* (Greten *et al.*, 2004) examined NF-κB inhibition by deletion of IKKβ in inflammatory cells compared with intestinal epithelial cells in a mouse model of colitis-associated cancer. They found that deletion of IKKβ in intestinal epithelial cells was associated with a dramatic decrease in tumor incidence and an increase in tumor cell apoptosis, while deletion in myeloid cells resulted in a decrease in tumor size without an effect on incidence and a reduction in cytokines that serve as tumor growth factors. Luo *et al.* (2004) examined the effect of NF-κB inhibition on the growth and metastasis of a murine model of colon adenocarcinoma. Utilizing an IκBα superrepressor resistant to degradation, they showed that inhibition of NF-κB activation *in vivo* resulted in tumor cell apoptosis and tumor regression. Murano *et al.* (2000) found a significant decrease in cytokines and attenuation of inflammation in mice with dextran sulphate sodium-induced colitis treated with p65 NF-κB subunit antisense oligonucleotide.

Overexpression of NF-κB has similarly been documented in pancreatitis and pancreatic cancer. Wang *et al.* (1999) examined several human pancreatic adenocarcinoma biopsy samples and human pancreatic tumor cell lines and identified constitutive activation of NF-κB in 16 of 24 (67%) pancreatic adenocarcinomas and 9 of 11 (82%) human pancreatic tumor cell lines. Other experiments have documented an increase in NF-κB in mouse and rat models of chemically-induced pancreatitis. Utilizing a mouse model of cerulein-induced pancreatitis, Ethridge *et al.* (2002b) showed that inhibition of NF-κB with NEMO (NF-κB essential modifier = IKKγ) binding domain (NBD) resulted in amelioration of the pancreatitis, thus supporting an essential role for this pathway in the pathogenesis of inflammation and cancer formation.

Interest in the role of NF-κB in tumor development and the role of NF-κB inhibition as an adjunct to chemotherapy and radiation stems from the fact that the transcription factor is activated in many tumors. Chemotherapeutic agents and radiation stimulate NF-κB activation, and this results in the production of anti-apoptotic proteins. Experimental inhibition or deletion of NF-κB attenuated inflammation and tumor growth and enhanced sensitivity of cancer cells to apoptosis when combined with standard chemotherapeutic agents and radiation.

## 4.3 Phosphatidylinositol 3-kinase (PI3K)

Another pathway playing a critical role in the balance between cell survival and apoptosis is the phosphatidylinositol 3-kinase (PI3K) pathway. PI3K, a ubiquitous lipid kinase activated by a wide variety of extracellular stimuli such as cytokines (e.g., TNF-α) and growth factors, is involved in the regulation of diverse cellular processes, such as cell growth and survival, actin cytoskeletal rearrangement, membrane ruffling, and vesicular trafficking (Wang *et al.*, 2002a); therefore, signaling through this pathway plays a pivotal role in the regulation of cellular growth, transformation, and tumorigenesis. Increased PI3K activity has been identified in as many as 86% of human colorectal cancers, with increasing activity correlating with increasing tumorigenic potential of the cancer cell lines examined (Wang *et al.*, 2002a; Kaleghpour *et al.*, 2004). The promotion of cell survival by PI3K and its subsequent contribution to tumorigenesis is thought to occur via the inhibition of proapoptotic signals and the induction of survival signals.

PI3K is a heterodimeric protein composed of a regulatory subunit (p85) and a catalytic subunit (p110) (Fig. 3). When its receptor is activated, PI3K catalyzes the phosphorylation of phosphatidylinositol 4-phosphate and phosphatidylinositol 4,5-phosphate, yielding $PIP_2$ and $PIP_3$ (Weaver and Ward, 2001; Wang *et al.*, 2002b; Sheng *et al.*, 2003). $PIP_3$ then binds protein kinase B (Akt) and phosphatidylinositide-dependent kinase-1 (PDK-1), resulting in their translocation to the plasma membrane, where PDK-1 phosphorylates and activates Akt kinase. Activated Akt kinase then phosphorylates glycogen synthase kinase-3 (GSK-3), rendering it inactive. Constitutively active GSK-3 is unphosphorylated and responsible for maintaining the cell cycle-activating transcription factors c-*myc*, c-*jun*, c-*myb* and cyclin D1 in their inactive (i.e., phosphorylated) state. Inactivation of GSK-3 via phosphorylation therefore allows cells to progress through the cell cycle. Additionally, Akt kinase phosphorylates the Bcl-2 antagonist of cell death (BAD), caspase 9, and forkhead transcription factor (FKHR), suppressing the pro-apoptotic function of these proteins. FKHRL1, belonging to a small subset of forkhead family of transcription factors, has the function of regulating p27[KIP1] gene expression when it is in its active, unphosphorylated state. Since the product of the p27[KIP1] gene is a Cdk inhibitor protein, inactivation of this inhibitor via phosphorylation and nuclear exclusion of FKHRL1 increases Cdk proteins, thus promoting cell survival (Weaver and Ward, 2001; Wang *et al.*, 2002b; Sheng *et al.*, 2003).

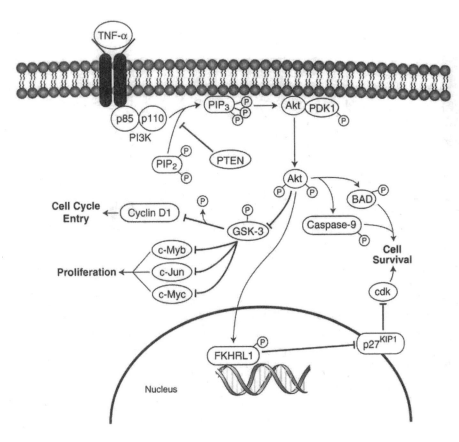

*Figure 3.* The PI3K pathway. p85/p110 = PI3K heterodimer; P = phosphorylation site; PIP$_2$ = phosphatidylinositol 4,5-phosphate; PIP$_3$ = phosphatidylinositol 3,4,5-phosphate; PDK = phosphatidylinositide-dependent kinase; GSK-3 = glycogen synthase kinase-3; FKHR-L1 = forkhead transcription factor; BAD = Bcl-2 antagonist of cell death.

Activation of the PI3K pathway is independently regulated by the tumor suppressor gene PTEN (phosphatase and tensin homolog deleted on chromosome ten), also known as MMAC (mutated in multiple advanced cancers). The product of the PTEN gene, a 3' phosphatase, acts as a tumor suppressor by degrading the PIP$_3$ product of PI3K activation, thus inhibiting PI3K pathway activation (Weaver and Ward, 2001). Mutation of this gene is associated with several neoplastic disorders, including Cowden's disease, Lhermitte-Duclos disease, and Bannayan-Zonana syndrome, all of which are associated with an increased incidence of colorectal polyposis and cancer, as well as neoplasia in other organ systems (Cantley and Neel, 1999; Kim *et al.*, 2004). PTEN$^{-/-}$ knockout mice are embryonic lethals; however, PTEN$^{+/-}$

heterozygous mice, possessing one normal and one defective copy of the PTEN gene, develop intestinal polyposis reminiscent of the human neoplastic disorders (Cantley and Neel, 1999; Kim *et al.*, 2004). It has been shown that restoration of PTEN expression in PTEN$^{-/-}$ glioblastoma multiforme, prostate, melanoma, and breast cancer cell lines can lead to tumor growth suppression (Cantley and Neel, 1999), and forced overexpression of PTEN in HT-29 colon cancer cells results in restoration of apoptosis (Arico *et al.*, 2001), supporting the role of PTEN as a tumor suppressor.

The link between the PI3K pathway and carcinogenesis has been explored by examining the differential expression of the various pathway components and the effects of their inhibition or overexpression in tumor tissue. Wang *et al.* (Wang *et al.*, 2002a) demonstrated that PI3K inhibition greatly enhanced sodium butyrate-mediated apoptosis of KM20 human colon cancer cells *in vitro* and *in vivo,* and that the PI3K inhibitor, wortmannin, alone inhibited KM20 xenograft growth *in vivo.* Semba *et al.* (2002) produced similar tumor cell apoptosis and suppression of tumor growth utilizing the PI3K inhibitor, LY294002, in multiple human colon cancer cell lines *in vitro* and *in vivo.* Sheng *et al.* (2003) demonstrated that ectopic expression of either active p110α or Akt-1 increased rat intestinal epithelial (RIE) cell proliferation *in vitro,* and *in vivo* experiments confirmed that this PI3K activation was associated with increased proliferative activity of the intestinal mucosa which could be attenuated by oral intake of the PI3K inhibitors.

## 4.4    Summary of pathways

While it has been shown that the COX-2, NF-κB, and PI3K pathways independently contribute to the induction of cell survival signals and the inhibition of apoptosis, a complex relationship exists between the three pathways (Fig. 4). Kim *et al.* (2002) found that treatment of cancer cell lines with TNF-α resulted in NF-κB-dependent transcriptional downregulation of PTEN, leading to activation of the PI3K/Akt pathway. Overexpression of NF-κB-inducing kinase (NIK) or the p65 subunit of NF-κB led to direct increases in phosphorylated Akt and its downstream target, GSK-3β. Ozes *et al.* (1999) noted inhibition of TNF-α-mediated NF-κB activation in cells treated with the PI3K inhibitor wortmannin, dominant-negative PI3K, or kinase-dead Akt. Moreover, Akt-mediated IKKα phosphorylation at threonine 23 was identified as a key interaction between these pathways, since mutation of this amino acid blocks activation of NF-κB. Further evidence for the functional crosstalk between these pathways is the fact that malignant cells with a high ratio of IKKα to IKKβ are the most sensitive to treatment with PI3K inhibitors (Gustin *et al.*, 2004). Jobin *et al.* (1998) found that infection of HT-29 colon cancer cells with an NF-κB superrepressor significantly decreased COX-2 mRNA and protein expression in response to TNF-α stimulation. Slogoff *et al.* (2004) described inhibition of late-phase NF-κB activation via COX-2 inhibition. It has also been demonstrated that Akt can modulate the stability of COX-2 mRNA (Shao *et al.*, 2000). Thus, it is evident that there is a complex relationship involving crosstalk between the three pathways that has yet to be fully elucidated.

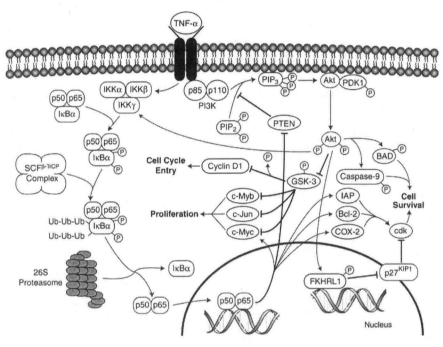

*Figure 4.* COX-2, NF-κB, and PI3K pathways. IKKα, β, γ = IκB kinase complex; p50, p65 = NF-κB heterodimer; IκBα = inhibitor of NF-κB α; E3-SCF$^{β-TrCP}$ complex = ubiquitin ligase complex; Ub = ubiquitination site; P = phosphorylation site; IAP = inhibitor of apoptosis protein; p85/p110 = PI3K heterodimer; P = phosphorylation site; PIP$_2$ = phosphatidylinositol 4,5-phosphate; PIP$_3$ = phosphatidylinositol 3,4,5-phosphate; PDK = phosphoinositide-dependent kinase; GSK-3 = glycogen synthase kinase-3; FKHR-L1 = forkhead transcription factor.

# 5.     IMPLICATIONS FOR FUTURE TREATMENT AND PREVENTION

## 5.1     Anti-inflammatory medications

Many epidemiologic, non-randomized studies have demonstrated a 30-50% reduction in the incidence and mortality from colorectal cancer in individuals taking nonsteroidal anti-inflammatory medications (NSAIDs) on a regular basis, raising interest in the use of these drugs as chemopreventive and chemotherapeutic agents (DuBois *et al.*, 1996; Thun *et al.*, 1991). NSAIDs are classified as either nonselective (affecting both COX-1 and COX-2) or selective (targeting only COX-2). The classes that specifically inhibit COX-2 activity, such as sulindac and celecoxib, are predominantly of interest in the prophylaxis and treatment of colorectal tumors as they decrease the probability of developing the untoward side effects of COX-1 inhibition, including gastritis and peptic ulcer disease.

Tumor inhibition by NSAIDS is believed to occur by at least two distinct cellular processes - the inhibition of angiogenesis and the restoration of apoptosis (Sun *et al.*, 2002). A reduction in two products of COX-2 activation, the proangiogenic factors $PGE_2$ and $PGI_2$, contribute to inhibition of angiogenesis (Ethridge *et al.*, 2002a). Restoration of apoptosis may occur as a direct result of COX inhibition, or through an additional mechanism of action of several NSAIDs (i.e., inhibition of NF-κB). This is thought to occur via inhibition of ATP binding to IKKβ, thus preventing phosphorylation of IκB and leading to a decrease in NF-κB translocation to the nucleus (Yamamoto and Gaynor, 2001).

The treatment of patients with FAP with NSAIDs has proven to decrease polyp incidence and cause polyp regression, often within the first three months of initiating treatment, and prospective studies on NSAID use in the general population have demonstrated a survival benefit for individuals taking aspirin, a NSAID, on a daily basis (DuBois *et al.*, 1996). Giardiello *et al.* (Giardiello *et al.*, 1993) conducted a double-blind, randomized, placebo-controlled trial of the effects of sulindac on polyp progression in patients with FAP. After 9 months, they found that polyp number had decreased by 44%, and polyp size had decreased by 35% in patients treated with sulindac, while the placebo group experienced an increase in the size and number of polyps. Labayle *et al.* (1991) performed a randomized, double-blind, placebo-controlled trial of sulindac in FAP patients who had had prior colectomy and ileoanal anastomosis. They confirmed a statistically significant decrease in the number of polyps in patients treated with sulindac, and no change in the placebo group. A prospective study by Thun *et al.* (1991) followed a population of greater than 650,000 persons for 6 years and found that the relative risk of colon cancer mortality among men taking aspirin less than once a month, when controlled for other cancer risk factors, was 0.84, compared to 0.48 for those taking aspirin more than 16 times per month. This represents an approximate 43% decrease in cancer mortality for those taking aspirin 16 times per month or more, reinforcing the potential role of NSAIDs in chemoprevention.

Despite promising results indicating a decreased risk of developing colorectal cancer or a reduction in size of established tumors with NSAID therapy, the potential side effects of administering these medications to healthy individuals as prophylaxis is currently a concern. For example, the COX-2 selective inhibitor valdecoxib (Vioxx) was recently withdrawn from the market after the three-year prospective, randomized, placebo-controlled clinical trial, APPROVe (Adenomatous Polyp Prevention on Vioxx), concluded that there was an increased risk for cardiovascular events (including myocardial infarction and stroke) for those taking the medication (Fitzgerald, 2004). New clinical studies are concentrating instead on the use of NSAIDs as adjuvant therapy for precancerous lesions expressing COX-2 (Thun *et al.*, 2002).

## 5.2    NF-κB inhibitors

The importance of NF-κB to tumor cell survival pathways has identified it as a novel target for cancer chemoprevention. A number of animal studies have demonstrated that experimental inhibition or knockout of NF-κB attenuates tumor growth and enhances the sensitivity of tumor cells to apoptosis when combined with other chemotherapeutic agents (Schwartz *et al.*, 1999; Ethridge *et al.*, 2002b; Luo *et al.*, 2004). Since a number of discrete steps are involved in the activation of NF-κB, as previously discussed, there are several potential methods to down-regulate NF-κB in target tissues. This has led to the development of a wide range of therapeutic agents, including salicylates, corticosteroids, antioxidants, flavonoids (quercetin, resveratrol), proteasome inhibitors (MG-132, -101, and -115, lactacystin, PS-341), synthetic peptides (SN-50), viral proteins (adenoviral E1A protein), nucleotides (antisense oligonucleotides, transcription factor decoys), and plasmids (IκBα expression plasmids), each possessing a different mechanism of action (Schwartz *et al.*, 1999).

Several classes of drugs that inhibit NF-κB either directly or indirectly are currently in clinical use. Glucocorticoids, including prednisone and dexamethasone, widely used as anti-inflammatory and immunosuppressive agents, are capable of inhibiting NF-κB via several different mechanisms.

Dexamethasone induces synthesis of IκBα mRNA, leading to upregulation of IκBα protein and cytoplasmic retention of p65 in monocytes. In endothelial cells, dexamethasone decreases NF-κB transcriptional activity without altering IκB (Thun *et al.*, 1991). Competition between NF-κB and the glucocorticoid receptor for limited amounts of coactivators can also lead to NF-κB inhibition. Sulfasalazine, mesalamine, and sulindac, three anti-inflammatory agents, each have different mechanisms to downregulate NF-κB activation (Yamamoto and Gaynor, 2001). Sulfasalazine, which combines a nonsteroidal moiety (5-aminosalicyclic acid or 5-ASA) and an antibacterial moiety (sulfapyridine), is currently used in the treatment of inflammatory bowel disease and rheumatoid arthritis. It inhibits NF-κB activation by suppressing IκB phosphorylation, thus preventing its degradation. Mesalamine prevents p65 phosphorylation without inhibiting IκB degradation. Sulindac is capable of inhibiting IKKα activity by an unknown mechanism, and has proven to induce apoptosis in COX-2 deficient HCT-15 colon cancer cells, thus suggesting that NF-κB, not COX-2 inhibition, is responsible for its effects in this cancer cell line (Yamamoto and Gaynor, 2001). Lastly, the immunosuppressive agents cyclosporine A (CsA) and tacrolimus (FK-506), in addition to their chief mechanism of cell cycle blockage via calcineurin inhibition, are capable of downregulating NF-κB. Cyclosporin acts as a non-competitive inhibitor of the 20S proteasome, preventing IκB degradation, while FK-506 specifically blocks the translocation of the c-Rel subunit of NF-κB to the nucleus (Yamamoto and Gaynor, 2001).

While inhibition of NF-κB alone is unlikely to result in adequate tumor regression, its use as an adjunct with existing chemotherapeutic agents and radiation is promising. Novel approaches to specific NF-κB inhibition continue to be developed, but a lack of specificity and numerous side effects currently limit their usefulness in humans despite promising results in animal studies.

## 5.3    PI3K pathway inhibitors

The importance of the PI3K pathway to cell cycle control, differentiation, and proliferation of tumor cells has led to the development of specific inhibitors targeting the pathway. Like the NF-κB pathway, a cascade of cellular events is responsible for PI3K signaling, and thus there are several intracellular targets for inhibition.

Several potential chemotherapeutic agents that inhibit PI3K activation or interfere with PI3K signaling are currently being evaluated in clinical trials. Rapamycin (sirolimus), a microbially derived antiproliferative agent currently used as a potent immunosuppressant agent in transplant patients, binds with high affinity to the mammalian target of rapamycin (mTOR), resulting in a decrease in the capacity of cellular translational machinery to meet the increased demand for protein synthesis needed for cell cycle progression (Sekulic *et al.*, 2000). It has recently been discovered that mTOR is normally phosphorylated as a result of PI3K pathway activation; thus, rapamycin exerts its primary effect by inhibiting a downstream effector of PI3K. Phase II clinical trials studying the effects of the rapamycin analogue CCI-779 as a chemotherapeutic agent have been promising. For example, in a recent study by Atkins *et al.* (2004), 26% of 111 patients with renal cell carcinoma refractory to chemotherapy experienced minor responses, seven patients experienced partial responses (at least 50% reduction in cancer load), and one experienced a complete response. Farnesyltransferase inhibitors such as FTI-277 and R115777 induce apoptosis of cancer cells *in vitro* by directly inhibiting PI3K activation, although the precise mechanism remains unclear (Atkins *et al.*, 2004). Clinical trials indicate that the compound R115777 may be the most effective in the treatment of myeloproliferative disorders (two complete responses and two partial responses out of a total of seven patients), while there has been some success with solid malignancies as well (4 partial responses out of 41 patients with metastatic breast cancer treated with R115777) (Brunner *et al.*, 2003). EGFR antagonists directly inhibit activation of PI3K by blocking the receptor's activation in response to TNF-α binding (Mendelsohn and Baselga, 2003). A recent phase II clinical study which combined the EGFR antagonist cetuximab with the chemotherapeutic agent irinotecan in the treatment of advanced colorectal carcinoma in 120 patients resulted in a response rate of 22.5% (Mendelsohn and Baselga, 2003).

Other PI3K inhibitors (wortmannin and LY294002) have been developed, but their use is limited by nonspecific activity and toxicity noted in preclinical trials (Weaver and Ward, 2001; Stein and Waterfield, 2000). Plasmids encoding PTEN or GSK-3 overexpression have been explored, but again, toxicity limits their use (Weaver and Ward, 2001; Talapatra and Thompson, 2001). While promising results have been obtained using PI3K inhibitors *in vitro*, a lack of specificity and systemic toxicity limit their use in the treatment of chronic inflammation and tumorigenesis at this time.

## 5.4     Novel experimental therapies

Conventional chemotherapeutic agents used in the treatment of patients with advanced GI and liver cancer confer limited survival benefit, since many cancer cells resist cell killing by upregulating cell survival pathways or inhibiting cell apoptotic pathways (Bold *et al.*, 1997). Sensitization of such resistant cells by blocking cell survival pathways or inducing apoptotic mechanisms, used in combination with standard cytotoxic chemotherapeutic agents, has thus become an important focus of cancer research (Schwartz *et al.*, 1999). Such innovative strategies for the treatment of GI cancers include post-transcriptional gene silencing utilizing small interfering RNA (siRNA) or antisense oligonucleotides, anti-cytokine vaccines, transcription factor decoys, and gene expression plasmid transfection (Hasuwa *et al.*, 2002; Tiscornia *et al.*, 2003). Many of these therapies target components of the PI3K, NF-κB, and COX-2 pathways, blocking cell survival pathways and inducing apoptosis when used in combination with standard chemotherapeutic agents and radiotherapy (Talapatra and Thompson, 2001; Hersey and Zhang, 2003). *In vitro* studies utilizing these agents in combination with chemotherapy have been quite promising, but a narrow therapeutic index and a lack of specificity currently limit use for many of them *in vivo* (Hersey and Zhang, 2003). Clinical trials currently in progress using antisense oligonucleotides to Bcl-2 in the treatment of melanoma, chronic lymphatic leukemia, small cell carcinoma of the lung, acute myeloid leukemia, and multiple myeloma, have produced promising initial results with low toxicity (Bold *et al.*, 1997; Hersey and Zhang, 2003). More novel therapeutic agents are expected to enter clinical trial as advances are made in delivery and specificity.

## 6. CONCLUSIONS

Increasing evidence supports the contribution of chronic inflammation to the development of GI and pancreatic cancers. Individuals with chronic inflammatory or infectious diseases (e.g., *H. pylori* gastritis, chronic pancreatitis, IBD) are far more likely to develop malignancy than their healthy counterparts, while treatment of the underlying inflammation or infection has been shown to significantly reduce the risk of cancer development. The production of cytokines, chemokines, and ROS in response to a persistent inflammatory stimulus results in an accumulation of cellular damage. Such stimulators also result in the activation of cell signaling pathways, such as COX-2, NF-κB, and PI3K, which lead to activation of cell survival pathways and inhibition of apoptosis. Although hindered by a lack of tissue specificity and numerous side effects, promising results have already been obtained utilizing novel inhibitors of signaling pathways activated in settings of chronic inflammation and malignancy.

# 7.    REFERENCES

Agoff, S.N. *et al.* (2000). The role of cyclooxygenase 2 in ulcerative colitis-associated neoplasia. *Am. J. Pathol.* **157**: 737-745.

Arico, S. *et al.* (2001). The tumor suppressor PTEN positively regulates macroautophagy by inhibiting the phosphatidylinositol 3-kinase/protein kinase B pathway. *J. Biol. Chem.* **276**: 35243-35246.

Atkins, M.B. *et al.* (2004). Randomized phase II study of multiple dose levels of CCI-779, a novel mammalian target of rapamycin kinase inhibitor, in patients with advanced refractory renal cell carcinoma. *J. Clin. Oncol.* **22**: 909-918.

Baldwin, Jr., A.S. (1996). The NF-kappa B and I kappa B proteins: new discoveries and insights. *Annu. Rev. Immunol.* **14**: 649-683.

Balkwill, F. and Mantovani, A. (2001). Inflammation and cancer: back to Virchow? *Lancet* **357**: 539-545.

Bing, R.J. *et al.* (2001). Nitric oxide, prostanoids, cyclooxygenase, and angiogenesis in colon and breast cancer. *Clin. Cancer Res.* **7**: 3385-3392.

Bold, R.J. *et al.* (1997). Apoptosis, cancer and cancer therapy. *Surg. Oncol.* **6**: 133-142.

Brunner, T.B. *et al.* (2003). Farnesyltransferase inhibitors: an overview of the results of preclinical and clinical investigations. *Cancer Res.* **63**: 5656-5668.

Cantley, L.C. and Neel, B.G. (1999). New insights into tumor suppression: PTEN suppresses tumor formation by restraining the phosphoinositide 3-kinase/AKT pathway. *Proc. Natl Acad. Sci. U. S. A.* **96**: 4240-4245.

Celik, E. *et al.* (2003). Case report: early arising Marjolin's ulcer in the scalp. *Ann. Burn Fire Dis.* **16**: 217-220.

Correa, P *et al.* (2000). Chemoprevention of gastric dysplasia: randomized trial of antioxidant supplements and anti-helicobacter pylori therapy. *J. Natl Cancer Inst.* **92**: 1881-1888.

Correa, P. (2003). Bacterial infections as a cause of cancer. *J. Natl Cancer. Inst.* **95**: E3.

Cotran, R.S. *et al.* (1999). *Pathologic Basis of Disease* (W.B. Saunders Company, Philadelphia).

Coussens, L.M. and Werb, Z. (2002). Inflammation and cancer. *Nature* **420**: 860-867.

DuBois, R.N. *et al.* (1996). Nonsteroidal anti-inflammatory drugs, eicosanoids, and colorectal cancer prevention. *Gastroenterol. Clin. North Am.* **25**: 773-791.

Dvorak, H.F. (1986). Tumors: wounds that do not heal. Similarities between tumor stroma generation and wound healing. *N. Engl. J. Med.* **315**: 1650-1659.

Eaden, J.A. *et al.* (2001). The risk of colorectal cancer in ulcerative colitis: a meta-analysis. *Gut* **48**: 526-535.

Ethridge, R.T. *et al.* (2002a). Cyclooxygenase-2 gene disruption attenuates the severity of acute pancreatitis and pancreatitis-associated lung injury. *Gastroenterology* **123**: 1311-1322.

Ethridge, R.T. *et al.* (2002b). Selective inhibition of NF-kappaB attenuates the severity of cerulein-induced acute pancreatitis. *J. Am. Coll. Surg.* **195**: 497-505.

Farrow, B. and Evers, B.M. (2002). Inflammation and the development of pancreatic cancer. *Surg. Oncol.* **10**: 153-169.

Farrow, B. *et al.* (2004). Inflammatory mechanisms contributing to pancreatic cancer development. *Ann. Surg.* **239**: 763-769.

Fitzgerald, G.A. (2004). Coxibs and cardiovascular disease. *N. Engl. J. Med.* **351:** 1709-1711.

Gasche, C. *et al.* (2001). Oxidative stress increases frameshift mutations in human colorectal cancer cells. *Cancer Res.* **61**: 7444-7448.

Giardiello, F.M. *et al.* (1993). Treatment of colonic and rectal adenomas with sulindac in familial adenomatous polyposis. *N. Engl. J. Med.* **328**: 1313-1316.

Greten, F.R. *et al.* (2004). IKKbeta links inflammation and tumorigenesis in a mouse model of colitis-associated cancer. *Cell* **118**: 285-296.

Gustin, J.A. *et al.* (2004). Cell type-specific expression of the IkappaB kinases determines the significance of phosphatidylinositol 3-kinase/Akt signaling to NF-kappa B activation. *J. Biol .Chem.* **279**: 1615-1620.

Hasuwa, H. *et al.* (2002). Small interfering RNA and gene silencing in transgenic mice and rats. *FEBS Lett.* **532**: 227-230.

Hersey, P. and Zhang, X.D. (2003). Overcoming resistance of cancer cells to apoptosis. *J. Cell Physiol.* **196**: 9-18.

Hussain, S.P. *et al.* (2000). Increased p53 mutation load in noncancerous colon tissue from ulcerative colitis: a cancer-prone chronic inflammatory disease. *Cancer Res.* **60**: 3333-3337.

Itzkowitz, S.H. and Yio, X. (2004). Inflammation and cancer IV. Colorectal cancer in inflammatory bowel disease: the role of inflammation. *Am. J. Physiol. Gastrointest. Liver Physiol.* **287**: G7-G17.

Jobin, C. *et al.* (1998). Specific NF-kappaB blockade selectively inhibits tumour necrosis factor-alpha-induced COX-2 but not constitutive COX-1 gene expression in HT-29 cells. *Immunology* **95**: 537-543.

Khaleghpour, K. *et al.* (2004). Involvement of the PI 3-kinase signaling pathway in progression of colon adenocarcinoma. *Carcinogenesis* **25**: 241-248.

Kim, S. *et al.* (2002). PTEN and TNF-alpha regulation of the intestinal-specific Cdx-2 homeobox gene through a PI3K, PKB/Akt, and NF-kappaB-dependent pathway. *Gastroenterology* **123**: 1163-1178.

Kim, S. *et al.* (2004). Down-regulation of the tumor suppressor PTEN by the tumor necrosis factor-alpha/nuclear factor-kappaB (NF-kappaB)-inducing kinase/NF-kappaB pathway is linked to a default IkappaB-alpha autoregulatory loop. *J. Biol. Chem.* **279**: 4285-4291.

Labayle, D. *et al.* (1991). Sulindac causes regression of rectal polyps in familial adenomatous polyposis. *Gastroenterology* **101**: 635-639.

Lichtenstein, G.R. (2002). Reduction of colorectal cancer risk in patients with Crohn's disease. *Rev. Gastroenterol. Disord.* **2** (Suppl. 2): S16-S24.

Lowenfels, A.B. *et al.* (1993). Pancreatitis and the risk of pancreatic cancer. International Pancreatitis Study Group. *N. Engl. J. Med.* **328**: 1433-1437.

Luo, J.L. *et al.* (2004). Inhibition of NF-kappaB in cancer cells converts inflammation-induced tumor growth mediated by TNFalpha to TRAIL-mediated tumor regression. *Cancer Cell* **6**: 297-305.

Mantovani, A. *et al.* (1992). The origin and function of tumor-associated macrophages. *Immunol. Today* **13**: 265-270.

May, M.J. and Ghosh, S. (1998). Signal transduction through NF-kappa B. *Immunol. Today* **19**: 80-88.

McCawley, L.J. and Matrisian, L.M. (2001). Tumor progression: defining the soil round the tumor seed. *Curr. Biol.* **11**: R25-R27.

Mendelsohn, J. and Baselga, J. (2003). Status of epidermal growth factor receptor antagonists in the biology and treatment of cancer. *J. Clin. Oncol.* **21**: 2787-2799.

Moore, R.J. *et al.* (1999). Mice deficient in tumor necrosis factor-alpha are resistant to skin carcinogenesis. *Nat. Med.* **5**: 828-831.

Murano, M. *et al.* (2000). Therapeutic effect of intracolonically administered nuclear factor kappa B (p65) antisense oligonucleotide on mouse dextran sulphate sodium (DSS)-induced colitis. *Clin. Exp. Immunol.* **120**: 51-58.

Oshima, M. *et al.* (1996). Suppression of intestinal polyposis in Apc delta716 knockout mice by inhibition of cyclooxygenase 2 (COX-2). *Cell* **87**: 803-809.

Ozes, O. N. *et al.* (1999). NF-kappaB activation by tumour necrosis factor requires the Akt serine-threonine kinase. *Nature* **401**: 82-85.

Parsonnet, J. *et al.* (1991). Helicobacter pylori infection in intestinal- and diffuse-type gastric adenocarcinomas. *J. Natl Cancer Inst.* **83**: 640-643.

Schwartz, S.A. *et al.* (1999). The role of NF-kappaB/IkappaB proteins in cancer: implications for novel treatment strategies. *Surg. Oncol.* **8**: 143-153.

Sekulic, A. *et al.* (2000). A direct linkage between the phosphoinositide 3-kinase-AKT signaling pathway and the mammalian target of rapamycin in mitogen-stimulated and transformed cells. *Cancer Res.* **60**: 3504-3513.

Semba, S. *et al.* (2002). The in vitro and in vivo effects of 2-(4-morpholinyl)-8-phenyl-chromone (LY294002), a specific inhibitor of phosphatidylinositol 3'-kinase, in human colon cancer cells. *Clin. Cancer Res.* **8**: 1957-1963.

Shao, J. *et al.* (2000). Regulation of constitutive cyclooxygenase-2 expression in colon carcinoma cells. *J. Biol. Chem.* **275**: 33951-33956.

Sheng, H. *et al.* (1997). Inhibition of human colon cancer cell growth by selective inhibition of cyclooxygenase-2. *J. Clin. Invest.* **99**: 2254-2259.

Sheng, H. *et al.* (2003). Phosphatidylinositol 3-kinase mediates proliferative signals in intestinal epithelial cells. *Gut* **52**: 1472-1478.

Shi, Q. *et al.* (1999). Constitutive and inducible interleukin 8 expression by hypoxia and acidosis renders human pancreatic cancer cells more tumorigenic and metastatic, *Clin. Cancer Res.* **5**: 3711-3721.

Slogoff, M.I. *et al.* (2004). COX-2 inhibition results in alterations in nuclear factor (NF)-kappaB activation but not cytokine production in acute pancreatitis. *J. Gastrointest. Surg.* **8**: 511-519.

Stein, R.C. and Waterfield, M.D. (2000). PI3-kinase inhibition: a target for drug development? *Mol. Med. Today* **6**: 347-357.

Stoicov, C. *et al.* (2004). Molecular biology of gastric cancer: Helicobacter infection and gastric adenocarcinoma: bacterial and host factors responsible for altered growth signaling. *Gene* **341**: 1-17.

Stolte, M. and Meining, A. (1998). Helicobacter pylori and Gastric Cancer. *Oncologist* **3**: 124-128.

Suganuma, M. *et al.* (1999). Essential role of tumor necrosis factor alpha (TNF-alpha) in tumor promotion as revealed by TNF-alpha-deficient mice. *Cancer Res.* **59**: 4516-4518.

Sun, Y. *et al.* (2002). Cyclooxygenase-2 overexpression reduces apoptotic susceptibility by inhibiting the cytochrome c-dependent apoptotic pathway in human colon cancer cells. *Cancer Res.* **62**: 6323-6328.

Talapatra, S. and Thompson, C.B. (2001). Growth factor signaling in cell survival: implications for cancer treatment. *J. Pharmacol. Exp. Ther.* **298**: 873-878.

Thun, M.J. *et al.* (1991). Aspirin use and reduced risk of fatal colon cancer. *N. Engl. J. Med.* **325**: 1593-1596.

Thun, M.J. *et al.* (2002). Nonsteroidal anti-inflammatory drugs as anticancer agents: mechanistic, pharmacologic, and clinical issues. *J. Natl Cancer Inst.* **94**: 252-266.

Tiscornia, G. *et al.* (2003). A general method for gene knockdown in mice by using lentiviral vectors expressing small interfering RNA. *Proc. Natl Acad. Sci. U. S. A.* **100**: 1844-1848.

Tricot, G. (2000). New insights into role of microenvironment in multiple myeloma. *Lancet* **355**: 248-250.

Uemura, N. *et al.* (1997). Effect of Helicobacter pylori eradication on subsequent development of cancer after endoscopic resection of early gastric cancer. *Cancer Epidemiol. Biomarkers Prev.* **6**: 639-642.

Uemura, N. *et al.* (2001). Helicobacter pylori infection and the development of gastric cancer. *N. Engl. J. Med.* **345**: 784-789.

Vidal-Vanaclocha, F. *et al.* (2000). IL-18 regulates IL-1beta-dependent hepatic melanoma metastasis via vascular cell adhesion molecule-1. *Proc. Natl Acad. Sci. U. S. A.* **97**: 734-739.

Wang, Q. *et al.* (2002a). Augmentation of sodium butyrate-induced apoptosis by phosphatidylinositol 3'-kinase inhibition in the KM20 human colon cancer cell line. *Clin. Cancer Res.* **8**: 1940-1947.

Wang, Q. *et al.* (2002b). Regulation of TRAIL expression by the phosphatidylinositol 3-kinase/Akt/GSK-3 pathway in human colon cancer cells. *J. Biol. Chem.* **277**: 36602-36610.

Wang, W. *et al.* (1999). The nuclear factor-kappa B RelA transcription factor is constitutively activated in human pancreatic adenocarcinoma cells. *Clin. Cancer Res.* **5**: 119-127.

Weaver, S.A. and Ward, S.G. (2001). Phosphoinositide 3-kinases in the gut: a link between inflammation and cancer? *Trends Mol. Med.* **7**: 455-462.

Yamamoto, Y. and Gaynor, R.B. (2001). Therapeutic potential of inhibition of the NF-kappaB pathway in the treatment of inflammation and cancer. *J. Clin. Invest.* **107**: 135-142.

# Chapter 3

# CYTOKINES, NF-κB, MICROENVIRONMENT, INTESTINAL INFLAMMATION AND CANCER

Arndt J. Schottelius[1] and Harald Dinter[2]

*Development Sciences, Genentech, Inc., 1 DNA Way, South San Francisco CA 94080[1] and Research Business Area Dermatology USA and Research Business Area Oncology USA, Berlex Biosciences, 2600 Hilltop Drive, Richmond CA 94806[2]*

Abstract:      Inflammation and cancer have been viewed as closely linked for many years. This link is not merely a loose association but causative. In colorectal cancer (CRC), chronic inflammation as observed in inflammatory bowel (IBD) disease is a key predisposing factor and IBD-associated CRC comprises five percent of all CRCs. Although the molecular mechanisms linking IBD with CRC are not well understood, recent results obtained in preclinical models point to the transcription factor NF-κB as a central player. On the one hand, NF-κB regulates the expression of various cytokines and modulates the inflammatory processes in IBD. On the other, NF-κB stimulates the proliferation of tumor cells and enhances their survival through the regulation of anti-apoptotic genes. Furthermore, it has been clearly established that most carcinogens and tumor promoters activate NF-κB, while chemopreventive agents generally suppress this transcription factor. Actually, several lines of evidence suggest that activation of NF-κB may cause cancer. These include the finding that NF-κB genes can be oncogenes, and that this transcription factor controls apoptosis, cell-cycle progression and proliferation, and possibly also cell differentiation.

Keywords:     colorectal cancer; chronic inflammation; NF-κB; macrophages; growth factors

# 1.    INTRODUCTION

Inflammation and cancer have been viewed as closely linked for many years. This link is not merely a loose association but causative. In fact, it is estimated that inflammation-associated processes caused by chronic infections contribute to about one-third of the world's cancers (Ames *et al.*, 1995). Oxidants produced by leukocytes and other phagocytic cells to fight bacteria and parasites protect the infected individual from death by infection but at the same time cause oxidative damage to the individual's own DNA. This damage, especially when accumulated over time, may cause multiple mutations ultimately leading to the development of cancer. Furthermore, once the cancer is established, multiple inflammatory processes can contribute to the growth and dissemination of cancer cells. For example, tumor-associated macrophages were shown to produce factors which stimulate tumor angiogenesis, promote metastases and enhance the invasiveness of tumors. Moreover, these macrophages produce mitogens such as epidermal growth factor (EGF), which can directly affect the proliferation of tumor cells (Bingle *et al.*, 2002; Leek and Harris, 2002). Thus, it is not surprising that increased density of tumor-associated macrophages is correlated with poor prognosis in some tumor types or in certain tumor stages (Lin and Pollard, 2004; Miyagawa *et al.*, 2002; Toomey ·*et al.*, 1999; Lackner *et al.*, 2004).

In colorectal cancer (CRC), chronic inflammation as observed in inflammatory bowel diseases (IBD) is a key predisposing factor. Five to ten percent of IBD patients develop colon cancer after 20 years and 12-20% after 30 years with the disease (Munkholm, 2003). IBD-associated CRC comprises five percent of all CRCs. Furthermore, ulcerative colitis, a subtype of IBD, besides Familial Adenomatous Polyposis and Hereditary Nonpolyposis Colorectal Cancer, is the most common condition predisposing to CRC (Itzkowitz and Yio, 2004). The importance of inflammatory processes in CRC is highlighted by a large number of studies demonstrating the efficacy of anti-inflammatory drugs in CRC. Nonselective, nonsteroidal, anti-inflammatory drugs (NSAIDs) were shown to decrease the mortality in CRC, and aspirin as well as cyclooxygenase-2 inhibitors reduced the risk of CRC (Thun *et al.*, 1993; Giovannucci *et al.*, 1994; Collet et al., 1999; Langman et al., 2001; Jolly *et al.*, 2002; Chan, 2003; Koehne and Dubois, 2004). Although the molecular mechanisms linking IBD with CRC are not well understood, recent results obtained in preclinical models point to the transcription factor NF-κB as a central player. On the one hand, NF-κB regulates the expression of various cytokines and modulates the inflammatory processes in IBD. On the other, NF-κB stimulates the proliferation of tumor cells and enhances their survival.

## 2.    CELLULAR MECHANISMS IN INFLAMMATORY BOWEL DISEASE AND THE ROLE OF NF-κB

IBD, which includes Crohn's disease (CD) and UC, is the main chronic inflammatory disease of the gastrointestinal tract in humans. Over the past years, evidence has been accumulating pointing to the central role of increased production of pro-inflammatory cytokines by inflammatory cells in the pathogenesis of IBD (Schottelius and Baldwin, 1999) (Fig. 1). This has been suggested by the increased expression of pro-inflammatory cytokines, such as interleukin (IL)-1, IL-6 and TNFα in the inflamed mucosa from patients with Crohn's disease (CD) and ulcerative colitis (UC). It has now been established that CD is driven by the production of the Th1 cytokines interleukin-12 (Monteleone, 1997), interleukin-18 (Reuter and Pizarro, 2004) and interferon-γ (Strober *et al.*, 2002), whereas UC is probably driven by the production of IL-13 (Bouma and Strober, 2003). However, the elements governing dysregulated cytokine production in IBD had remained less clear until recently.

Several studies have demonstrated that NF-κB is activated in IBD suggesting that this transcription factor, when excessively activated, could be the driver for dysregulated cytokine production observed in IBD (Schottelius and Baldwin, 2004). NF-κB p65 has been found to be strongly activated in animal models of IBD, i.e. 2,4,6-trinitrobenzene sulphonic acid (TNBS)-induced colitis, dextran sulfate sodium induced colitis and in colitis of IL-10-deficient mice (Neurath *et al.*, 1996; Spiik *et al.*, 2002). Remarkably, local administration of p65 antisense phosphorothioate oligonucleotides abrogated clinical and histological signs of colitis more efficiently than glucocorticoids did.

Furthermore, evidence for the activation of NF-κB in human IBD has been found in lamina propria macrophages displaying activated p50, c-Rel, and especially p65. Significant upregulation of p65 protein levels in lamina propria macrophages and endothelial cells from patients with CD was accompanied by increased production of proinflammatory cytokines such as IL-1β, IL-6, and TNFα. Importantly, treatment of these cells with antisense

70

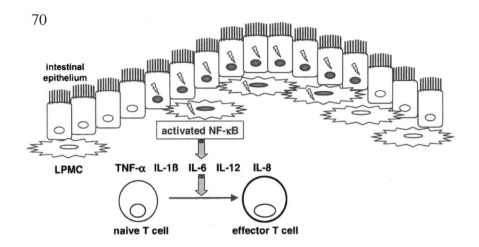

*Figure 1.* The pathophysiological hallmark of chronic intestinal inflammation and inflammatory bowel disease is the dysregualted secretion of pro-inflammatory cytokines produced by lamina propria mononuclear cells (LPMC) and T cells. One of the drivers of this dysregulated secretion of cytokines is the activation of the transcription factor NF-κB in activated epithelial cells and LPMC (dark nuclei).

p65 oligonucleotides *in vitro* reduced the production of pro-inflammatory cytokines (Neurath *et al.*, 1996). Schreiber and colleagues (Schreiber *et al.*, 1998) have also demonstrated increased p65 levels in nuclear extracts of lamina propria biopsies from CD patients.

In a study by Rogler *et al.* (1998), activated NF-κB was detected in macrophages and epithelial cells in the inflamed mucosa of IBD patients *in situ*. Here, positive p65 staining could be correlated with disease severity. While some studies had described a predominant activation of NF-κB in CD over UC (Schreiber *et al.*, 1998), other work did not detect a difference in NF-κB activation between the forms of IBD or non-specific colitis (Rogler *et al.*, 1998). This finding has led scientists to the conclusion that increased activation of NF-κB may represent an important step in the pathogenesis of any kind of mucosal inflammation. While some evidence exists for a role for NF-κB in intestinal inflammation in mucosal endothelial cells (Neurath *et al.*, 1996), or mucosal T cells and lymphocytes, there is clear proof for its role in inflammation in lamina propria macrophages (Neurath *et al.*, 1996; Rogler *et al.*, 1998; Schreiber *et al.*, 1998) and to a lesser extent in intestinal epithelial cells (Rogler *et al.*, 1998). The critical role of the NF-κB pathway in CD is further evidenced by studies demonstrating that the CARD15 (=NOD2) gene predisposes to CD (Girardin *et al.*, 2003; Lesage *et al.*,

2002). Both, intestinal epithelial cells and macrophages overexpress CARD15 in CD, which leads to the activation of NF-κB (Berrebi *et al.*, 2003; Ogura *et al.*, 2001).

As could be shown experimentally *ex vivo*, the initial activation of NF-κB at the initiation sites of inflammation will most likely trigger a further increase in production of pro-inflammatory cytokines which will feed back to activate NF-κB (Wang *et al.*, 1998). This eventually leads to the recruitment of inflammatory cells such as T cells, neutrophils, and macrophages, resulting in the amplification and chronicity of intestinal inflammation (Schottelius and Baldwin, 1999).

The presence of commensal bacteria in the gut appears to be of crucial importance in the pathogenesis of IBD (Podolsky, 2002; Sartor, 2003). Rakoff-Nahoum *et al.* have recently demonstrated that these bacteria, especially their flagellins, are recognized by toll-like receptors (TLR) under normal steady-state conditions, and that this interaction plays a crucial role in the maintenance of intestinal epithelial homeostasis (Rakoff-Nahoum *et al.*, 2004; Lodes *et al.*, 2004). Activation of the NF-κB pathway mediated by TLR signaling triggers a cell-survival response that protects against intestinal injury as indicated by experiments with mice deficient in both TLR2 and TLR4, which show increased susceptibility to dextran sulfate sodium (DSS)-induced colitis (Rakoff-Nahoum *et al.*, 2004). This increase in DSS-induced injury was also seen in mice deficient in the central adaptor protein needed for TLR signaling, MyD88 (Rakoff-Nahoum *et al.*, 2004). In this study, it was demonstrated that under physiological conditions, commensal bacteria activate TLRs, and that the resulting TLR activity provided protection from colitis-associated damage. These effects could best be explained in a model, in which the commensal intestinal flora activates TLRs on the luminal surface of intestinal epithelial cells. However, in the context of mucosal inflammation, which would permeabilize the epithelial tight junctions, bacterial antigens would get access also to the basolateral surface of the epithelial cells and activate its TLRs (Hershberg, 2002). TLR-activation would then trigger intracellular signaling pathways, such as the IKKβ/NF-κB cascade, which is the major signaling pathway downstream of TLRs and MyD88 (Beutler, 2004). Activated TLRs would thus mediate a cell-autonomous cell-survival response through NF-κB that protects the intestinal epithelium from diverse insults. These results are supported by an earlier study demonstrating that ablation of NF-κB activation in colonic epithelium results in increased susceptibility to ischemic injury (Chen *et al.*, 2003).

## 3. CELLULAR MECHANISMS OF CANCER AND THE ROLE OF NF-κB

It has been clearly established that most carcinogens and tumor promoters activate NF-κB, while chemopreventive agents generally suppress this transcription factor. This suggests a strong link between NF-κB and carcinogenesis. Actually, several lines of evidence suggest that activation of NF-κB may cause cancer. These include the finding that NF-κB genes can be oncogenes, and that this transcription factor controls apoptosis, cell-cycle progression and proliferation, and possibly also cell differentiation (Orlowski and Baldwin, 2002). However, cytokines, chemotherapeutic agents, and radiation, all inducing apoptosis, have also been demonstrated to activate NF-κB (Beg and Baltimore, 1996; Wang *et al.*, 1996; Wang *et al.*, 1999). Activation of NF-κB in these instances can be viewed as a defense mechanism of the cell that can induce desensitization, chemoresistance, and radioresistance and thus inhibit the ability of cancer therapy to induce cell death (Baldwin, 2001).

### 3.1 NF-κB as an oncogene

Specific members of the NF-κB family have been shown to be oncogenic. The c-*rel* gene has been demonstrated to consistently transform cells in culture (Gilmore *et al.*, 2004). Amplifications of c-*rel* are frequently seen in Hodgkin´s lymphomas and certain forms of B-cell lymphomas (Gilmore *et al.*, 2004). Moreover, v-*rel*, a viral homologue of c-Rel causes aggressive tumors in chickens (Rayet and Gelinas, 1999).

Several oncogene products mediate their effect through NF-κB activation. Oncogenic Ras, which is found to be constitutively active in several tumor types (Mayo *et al.*, 2001; Balmain and Pragnell, 1983) including prostate (Kim *et al.*, 2002) and colon cancer, can activate this transcription factor. Other examples include c-Myc, which mediates tumorigenesis (Kim *et al.*, 2000) and Pim-2, an oncogenic kinase, which promotes cell survival by NF-κB activation (Fox *et al.*, 2003). LMP-1, the protein that mediates the effects of EBV to cause malignancies such as Burkitt´s lymphoma, Hodgkin´s disease or gastric carcinoma, has also been identified to be a potent activator of NF-κB (Thornburg *et al.*, 2003).

Consistent with its potential role in transformation and tumorigenesis, NF-κB has been found to be constitutively active in most cell lines of hematopoietic cancers or solid tumors (Garg and Aggarwal, 2002). Constitutively active NF-κB has also been detected in tumor tissues, e.g., in breast cancer (Nakashatri *et al.*, 1997; Sovak *et al.*, 1997; Cogswell *et al.*, 2000), prostate cancer (Palayoor *et al.*, 1999), multiple myeloma (Feinman *et al.*, 1999), acute lymphocytic leukemia (Kordes *et al.*, 2000), Philadelphia -chromosome-positive acute lymphoblastic leukemia (Munzert *et al.*, 2004), acute myelogenous leukemia (Griffin, 2001), and in chronic myelogenous leukemia (Baron *et al.*, 2002). While it is not totally clear what causes the constitutive NF-κB activity in these types of tumors, some possible mechanisms have been described. For example, the inhibitor of NF-κB, IκBα, is mutated in Hodgkin's lymphoma (Cabannes *et al.*, 1999) resulting in the constitutive activation of NF-κB which drives proliferation and survival of these cells (Bargou *et al.*, 1997). These data indicate that IκBα can function as a tumor suppressor.

Furthermore, in colorectal cancer, increased levels of NF-κB protein have been observed which correlate with tumor progression (Kojima *et al.*, 2004). These observations are supported by recent studies suggesting NF-κB to play an important role in the transition from colorectal adenoma with low dysplasia to adenocarcinoma (Yu *et al.*, 2003).

## 3.2      NF-κB has anti-apoptotic activity

The fact that NF-κB activation can block cell-death pathways has been demonstrated in numerous studies (Baldwin, 2001). It was shown that the activation of this transcription factor is required to protect cells from the apoptotic cascade induced by TNFα and other stimuli. This anti-apoptotic effect can be explained by the ability of NF-κB to induce the expression of anti-apoptotic proteins such as caspase inhibitors (TRAF1 and 2, cIAP1 and 2, XIAP) and mitochondria membrane stabilizing proteins (Bcl-XL) (LaCasse *et al.* 1998; Sevilla *et al.*, 2001; Wang *et al.*, 1998). Importantly, NF-κB's ability to antagonize p53, possibly through cross-competition for transcriptional co-activators, provides an additional mechanism for the anti-apoptotic properties of NF-κB (Webster and Perkins, 1999). Inactivation of NF-κB by the IκBα superrepressor, a degradation-resistant mutant of IκBα, leads to induction of apoptosis in H-ras transformed tumor cells (Mayo *et al.*, 1997), suggesting a role for NF-κB activation in suppressing transformation-associated apoptosis.

Evidence for NF-κB as a protective factor in the intestinal mucosa comes from studies demonstrating that the inhibition of NF-κB activity enhances apoptosis of intestinal epithelial cells under inflammatory conditions (Potoka *et al.*, 2002). IKKβ removal from enterocytes results in severe apoptotic damage to the reperfused intestinal mucosa following intestinal ischemia, further underscoring the tissue-protective role of the NF-κB pathway (Chen *et al.*, 2003).

A very recent study by Greten *et al.* (2004) has provided the missing evidence required for establishing the NF-κB pathway as a link between chronic inflammation and tumorigenesis. Using a colitis-associated cancer model, they demonstrated that inhibition of NF-κB activation in colonic epithelial cells (via deletion of IKKβ) leads to a dramatic decrease in tumor incidence. Tumor size, however, was not affected. Thus, NF-κB seems to play a role in suppressing apoptosis in the early stages of tumorigenesis. Furthermore, in a model of inflammation-induced growth of colorectal tumors, NF-κB is necessary for tumor growth with inhibition of NF-κB activity results in tumor regression (Luo *et al.*, 2004).

The anti-apoptotic effect of NF-κB was also demonstrated in a model of cell-bound TNFα-mediated liver apoptosis (Maeda *et al.*, 2003). Furthermore, in the mdr2-knock-out mouse strain which develops hepatocellular carcinoma, suppression of NF-κB activation through anti-TNFα antibody treatment resulted in the apoptosis of transformed hepatocytes and inhibition of progression to carcinoma (Pikarsky *et al.*, 2004).

## 3.3     NF-κB induces proliferation of tumor cells

Evidence for a role for NF-κB as a promoter of cell proliferation comes from studies demonstrating the crucial role of this transcription factor in inducing cell cycle progression. This occurs in response to stimuli such as EGF, a growth factor for many solid tumors, which has been shown to activate NF-κB in EGF-receptor-positive breast cancer (Biswas *et al.*, 2000) and HER2, which is sometimes overexpressed in prostate, breast and other cancers, and can mediate its effects, at least partially, through the activation of NF-κB (Bhat-Nakshatri *et al.*, 2002; Myers *et al.*, 1996).

Furthermore, NF-κB has been shown to control growth through transcriptional regulation of certain cell cycle proteins such as cyclin D1, that are needed for the transition of cells from $G_1$ to S phase (Hinz *et al.*, 1999). Moreover, cytokines which can act as growth factors for tumor cells are regulated by NF-κB (Balkwill and Mantovani, 2001). These cytokines and chemokines are produced by tumor cells (Burke *et al.*, 1996) and/or the tumor-associated leukocytes and platelets. Many of these cytokines and chemokines are inducible by hypoxia, which in contrast to normal tissue can be observed in tumors (Koong *et al.*, 2000). A possible explanation for the induction of pro-inflammatory cytokines and chemokines in the state of hypoxia may be the induction of NF-κB, which is also activated in hypoxia (Koong *et al.*, 1994). Cytokines and colony-stimulating factors produced by tumor cells can prolong the survival of tumor-associated macrophages, which can be found in most, if not all tumors (Mantovani *et al.*, 1992). These cells also secrete growth and angiogenic factors as well as proteases that are able to degrade the extracellular matrix and are thus capable of stimulating tumor-cell proliferation, promoting angiogenesis, and of favoring invasion and metastasis (Mantovani *et al.*, 1992).

Among the long list of pro-inflammatory cytokines produced in tumors are TNFα, IL-1 and IL-6. TNFα is produced in a variety of hematopoetic and solid cancers, including colon cancer (Naylor *et al.*, 1990). There is accumulating evidence that TNFα, as one of the major mediators of inflammation (Schottelius *et al.*, 2004), also directly contributes to malignant progression (Balkwill and Mantovani, 2001). It has very recently been shown in a colon cancer model that metastatic growth depends on this master cytokine produced by host hematopoietic cells, and on the activation of NF-κB in the tumor cells (Luo *et al.*, 2004). Importantly, TNFα can also act as a growth factor in a mouse model of colitis-associated cancer (Greten *et al.*, 2004). Furthermore, TNFα has been shown to be a growth factor for Hodgkin's lymphoma, cutaneous T cell lymphoma, and gliomas (Pahl, 1999). Among the many effects of TNFα on cancer growth is its ability to induce angiogenic factors, including VEGF, the main such factor for colon cancer (Arii *et al.*, 1999; Bottomley *et al.*, 1999; Kollias *et al.*, 1999). Moreover, IL-1β has been shown to induce VEGF in human colon cancer (Akagi *et al.*, 1999) and IL-6 is also an inducer of VEGF expression in a variety of cell types (Cohen *et al.*, 1996). Importantly, all of the cytokines discussed above are transcriptionally regulated by NF-κB thus inducing their proliferative effects through this transcription factor (Baldwin, 1996; Osborn *et al.*, 1989).

## 3.4 NF-κB enhances tumor cell metastasis and cell adhesion

Among the hallmarks of cancer progression are invasiveness, increased angiogenesis and metastasis. NF-κB is involved in all three of these events. Invasiveness and metastasis is influenced by the expression of adhesion molecules. NF-κB was shown to regulate the expression of the adhesion molecules ICAM-1, VCAM-1 and E-Selectin (Roebuck and Finnegan, 1999; Iademarco *et al.*, 1992; Whelan *et al.*, 1991). Their increased expression, especially that of ICAM, is of clinical significance since it is associated with poor prognosis and reduced disease-free intervals in some type of cancers (Shin *et al.*, 2004; O'Hanlon *et al.*, 2002; Maruo *et al.*, 2002; Mulder *et al.*, 1997). Furthermore, in a model of breast cancer progression, Huber and colleagues demonstrated that NF-κB is essential for epithelial-mesenchymal transition and metastasis of tumor cells (Huber *et al.*, 2004). In part, metastasis may be driven by the NF-κB-induced expression of the chemokine receptor CXCR4 (Helbig *et al.*, 2003) and by NF-κB modulating the expression of the extracellular matrix protein tenascin-C (Mettouchi *et al.*, 1997). Of significance for the metastatic process is the induction of metalloprotease expression, i.e., of MMP2 and 9, by NF-κB (Yamanaka *et al.*, 2004; Hah and Lee, 2003; Philip *et al.*, 2001). The presence of these cell-surface proteases allows the tumor cells to degrade extracellular matrix and basement membranes and thus to enter the circulation and later to extravasate at a different site to cause metastatic growth.

NF-κB increases tumor angiogenesis by at least two mechanisms. Firstly, it induces the expression of the chemokine Growth Regulated Oncogene-alpha (Gro-α) and, secondly, of cyclooxygenase 2 (Cox-2) (Loukinova *et al.*, 2001; Charalambous *et al.*,2003; Liu *et al.*, 2003). Gro-α has been implicated in angiogenesis. Its continuous expression can enhance tumor growth by stimulating the outgrowth of microvessels into the tumor (Haghnegahdar *et al.*, 2000). The expression of the pro-angiogenic cyclooxygenase enzymes is upregulated in aggressive forms of CRC and may be responsible for the poor prognosis of these types of colorectal cancer (Tsujii *et al.*, 1998; Zhan *et al.*, 2004; Konno *et al.*, 2002). The most conclusive and direct evidence for the role of NF-κB in tumor progression comes from animal studies demonstrating that NF-κB activity is correlated with growth and angiogenesis in a melanoma mouse model. Furthermore, overexpression of the NF-κB inhibitor IκBα in tumor cells decreased the frequency of metastases in this model (Huang *et al.*, 2000).

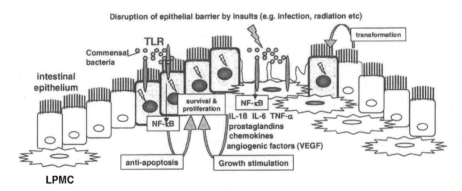

*Figure 2.* Tumorigenesis in the intestinal epithelium is promoted by two NF-κB pathways: following epithelial injury, the intestinal flora can trigger the NF-κB pathway in macrophages which then secrete pro-inflammatory factors such as prostaglandins, chemokines and cytokines. These factors promote the survival of transformed epithelial cells (darker cells). Furthermore, the intestinal flora can independently activate the NF-κB pathway through binding to TLRs on the surface of epithelial cells and through increased expression of anti-apoptotic genes. Moreover, NF-κB activation in already transformed intestinal epithelial cells stimulates their proliferation and enhances their survival. Activation of these two pathways may result in tumorigenesis and thus could explain the increased incidence of cancer in patients with IBD.

## 4.    AN NF-κB-BASED MODEL LINKING INFLAMMATORY BOWEL DISEASE TO COLORECTAL CANCER

As described above, ample evidence now exists suggesting that NF-κB may mediate tumorigenesis. Furthermore, the role of NF-κB as a key signal transducer in inflammation is clearly established. Considering data from recent studies (Greten *et al.*, 2004; Rakoff-Nahoum *et al.*, 2004), a model in which two NF-κB pathways converge to promote tumor formation in the bowel can be developed further: following epithelial injury, the intestinal flora can trigger the NF-κB pathway in macrophages which then produce and activate key pro-inflammatory factors such as prostaglandins, chemokines, cytokines, COX-2 and nitric oxide (NO) synthase 2, as observed in IBD (Fig. 2). The observed enhanced epithelial cell turnover in the colonic mucosa of IBD patients combined with the oxidative stress caused by the inflammation, increases the likelihood of epithelial cell transformation and carcinogenesis. In addition, the cytokines and chemokines produced by macrophages promote the survival of transformed epithelial cells. This pathway is complemented by a cell-autonomous pathway, in which the intestinal flora constitutively activates the NF-κB pathway through TLRs on epithelial cells and under normal conditions would thus support their survival and protection from injury. When this pathway is stimulated in already transformed epithelial cells, however, it accelerates the development of tumors in a cell-autonomous fashion. This would explain why deletion of IKKβ and blockade of the NF-κB pathway in intestinal epithelial cells leads to a dramatic decrease in tumor incidence (Greten *et al.*, 2004). Therefore, activation of these two pathways can result in tumorigenesis and thus could be responsible for the increased incidence of cancer in patients with IBD.

## 5.    OUTLOOK: CLINICAL USE OF NF-κB INHIBITORS

As pointed out above, epidemiological studies indicate that the regular administration of NSAIDs lowers mortality from sporadic colorectal cancer and leads to regression of adenomas in patients with Familial Adenomatous Polyposis (FAP) (Oshima and Taketo, 2002; Yamamoto and Gaynor, 2001). Indeed, NSAIDs reduce the risk of colorectal cancer by 75% to 81% (Eaden *et al.*, 2000). The ability of NSAIDs to inhibit COX activity to prevent prostaglandin synthesis is the most commonly accepted mechanism to account for the anti-inflammatory effects of NSAIDs and the prevention of colon cancer (Gupta and Dubois, 2001; Vane, 1994). However, a number of studies suggest, that the ability of NSAIDs to inhibit the NF-κB pathway is responsible for the anti-inflammatory properties of these compounds (Kopp and Ghosh, 1994; Yamamoto *et al.*, 1999; Yin *et al.*, 1998). Sodium salicylates inhibit NF-κB through a mechanism involving inhibition of IκBα phosphorylation (Kopp and Ghosh, 1994; Pierce *et al.*, 1996), which appears to require the activation of mitogen-activated protein kinase p38 (Schwenger *et al.*, 1998). It has been demonstrated that aspirin and sodium salicylate specifically inhibit IKKβ *in vitro* and *in vivo* at concentrations found in the serum of patients treated for chronic inflammatory diseases (Yin *et al.*, 1998). More recent studies have identified sulfasalazine, which is effectively used in the therapy of IBD, as a direct inhibitor of IKKα and β (Weber *et al.*, 2000). Also mesalamine, a derivative of 5-aminosalicylic acid, has been shown to block TNFα-stimulated NF-κB activation by inhibiting degradation of IκBα (Kaiser *et al.*, 1999). Sulindac, an NSAID structurally related to indomethacin, and its metabolites can inhibit IKK activity (Yamamoto *et al.*, 1999). Additionally, sulindac and aspirin induce apoptosis in HCT-15 cells, a colon carcinoma cell line that is defective in the generation of prostaglandins (Yamamoto *et al.,* 1999). These results implicate the inhibition of NF-κB in the anti-inflammatory as well as the growth-inhibitory properties of certain NSAIDs (Yamamoto and Gaynor, 2001) and underscores the notion that NF-κB may be a good target in cancer therapy. Surprisingly, Stark *et al.* (2001) have described increased NF-κB activation and the induction of apoptosis after continuous treatment of colorectal cancer cells with aspirin. These effects were specific to colon cancer cells and were not observed in other cancer cell types (Din *et al.*, 2004). These data demonstrate that the effects of aspirin on the NF-κB pathway may depend on the context of cells and treatment regimen and that, under some circumstances, NF-κB may also mediate apoptotic effects. Interestingly, NF-κB activation is also seen after treatment of myeloid and lymphoid cells with doxorubicin and its analogues and this activation was required for the cytotoxic effects of doxorubicin, giving NF-κB a pro-apoptotic role in this context (Ashikawa *et al.*, 2004).

A number of studies investigating the potential of NF-κB inhibitors in combination with chemo- and radiation therapy provide growing evidence that inhibition of the NF-κB pathway may prove to be an effective adjuvant therapy in colon cancer, but might be less effective in other forms of cancer. These studies were inspired by the knowledge of NF-κB being a suppressor of apoptosis and the observation that this transcription factor was activated by several apoptosis-inducing drugs as well as ionizing radiation. Baldwin and colleagues found that the inducible chemoresistance to CPT-11 (irinotecan) in the colorectal cancer cell line LOVO as well as LOVO tumors could be overcome by transient inhibition of NF-κB using adenoviral delivery of the superrepressor (Baldwin, 2001; Cusack, *et al.*, 2000). Also, the use of the proteasome inhibitor PS-341 as a systemic inhibitor of NF-κB in conjunction with CPT-11 treatment led to significantly improved chemotherapeutic responses in colorectal cancer cell lines and xenografts through an increase in apoptosis of cancer cells (Cusack *et al.*, 2001). Similarly, a 84% reduction in initial tumor volume was obtained in LOVO xenografts receiving radiation and PS-341 (Russo *et al.*, 2001) where the radiosensitivity of colon cancer cells is enhanced by inhibition of NF-κB after adenoviral infection with a degradation resistant form of IκBα (Mukogawa *et al.*, 2003).

However, the induction of apoptosis by some chemotherapeutic compounds appears to be dependent on the presence of functional p53 (Wu and Ding, 2002; Lorenzo *et al.*, 2002) and this tumor suppressor gene has been shown to require NF-κB for the induction of apoptosis (Ryan *et al.*, 2000). Thus, depending on the mode of activation, NF-κB can also have pro-apoptotic effects, potentially limiting the effectiveness of NF-κB inhibition as adjuvant cancer therapy to such compounds that do not require functional p53 and to tumors with defective p53 (Haefner, 2002). For example in the case of NF-κB inhibition by PS-341, wild-type p53 is apparently not needed for the enhanced apoptotic response (Cusack *et al.*, 2001).

Interestingly, evidence now exists for the ability of NF-κB to transcriptionally regulate the multidrug resistance 1 (MDR1) gene in colon cancer cells (Bentires-Alj *et al.*, 2003). Thus, in addition to inhibiting apoptosis, this transcription factor seems to also promote survival of cancer cells under chemotherapy by the induction of MDR1 expression.

Clinical trials with NF-κB inhibitors, such as thalidomide and PS-341 have so far demonstrated efficacy of these agents as monotherapy for hematological malignancies (Orlowski and Baldwin, 2002). Conclusions regarding the efficacy of NF-κB inhibitors in cancer, however, should not be drawn based on the data obtained with PS-341 and thalidomide in clinical trials, since these compounds are likely to also function through mechanisms other than blocking NF-κB activity, e.g., the interruption of growth signaling pathways (Hideshima *et al.*, 2001). A general concern regarding clinical use of NF-κB specific inhibitors is the lack of knowledge of the specific roles of the various NF-κB subunits and regulators. It might be possible, that the function of NF-κB in leukemia and lymphomas might differ from the function in solid tumors (Orlowski and Baldwin, 2002). Furthermore, as discussed above, within a tumor cell, NF-κB can have pro-apoptotic and anti-apoptotic activity. The immune system regulated by NF-κB can support tumorigenesis but can also kill tumor cells. Therefore, the efficacy of NF-κB inhibitors in cancer therapy will most likely depend on the targeted tumor type and/or tumor stage.

Nevertheless, the NF-κB signaling pathway is increasingly being recognized by the pharmaceutical industry as a target for anti-inflammatory and anti-cancer drugs (Haefner, 2002). It is therefore conceivable that small molecular NF-κB inhibitors specifically targeting central molecules in the NF-κB pathway such as IKK will be tested in cancer models either as monotherapy or as adjuvant therapy with established chemotherapeutic drugs or radiation therapy. With IKKβ now being identified as the link between chronic inflammation and colitis-associated cancer, pharmacological inhibition of IKKβ may be effective in preventing this type of cancer (Greten *et al.*, 2004). Considering the crucial role of IKKβ in innate immune responses and also in suppressing certain kinds of cancer (Dajee *et al.*, 2003), the long-term use of such drugs will have to be closely monitored. The challenge of future research will be to elucidate the specific NF-κB pathways and roles of NF-κB subunits in different cancer types, which should pave the way for more specific and safer NF-κB inhibitors in the treatment of cancer.

# 6.    REFERENCES

Akagi, Y. *et al.* (1999). Regulation of vascular endothelial growth factor expression in human colon cancer by interleukin-1beta. *Br. J. Cancer* **80**: 1506-1511.

Ames, B.N. *et al.* (1995). The causes and prevention of cancer. *Proc. Natl Acad. Sci. USA* **92**: 5258-5265.

Arii, S. *et al.* (1999). Implication of vascular endothelial growth factor in the development and metastasis of human cancers. *Hum.Cell* **12**: 25-30.

Ashikawa, K. *et al.* (2004). Evidence that activation of nuclear factor-kappaB is essential for the cytotoxic effects of doxorubicin and its analogues. *Biochem. Pharmacol.* **67**: 353-364.

Baldwin, A.S., Jr. (1996). The NF-kappa B and I kappa B proteins: new discoveries and insights. *Annu. Rev. Immunol.* **14**: 649-683.

Baldwin, A.S., Jr. (2001). Control of oncogenesis and cancer therapy resistance by the transcription factor NF-kappaB. *J. Clin. Invest.* **107**: 241-246.

Baldwin, A.S., Jr. (2001). Series Introduction: The transcription factor NF-kappaB and human disease. *J. Clin. Invest.* **107**: 3-6.

Balkwill, F. and Mantovani, A. (2001). Inflammation and cancer: back to Virchow? *Lancet* **357**: 539-545.

Balmain, A. and Pragnell, I.B. (1983). Mouse skin carcinomas induced *in vivo* by chemical carcinogens have a transforming Harvey-ras oncogene. *Nature* **303**: 72-74.

Bargou, R.C. *et al.* (1997). Constitutive Nuclear Factor-kappa B-RelA Activation Is Required for Proliferation and Survival of Hodgkin's Disease Tumor Cells. *J. Clin. Invest.* **100**: 2961-2969.

Baron, F. *et al.* (2002). Leukemic target susceptibility to natural killer cytotoxicity: relationship with BCR-ABL expression. *Blood* **99**: 2107-2113.

Beg, A.A. and Baltimore D. (1996). An essential role for NF-kappaB in preventing TNF-alpha-induced cell death. *Science* **274**: 782-784.

Bentires-Alj, M. *et al.* (2003). NF-kappaB transcription factor induces drug resistance through MDR1 expression in cancer cells. *Oncogene* **22**: 90-97.

Berrebi, D. *et al.* Card15 gene overexpression in mononuclear and epithelial cells of the inflamed Crohn's disease colon. *Gut* **52**: 840-846.

Beutler, B. (2004). Inferences, questions and possibilities in Toll-like receptor signaling. *Nature* **430**: 257-263.

Bhat-Nakshatri, P. *et al.* (2002). Identification of signal transduction pathways involved in constitutive NF-kappaB activation in breast cancer cells. *Oncogene* **21**: 2066-2078.

Bingle, L. *et al.* (2002). The role of tumour-associated macrophages in tumour progression: implications for new anticancer therapies. *J. Pathol.* **196**: 254-265.

Biswas, D.K. *et al.* Epidermal growth factor-induced nuclear factor kappa B activation: A major pathway of cell-cycle progression in estrogen-receptor negative breast cancer cells. *Proc. Natl Acad. Sci. U.S.A.* **97**: 8542-8547.

Bottomley *et al.* (1999) Peripheral blood mononuclear cells from patients with rheumatoid arthritis spontaneously secrete vascular endothelial growth factor (VEGF): specific up-regulation by tumour necrosis factor-alpha in synovial fluid. *Clin. Exp. Immunol.* **117**: 171-176.

Bouma, G. and Strober W. (2003). The immunological and genetic basis of inflammatory bowel disease. *Nat. Rev. Immunol.* **3**: 521-533.

Burke, F. *et al.* (1996). A cytokine profile of normal and malignant ovary. *Cytokine* **8**: 578-585.

Cabannes, E. *et al.* (1999). Mutations in the IkappaBalpha gene in Hodgkin's disease suggest a tumour suppressor role for IkappaBalpha. *Oncogene* **18**: 3063-3070.

Chan, T.A. (2003). Cyclooxygenase inhibition and mechanisms of colorectal cancer prevention. *Curr. Cancer Drug Targets* **3**: 455-463.

Charalambous, M.P. *et al.* (2003). Upregulation of cyclooxygenase-2 is accompanied by increased expression of nuclear factor-kappa B and IkappaBkinase-alpha in human colorectal cancer epithelial cells. *Br. J. Cancer* **88**: 1598-1604.

Chen, L.W. *et al.* (2003). The two faces of IKK and NF-kappaB inhibition: prevention of systemic inflammation but increased local injury following intestinal ischemia-reperfusion. *Nat. Med.* **9**: 575-581.

Cogswell, P.C. *et al.* (2000). Selective activation of NF-kappa B subunits in human breast cancer: potential roles for NF-kappa B2/p52 and for Bcl-3. *Oncogene* **19**: 1123-1131.

Cohen, T. *et al.* (1996). Interleukin 6 induces the expression of vascular endothelial growth factor. *J. Biol. Chem.* **271**: 736-741.

Collet, J.P. *et al.* (1999). Colorectal cancer prevention by non-steroidal anti-inflammatory drugs: effects of dosage and timing. *Br. J. Cancer* **81**: 62-68.

Cusack, J.C., Jr. *et al.* (2000). Inducible chemoresistance to 7-ethyl-10-[4-(1-piperidino)-1-piperidino]carbonyloxycamptothecin (CPT-11) in colorectal cancer cells and a xenograft model is overcome by inhibition of nuclear factor-kappaB activation. *Cancer Res.* **60**: 2323-2330.

Cusack, J.C., Jr. *et al.* (2001). Enhanced chemosensitivity to CPT-11 with proteasome inhibitor PS-341: implications for systemic nuclear factor-kappaB inhibition. *Cancer Res.* **61**: 3535-3540.

Dajee, M. *et al.* (2003). NF-kappaB blockade and oncogenic Ras trigger invasive human epidermal neoplasia. *Nature* **421**: 639-643.

Din, F.V. *et al.* (2004). Evidence for colorectal cancer cell specificity of aspirin effects on NF-kappa B signaling and apoptosis. *Br. J. Cancer* **91**: 381-388.

Eaden, J. *et al.* (2000). Colorectal cancer prevention in ulcerative colitis: a case-control study. *Aliment. Pharmacol. Ther.* **14**: 145-153.

Feinman, R. *et al.* (1999). Role of NF-kappaB in the rescue of multiple myeloma cells from glucocorticoid-induced apoptosis by Bcl-2. *Blood* **93**: 3044-3052.

Fox, C.J. *et al.* (2003). The serine/threonine kinase Pim-2 is a transcriptionally regulated apoptotic inhibitor. *Genes Dev.* **17**: 1841-1854.

Garg, A. and Aggarwal B.B. (2002). Nuclear transcription factor-kappaB as a target for cancer drug development. *Leukemia* **16**: 1053-1068.

Gilmore, T.D. *et al.* (2004). RELevant gene amplification in B-cell lymphomas? *Blood* **103**: 3243-3244.

Giovannucci, E. *et al.* (1994). Aspirin use and the risk for colorectal cancer and adenoma in male health professionals. *Ann. Intern. Med.* **121**: 241-246.

Girardin, S.E. *et al.* (2003). Lessons from Nod2 studies: towards a link between Crohn's disease and bacterial sensing. *Trends Immunol.* **24**: 652-658.

Greten, F.R. *et al.* (2004). IKKbeta links inflammation and tumorigenesis in a mouse model of colitis-associated cancer. *Cell* **118**: 285-296.

Griffin, J.D. (2001). Leukemia stem cells and constitutive activation of NF-kappaB. *Blood* **98**: 2291.

Gupta, R.A. and Dubois R.N. (2001). Colorectal cancer prevention and treatment by inhibition of cyclooxygenase-2. *Nat. Rev. Cancer* **1**: 11-21.

Haefner, B. (2002). NF-kappaB: arresting a major culprit in cancer. *Drug Discov. Today* **7**: 653-663.

Haghnegahdar, H. *et al.* (2000). The tumorigenic and angiogenic effects of MGSA/GRO proteins in melanoma. *J. Leukoc. Biol.* **67**: 53-62.

Hah, N. and Lee S.T. (2003). An absolute role of the PKC-dependent NF-kappaB activation for induction of MMP-9 in hepatocellular carcinoma cells. *Biochem. Biophys. Res. Commun.* **30**: 428-433.

Helbig, G. *et al.* (2003). NF-kappaB promotes breast cancer cell migration and metastasis by inducing the expression of the chemokine receptor CXCR4. *J. Biol. Chem.* **278**: 21631-21638.

Hershberg, R.M. (2002). The epithelial cell cytoskeleton and intracellular trafficking: V. Polarized compartmentalization of antigen processing and Toll-like receptor signaling in intestinal epithelial cells. *Am. J. Physiol. Gastrointest. Liver Physiol.* **283**: G833-G839.

Hideshima, T. *et al.* (2001). The proteasome inhibitor PS-341 inhibits growth, induces apoptosis, and overcomes drug resistance in human multiple myeloma cells. *Cancer Res.* **61**: 3071-3076.

Hinz, M. *et al.* (1999). NF-kappaB function in growth control: regulation of cyclin D1 expression and G0/G1-to-S-Phase transition. *Mol. Cell. Biol.* **19**: 2690-2698.

Huber, M.A. *et al.* (2004). NF-kappaB is essential for epithelial-mesenchymal transition and metastasis in a model of breast cancer progression. *J. Clin. Invest.* **114**: 569-581.

Iademarco, M.F. *et al.* (1992). Characterization of the promoter for vascular cell adhesion molecule-1 (VCAM-1). *J. Biol. Chem.* **267**: 16323-16329.

Itzkowitz, S.H. and Yio, X. (2004). Inflammation and cancer IV. Colorectal cancer in inflammatory bowel disease: the role of inflammation. *Am. J. Physiol. Gastrointest. Liver Physiol.* **287**: G7-G17.

Jolly, K. *et al.* (1999). NSAIDs and gastrointestinal cancer prevention. *Drugs* **62**: 945-956.

Kaiser, G.C. *et al.* (1999). Mesalamine blocks tumor necrosis factor growth inhibition and nuclear factor kappaB activation in mouse colonocytes. *Gastroenterology* **116**: 602-609.

Kim, B.Y. *et al.* (2002). Constitutive activation of NF-kappaB in Ki-ras-transformed prostate epithelial cells. *Oncogene* **21**: 4490-4497.

Kim, D.W. *et al.* (2000). The RelA NF-kappaB subunit and the aryl hydrocarbon receptor (AhR) cooperate to transactivate the c-myc promoter in mammary cells. *Oncogene* **19**: 5498-5506.

Koehne, C.H. and Dubois, R.N. (2004). COX-2 inhibition and colorectal cancer. *Semin. Oncol.* **31** (Suppl. 7): 12-21.

Kojima, M. *et al.* (2004). Increased nuclear factor-kappaB activation in human colorectal carcinoma and its correlation with tumor progression. *Anticancer Res.* **24**: 675-681.

Kollias, G. *et al.* (1999). On the role of tumor necrosis factor and receptors in models of multiorgan failure, rheumatoid arthritis, multiple sclerosis and inflammatory bowel disease. *Immunol. Rev.* **169**: 175-194.

Konno, H. *et al.* (2002). Cyclooxygenase-2 expression correlates with uPAR levels and is responsible for poor prognosis of colorectal cancer. *Clin. Exp. Metastasis* **19**: 527-534.

Koong, A.C. *et al.* (1994). Hypoxic activation of nuclear factor-kappa B is mediated by a Ras and Raf signaling pathway and does not involve MAP kinase (ERK1 or ERK2). *Cancer Res.* **54**: 5273-5279.

Koong, A.C. *et al.* (2000). Candidate genes for the hypoxic tumor phenotype. *Cancer Res.* **60**: 883-887.

Kopp, E. and Ghosh S. (1994). Inhibition of NF-kappa B by sodium salicylate and aspirin. *Science* **265**: 956-959.

Kordes, U. *et al.* (2000). Transcription factor NF-kappaB is constitutively activated in acute lymphoblastic leukemia cells. *Leukemia* **14**: 399-402.

LaCasse, E.C. *et al.* (1998). The inhibitors of apoptosis (IAPs) and their emerging role in cancer. *Oncogene* **17**: 3247-3259.

Lackner, C. *et al.* (2004). Prognostic relevance of tumour-associated macrophages and von Willebrand factor-positive microvessels in colorectal cancer. *Virchows Arch.* **445**: 160-167.

Langman, M.J. *et al.* (2001). Effect of anti-inflammatory drugs on overall risk of common cancer: case-control study in general practice research database. *Br. Med. J.* **320**: 1642-1646.

Leek, R. D. and Harris A.L. (2002). Tumor-associated macrophages in breast cancer. *J. Mammary Gland Biol. Neoplasia* 7: 177-189.

Lesage, S. *et al.* (2002) CARD15/NOD2 mutational analysis and genotype-phenotype correlation in 612 patients with inflammatory bowel disease. *Am. J. Hum. Genet.* **70**: 845-857.

Lin, E. Y. and Pollard J.W. (2004). Macrophages: modulators of breast cancer progression. *Novartis Found Symp.* **256**: 158-168.

Liu, W. *et al.* (2003). Cyclooxygenase-2 is up-regulated by interleukin-1beta in human colorectal cancer cells via multiple signaling pathways. *Cancer Res.* **63**: 3632-3636.

Lodes, M.J. *et al.* (2004). Bacterial flagellin is a dominant antigen in Crohn disease. *J. Clin. Invest.* **113**: 1296-1306.

Lorenzo, E. *et al.* (2002). Doxorubicin induces apoptosis and CD95 gene expression in human primary endothelial cells through a p53-dependent mechanism. *J. Biol. Chem.* **277**: 10883-10892.

Loukinova, E. *et al.* (2001). Expression of proangiogenic chemokine Gro 1 in low and high metastatic variants of Pam murine squamous cell carcinoma is differentially regulated by IL-1alpha, EGF and TGF-beta1 through NF-kappaB dependent and independent mechanisms. *Int. J. Cancer*: 637-644.

Luo, J.L. *et al.* (2004). Inhibition of NF-kappaB in cancer cells converts inflammation-induced tumor growth mediated by TNFalpha to TRAIL-mediated tumor regression. *Cancer Cell* **6**: 297-305.

Maeda, S. *et al.* (2003) IKKbeta is required for prevention of apoptosis mediated by cell-bound but not by circulating TNFalpha. *Immunity* **19**: 725-737.

Mantovani, A. *et al.* (1992). The origin and function of tumor-associated macrophages. *Immunol. Today* **13**: 265-270.

Mantovani, A. *et al.* (1992). Cytokine regulation of endothelial cell function. *FASEB J.* **6**: 2591-2599.

Maruo, Y. *et al.* (2002). ICAM-1 expression and the soluble ICAM-1 level for evaluating the metastatic potential of gastric cancer. *Int. J. Cancer* **100**: 486-490.

Mayo, M.W. *et al.* (2001). Ras regulation of NF-kappa B and apoptosis. *Methods Enzymol.* **333**: 73-87.

Mayo, M.W. *et al.* (1997). Requirement of NF-kappaB activation to suppress p53-independent apoptosis induced by oncogenic Ras. *Science* **278**: 1812-1815.

Mettouchi, A. *et al.* (1997). The c-Jun-induced transformation process involves complex regulation of tenascin-C expression. *Mol. Cell Biol.* **17**: 3202-3209.

Miyagawa, S. *et al.* (2002). Morphometric analysis of liver macrophages in patients with colorectal liver metastasis. *Clin. Exp. Metastasis* **19**: 119-125.

Monteleone, G. (1997). Interleukin 12 is expressed and actively released by Crohn's disease intestinal lamina propria mononuclear cells. *Gastroenterology* **112**: 1169-1178.

Mukogawa, T. *et al.* (2003). Adenovirus-mediated gene transduction of truncated IkappaBalpha enhances radiosensitivity in human colon cancer cells. *Cancer Sci.* **94**: 745-750.

Mulder, W.M. *et al.* (1997). Low intercellular adhesion molecule 1 and high 5T4 expression on tumor cells correlate with reduced disease-free survival in colorectal carcinoma patients. *Clin. Cancer Res.* **3**: 1923-1930.

Munkholm, P. (2003). Review article: the incidence and prevalence of colorectal cancer in inflammatory bowel disease. *Aliment. Pharmacol. Ther.* **18** (Suppl. 2): 1-5.

Munzert, G. *et al.* (2004). Constitutive NF-kappab/Rel activation in Philadelphia chromosome positive (Ph+) acute lymphoblastic leukemia (ALL). *Leuk. Lymphoma* **45**: 1181-1184.

Myers, R.B. *et al.* (1996). Elevated serum levels of p105(erbB-2) in patients with advanced-stage prostatic adenocarcinoma. *Int. J. Cancer* **69**: 398-402.

Nakshatri, H. *et al.* (1997). Constitutive activation of NF-kappaB during progression of breast cancer to hormone-independent growth. *Mol. Cell. Biol.* **17**: 3629-3639.

Naylor, M.S. *et al.* (1990). Investigation of cytokine gene expression in human colorectal cancer. *Cancer Res.* **50**: 4436-4440.

Neurath, M.F. *et al.* (1998) Cytokine gene transcription by NF-kappaB family members in patients with inflammatory bowel disease. *Ann. N. Y. Acad. Sci.* **859**: 149-159.

Neurath, M.F. *et al.* (1996). Local administration of antisense phosphorothioate oligonucleotides to the p65 subunit of NF-kappaB abrogates established experimental colitis in mice. *Nat. Med.* **2**: 998-1004.

O'Hanlon, D.M. *et al.* (2002). Soluble adhesion molecules (E-selectin, ICAM-1 and VCAM-1) in breast carcinoma. *Eur. J. Cancer* **38**: 2252-2257.

Ogura, Y. *et al.* (2001). A frameshift mutation in NOD2 associated with susceptibility to Crohn's disease. *Nature* **411**: 603-606.

Orlowski, R.Z. and Baldwin, A.S., Jr. (2002) NF-kappaB as a therapeutic target in cancer. *Trends Mol. Med.* **8**: 385-389.

Osborn, L.S. *et al.* (1989). Tumor necrosis factor alpha and interleukin 1 stimulate the human immunodeficiency virus enhancer by activation of the nuclear factor kappa B. *Proc. Natl Acad. Sci. U.S.A.* **86**: 2336-2340.

Oshima, M. and Taketo, M.M. (2002). COX selectivity and animal models for colon cancer. *Curr. Pharm. Des.* **8**: 1021-1034.

Pahl, H.L. (1999). Activators and target genes of Rel/NF-kappaB transcription factors. *Oncogene* **18**: 6853-6866.

Palayoor, S.T. *et al.* (1999). Constitutive activation of IkappaB kinase alpha and NF-kappaB in prostate cancer cells is inhibited by ibuprofen. *Oncogene* **18**: 7389-7394.

Philip, S. *et al.* (2001). Osteopontin stimulates tumor growth and activation of promatrix metalloproteinase-2 through nuclear factor-kappaB-mediated induction of membrane type 1 matrix metalloproteinase in murine melanoma cells. *J. Biol. Chem.* **276**: 44926-44935.

Pierce, J.W. *et al.* (1996). Salicylates inhibit IkappaB-alpha phosphorylation, endothelial-leukocyte adhesion molecule expression, and neutrophil transmigration. *J. Immunol.* **156**: 3961-3969.

Pikarsky, E. *et al.* (2004). NF-kappaB functions as a tumour promoter in inflammation-associated cancer. *Nature* **431**: 461-466.

Podolsky, D.K. (2002). Inflammatory bowel disease. *New Engl. J. Med.* **347**: 417-429.

Potoka, D.A. *et al.* (2002). NF-kappaB inhibition enhances peroxynitrite-induced enterocyte apoptosis. *J. Surg. Res.* **106**: 7-14.

Rakoff-Nahoum, S. *et al.* (2004). Recognition of commensal microflora by toll-like receptors is required for intestinal homeostasis. *Cell* **118**: 671-674.

Rayet, B. and Gelinas C. (1999). Aberrant rel/nfkb genes and activity in human cancer. *Oncogene* **18**: 6938-47.

Reuter, B.K. and Pizarro, T.T. (2004). Commentary: the role of the IL-18 system and other members of the IL-1R/TLR superfamily in innate mucosal immunity and the pathogenesis of inflammatory bowel disease: friend or foe? *Eur. J. Immunol.* **34**: 2347-2355.

Roebuck, K.A. and Finnegan, A. (1999). Regulation of intercellular adhesion molecule-1 (CD54) gene expression. *J. Leukoc. Biol.* **66**: 876-888.

Rogler, G. *et al.* (1998). Nuclear factor kappaB is activated in macrophages and epithelial cells of inflamed intestinal mucosa. *Gastroenterology* **115**: 357-369.

Russo, S.M. *et al.* (2001). Enhancement of radiosensitivity by proteasome inhibition: implications for a role of NF-kappaB. *Int. J. Radiat. Oncol. Biol. Phys.* **50**: 183-193.

Ryan, K.M. *et al.* (2000). Role of NF-kappaB in p53-mediated programmed cell death. *Nature* **404**: 892-897.

Sartor, R.B. (2003). Innate immunity in the pathogenesis and therapy of IBD. *J. Gastroenterol.* **38** (Suppl. 15): 43-47.

Schottelius, A.J. and Baldwin, A.S., Jr. (1999). A role for transcription factor NF-kappa B in intestinal inflammation. *Int. J. Colorectal. Dis.* **14**: 18-28.

Schottelius, A.J. *et al.* (2004). Biology of tumor necrosis factor-alpha- implications for psoriasis. *Exp. Dermatol.* **13**: 193-222.

Schreiber, S. *et al.* (1998). Activation of nuclear factor kappa B inflammatory bowel disease. *Gut*: 477-484.

Schwenger, P. *et al.* (1998). Activation of p38 mitogen-activated protein kinase by sodium salicylate leads to inhibition of tumor necrosis factor-induced IkappaB alpha phosphorylation and degradation. *Mol.Cell. Biol.* **18**: 78-84.

Sevilla, L. *et al.* (2001). Transcriptional regulation of the bcl-x gene encoding the anti-apoptotic Bcl-xL protein by Ets, Rel/NFkappaB, STAT and AP1 transcription factor families. *Histol. Histopathol.* **16**: 595-601.

Shin, H.S. *et al.* (2004). The relationship between the serum intercellular adhesion molecule-1 level and the prognosis of the disease in lung cancer. *Korean J. Intern. Med.* **19**: 48-52.

Sovak, M.A. *et al.* (1997). Aberrant Nuclear Factor-kappa B/Rel Expression and the Pathogenesis of Breast Cancer. *J. Clin. Invest.* **100**: 2952-2960.

Spiik, A.K. *et al.* (2002). Abrogated lymphocyte infiltration and lowered CD14 in dextran sulfate induced colitis in mice treated with p65 antisense oligonucleotides. *Int. J. Colorectal Dis.* **17**: 223-232.

Stark, L.A. *et al.* (2001) Aspirin-induced activation of the NF-kappaB signaling pathway: a novel mechanism for aspirin-mediated apoptosis in colon cancer cells. *FASEB J.* **15**: 1273-1275.

Strober, W. *et al.* (2002). The immunology of mucosal models of inflammation. *Annu. Rev. Immunol.* **20**: 495-549.

Thornburg, N. *et al.* (2003). Activation of nuclear factor-kappaB p50 homodimer/Bcl-3 complexes in nasopharyngeal carcinoma. *Cancer Res.* **63**: 8293-8301.

Thun, M.J. *et al.* (1999). Aspirin use and risk of fatal cancer. *Cancer Res.* **53**: 1322-1327.

Toomey, D. *et al.* (1999). Phenotyping of immune cell infiltrates in breast and colorectal tumours. *Immunol. Invest.* **28**: 29-41.

Tsujii, M. *et al.* (1998). Cyclooxygenase regulates angiogenesis induced by colon cancer cells. *Cell* **93**: 705-716.

Vane, J. (1994). Towards a better aspirin. *Nature* **367**: 215-216.

Wang, C.Y. *et al.* (1999). Control of inducible chemoresistance: enhanced anti-tumor therapy through increased apoptosis by inhibition of NF-kappaB. *Nat. Med.* **5**: 412-417.

Wang, C.Y. *et al.* (1996). TNF- and cancer therapy-induced apoptosis: potentiation by inhibition of NF-kappaB. *Science* **274**: 784-787.

Wang, C.Y. *et al.* (1998). NF-kappaB antiapoptosis: induction of TRAF1 and TRAF2 and c-IAP1 and c-IAP2 to suppress caspase-8 activation. *Science* **281**: 1680-1683.

Wang, L. *et al.* (2003). IL-6 induces NF-kappaB activation in the intestinal epithelia. *J. Immunol.* **171**: 3194-3201.

Weber, C.K. *et al.* (2000). Suppression of NF-kappaB activity by sulfasalazine is mediated by direct inhibition of IkappaB kinases alpha and beta. *Gastroenterology* **119**: 1209-1218.

Webster, G.A. and Perkins, N.D. (1999). Transcriptional cross talk between NF-kappaB and p53. *Mol. Cell. Biol.* **19**: 3485-3495.

Whelan, J. *et al.* (1991). An NF-kappa B-like factor is essential but not sufficient for cytokine induction of endothelial leukocyte adhesion molecule 1 (ELAM-1) gene transcription. *Nucleic Acids Res.* **19**: 2645-2653.

Wu, G.S. and Ding, Z. (2002). Caspase 9 is required for p53-dependent apoptosis and chemosensitivity in a human ovarian cancer cell line. *Oncogene* **21**: 1-8.

Yamamoto, Y. and Gaynor, R.B. (2001). Therapeutic potential of inhibition of the NF-kappaB pathway in the treatment of inflammation and cancer. *J. Clin. Invest.* **107**: 135-42.

Yamamoto, Y. *et al.* (1999). Sulindac inhibits activation of the NF-kappaB pathway. *J. Biol. Chem.* **274**: 27307-27314.

Yamanaka, N. *et al.* (2004). Interleukin-1beta enhances invasive ability of gastric carcinoma through nuclear factor-kappaB activation. *Clin. Cancer Res.* **10**: 1853-1859.

Yin, M.J. *et al.* (1998). The anti-inflammatory agents aspirin and salicylate inhibit the activity of IkappaB kinase-beta. *Nature* **396**: 77-80.

Yu, H.G. *et al.* (2003). Increased expression of RelA/nuclear factor-kappa B protein correlates with colorectal tumorigenesis. *Oncology* **65**: 37-45.

Zhan, J. *et al.* (2004). Relationship between COX-2 expression and clinicopathological features of colorectal cancers. *Chin. Med. J.* (Engl.) **117**: 1151-54.

Chapter 4

# REGULATION OF NF-κB TRANSCRIPTIONAL ACTIVITY

Linda Vermeulen, Wim Vanden Berghe and Guy Haegeman
*Laboratory for Eukaryotic Gene Expression and Signal Transduction (LEGEST), Department of Molecular Biology, Ghent University, K. L. Ledeganckstraat 35, 9000 Gent, Belgium*

Abstract:     Nuclear factor κB (NF-κB) is regarded as a key regulator of inflammation; hence, several inflammatory diseases result from deregulation of NF-κB signaling. There is, however, also increasing evidence for a preponderant role of NF-κB in tumor development and progression. Constitutive activation of NF-κB activity by signaling defects, mutations or chromosomal rearrangements can be found in a wide variety of cancers. Additionally, a causal link between inflammation and cancer has been noted, which makes NF-κB an interesting target for development of both anti-inflammatory and anti-cancer therapeutics. Here, we review current knowledge of NF-κB signal transduction, focusing on the regulation of its transcriptional activity by post-translational modification of the NF-κB subunits.

Keywords:   NF-κB; signal transduction; acetylation; phosphorylation; inflammation; cancer

# 1. INTRODUCING NF-κB

NF-κB comprises a family of inducible transcription factors that serve as important regulators of immune and inflammatory responses. In addition, the relevance of NF-κB to the pathogenesis and treatment of cancer is becoming more evident. The homo- or heterodimeric NF-κB complexes are composed of members of the Rel family of proteins, which all contain an N-terminal Rel homology domain (RHD). According to their modular structure, Rel family members can be divided in 2 groups. The first one contains p65 (RelA), cRel and RelB. These proteins represent the transactivation function of the complexes, since they all posses one or more transactivation domain. The second subgroup, lacking transactivation domains, is produced cotranslationally or upon processing of precursor proteins (p100 to p52, p105 to p50). Activation of NF-κB is regulated by a variety of IκB proteins (IκBα, IκBβ, IκBγ, IκBε, BCL-3). They share C-terminal ankyrin repeats, which are also found in the p100 and p105 precursor proteins. In most cells, the majority of NF-κB complexes are retained in the cytoplasm by IκB molecules, which mask nuclear localization sequences. Translocation of NF-κB to the nucleus and engagement of NF-κB enhancer sequences generally results from signal-induced phosphorylation of IκB by the IκB kinase (IKK) complex (reviewed in Israel, 2000). Following subsequent ubiquitination, the inhibitor gets degraded by the 26S proteasome. Among the IκB molecules, IκBα is the only one which displays nucleocytoplasmic shuttling. NF-κB complexes bound to IκBα can freely translocate to the nucleus, where an efficient export machinery assures that only very low amounts of NF-κB can be found in the nucleus of unstimulated cells. Additionally, IκBα can actively relieve DNA-bound NF-κB complexes and send them back to the cytoplasm, hereby playing an important role in the termination of the signal. Full transcriptional activation of NF-κB in the nucleus is ensured by additional post-translational modification (phosphorylation/acetylation) of the transcription factor (Chen and Greene, 2004; Schmitz *et al.*, 2001; Vermeulen *et al.*, 2002). Genes activated by NF-κB include cytokines, chemokines, adhesion molecules and receptors involved in immune recognition. Deregulation of expression of these molecules is associated with a large variety of inflammatory and autoimmune diseases like rheumatoid arthritis, asthma and inflammatory bowel disease. Various scientists have suggested a causal link between inflammation and cancer (Farrow *et al.*, 2004; Greten *et al.*, 2004). However, the exact mechanism by which inflammation may promote tumorigenesis has not been entirely revealed, yet.

Constitutive NF-κB activity has been found in several breast cancers, tumor cell lines and lymphoid malignancies (Biswas *et al.*, 2004; Karin *et al.*, 2002). The first evidence that linked NF-κB to hematopoietic cancers came from studies with the avian REV-T retrovirus oncoprotein v-Rel (a viral mutant of c-Rel) that causes B-cell lymphomas in young birds. Other viruses that have evolved to affect NF-κB regulation and lead to viral transformation are human T-cell leukemia virus type 1 and Epstein-Barr virus (reviewed in Hiscott *et al.*, 2001). In addition, genetic alterations like amplification, deletion or chromosomal rearrangements of regions encoding NF-κB or IκB family members are found in several lymphomas (reviewed in Karin *et al.*, 2002). Furthermore, NF-κB is directly involved in protecting cells from undergoing apoptosis in response to DNA damage or cytokine treatment through the induction of anti-apoptotic genes. Unfortunately, many chemotherapeutics or radiation used in the treatment of cancer also induces NF-κB. This undesired property leads to anti-apoptotic signals which actually counteract the activity of the anti-cancer therapies.

Taken together, all these findings suggest that NF-κB inhibitors could be developed into a new class of anti-cancer therapeutics. It is therefore of extreme importance to fully dissect the mechanisms of activation and post-translational regulation of NF-κB to be able to design specific drugs.

## 2. REGULATING NF-κB TRANSCRIPTIONAL ACTIVITY

Although the primary mechanism of regulation of NF-κB activity is the liberation of the transcription factor from its inhibitor IκB leading to nuclear translocation, the transcriptional activity of NF-κB in the nucleus (that is the ability to recruit the transcriptional apparatus and stimulate target gene expression) is ensured by additional post-translational modification (i.e. phosphorylation, acetylation etc.) of the transcription factor itself and its surrounding chromatin environment.

To date, it has not been determined if altered post-translational regulation of either NF-κB family member lies at the basis of any of the diseases which involves deregulation of NF-κB.

## 2.1      Regulation by phosphorylation

### 2.1.1      p65 (RelA)

Phosphorylation of p65, the transactivating subunit of the most common NF-κB complex p50/p65, has been widely studied. In response to different stimuli, five phosporylated Ser residues have been identified (Figure 1).

Ser276 situated in the RHD can be phosphorylated both by PKAc and MSK1 (mitogen- and stress-induced protein kinase-1). PKAc, included in some fractions of the NF-κB/IκB complex, is held inactive by IκB. Upon LPS treatment, PKAc becomes activated after degradation of IκB and is able to phosphorylate Ser276 (Zhong *et al.*, 1997). MSK1, a nuclear kinase that is itself activated by both ERK and p38 kinases, phosphorylates p65 at the same site in response to TNF treatment (Vermeulen *et al.*, 2003). Conformational changes in p65 triggered by Ser276 phosphorylation enable binding to CBP/p300 cofactors. These proteins stimulate gene expression via their intrinsic histone acetyl transferase (HAT) activity (see 2.2) (Zhong *et al.*, 1998).

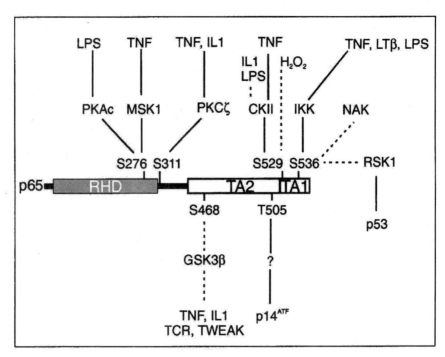

*Figure 1.* p65 phosphorylation

In endothelial cells where constitutive Ser276 phosphorylation was found, overexpression studies point to a possible role for PKCζ in the phosphorylation of the p65 RHD (Anrather *et al.*, 1999). Later, the role of PKCζ in p65 phosphorylation was confirmed using PKCζ$^{-/-}$ embryonal fibroblasts. The lack of functional PKCζ clearly inhibited cytokine-induced phosphorylation and transcriptional activity of p65 (Leitges *et al.*, 2001). Recently, Ser311 was identified as the PKCζ target. Its phosphorylation is essential for p65/CBP interaction and recruitment of CBP and RNA polymerase II to the NF-κB-dependent IL-6 promoter (Duran *et al.*, 2003).

Recently, Ser468 was also detected to be phosphorylated in response to TNF, IL-1 or phorbolester plus ionomycin treatment and T-cell receptor co-stimulation (Buss *et al.*, 2004a; Mattioli *et al.*, 2004b). In contrast to p65 phosphorylation at other sites, Ser468 phosphorylation appears to regulate NF-κB dependent gene expression in a negative way (Buss *et al.*, 2004a). Ser468 is one of the four GSK3β concensus phosphorylation sites that were detected in the C-terminal portion of p65, which are phosphorylated in vitro by GSK3β (Schwabe and Brenner, 2002). Furthermore, NF-κB-dependent transcription is impared in GSK3β$^{-/-}$ cells. Depletion of GSK3β did not alter IκB phosphorylation nor p65 nuclear translocation, but clearly decreased NF-κB/DNA-binding activity (Hoeflich *et al.*, 2000). Recently, we found that GSK3β also plays an important role in signaling from TWEAK (a TNF-family member) to NF-κB (De Ketelaere *et al.*, 2004). However, in response to TWEAK, GSK3β positively regulates NF-κB-dependent gene expression.

In response to TNF treatment, p65 can be phosphorylated in HeLa cells at Ser529 by a casein kinase II (CKII) fraction that is itself part of the NF-κB/IκB complex (Wang and Baldwin, 1998; Wang *et al.*, 2000). IL-1 can also mediate p65 phosphorylation through CKII (Bird *et al.*, 1997). In addition, phosphorylation of Ser529 was observed when KBM-5 cells were treated with $H_2O_2$ (Takada *et al.*, 2003). By comparing EMT-6 clones with different ability to induce the NOSII gene upon IL-1β or LPS treatment, it was found that absence of CKII-mediated p65 phosphorylation was responsible for a decreased NF-κB-mediated activation of the NOSII gene in some of these cells (Chantome *et al.*, 2004).

Phosphorylation of Ser536 is mediated by the IKK complex (Sakurai *et al.*, 1999). Dependent on the cell line and treatment, Ser 536 phosphorylation is either transient or sustained. In HeLa cells, phosphorylation is maximal at 5 minutes of TNF treatment. It was suggested that p65 is dephosphorylated once it enters the nucleus (Sakurai *et al.*, 2003). Cytoplasmic Ser536 phosphorylation also takes place after T-cell costimulation within an intact NF-κB/IκBα complex. Prior phosphorylation of IκBα is required. Reconstitution experiments in p65$^{-/-}$ MEF cells showed that Ser536 phosphorylation negatively regulates the kinetics of nuclear import during the shuttling of NF-κB/IκBα complexes. Concomitantly, cells expressing the Ser536 mutant form of p65 showed significantly higher amounts of IκBα in the nucleus, suggesting a contribution of Ser536 for cytoplasmic retention of IκBα (Mattioli *et al.*, 2004a). Recently, it was suggested that Ser536 phosphorylation enhances interaction with the TATA-binding protein-associated factor II31 (TAFII31), a component of TFIID of the basal transcription machinery. In the absence of phosphorylation, p65 favours binding of the corepressor amino-terminal enhancer of split (AES) (Buss *et al.*, 2004b). Other stimuli that induce Ser536 phosphorylation through the IKK complex are LPS (Yang *et al.*, 2003) and lymphotoxin β (LTβ) (Jiang *et al.*, 2003). In vitro, NAK (NF-κB-activating kinase), an IKK-related protein kinase was also found to phosphorylate Ser536 (Fujita *et al.*, 2003). Recently, Ser536 has been identified as a site that is phosphorylated by RSK1 as well. This happens in response to DNA damage through signaling by the tumor suppressor p53. p53-mediated activation of NF-κB does not occur via the classical activation pathway. Neither inducible degradation of IκB, nor the activation of the IKK complex is involved in this process. The lower affinity of RSK1-phosphorylated p65 for IκBα decreases IκBα-mediated nuclear export of shuttling forms of NF-κB, thereby promoting NF-κB/DNA-binding (Bohuslav *et al.*, 2004). It has also been suggested that intact Ser529 and Ser536 residues are necessary for an Akt-mediated increase in p65 transcriptional activity, although no kinase assays were performed to prove this (Madrid *et al.*, 2001). The contribrution of the Akt/PI3K pathway to either NF-κB translocation or p65 transcriptional activation is still controversial and has been discussed in detail in Vermeulen *et al.*, 2002. With respect to regulation of p65 transcriptional activity, Sizemore and colleagues observed specific inhibition of IL-1-induced p65 phosphorylation by PI3K inhibitors in HepG2 cells (Sizemore *et al.*, 1999). Later, they and others showed that this effect depends on IKK (Madrid *et al.*, 2000; Sizemore *et al.*, 2002) and p38 kinase activity (Madrid *et al.*, 2001).

Alternatively, phosphorylation can inhibit p65 transcriptional activity. Upon activation of the tumor suppressor gene ARF, Thr505 phosphorylation triggers association with the HDAC1 corepressor protein. Simultaneously, expression of TNF-induced anti-apoptotic genes, like Bcl-xL, are repressed (Rocha *et al.*, 2003).

Overexpression of CaMKIV also enables phosphorylation in the C-terminal domain (Jang *et al.*, 2001), whereas phosphorylation of the transactivation domain 2 (TA2) is visible upon PMA (phorbol myristate acetate) treatment (Schmitz *et al.*, 1995); however, the exact phosphorylation sites have not been identified.

Finally, it should be noted that the entire p65 phosphorylation status is not only determined by kinase activities, but results from the interplay of both kinases and phosphatases. Indeed, protein phosphatase 2A (PP2A) is physically associated with p65 in unstimulated melanocytes and is thus able to dephosphorylate p65 after IL-1 stimulation (Yang *et al.*, 2001). PP4 also interacts with p65 in cervical carcinoma cells. Overexpression of PP4 has been shown to activate NF-κB by p65 dephosphorylation. Phospho-Thr435 has been suggested as a target for PP4 (Yeh *et al.*, 2004).

### 2.1.2 Other NF-κB family members

Investigations into the effect of phosphorylation on the transactivation capacity of cRel or RelB have been rare. cRel-TD kinase, a 66 kDa Ser/Thr kinase has been identified to bind cRel both *in vitro* and *in vivo*. Ser451 in the C-terminal part of cRel was suggested to be the target of this kinase which has not been further characterized up until now. Mutation of Ser451 or deletion of the surrounding consensus sequence inhibited transcriptional activity of c-Rel (Fognani *et al.*, 2000). In the case of RelB, phosphorylation has not been found to alter its transcriptional activity. Instead, phosphorylation is involved in RelB degradation (Marienfeld *et al.*, 2001) and Ser368 has been shown to be crucial in dimerisation and p100 stabilization (Maier *et al.*, 2003).

## 2.2 Regulation by acetylation

Phosphorylation of p65 Ser276 and Ser311 is important for the recruitment of CBP/p300 cofactors. CBP and p300 are histone acetyl transferases (HATs). The levels of histone acetylation have been correlated with the transcription status of many genes. Transcriptionally active euchromatin is often bound to hyperacetylated histones (Jenuwein and Allis, 2001). Long-standing models have suggested that histone phosphorylation and/or acetylation disrupts electrostatical interaction between neighbouring histones or between the basic histone tails and the negatively charged DNA (Wolffe and Hayes, 1999). As a consequence, the accessibility of the underlying genome for nuclear factors is increased. Alternatively, reversible modification of histone tails might encode a histone 'language' that is specifically recognized by other proteins or protein modules to elicit appropriate downstream responses (Cheung *et al.*, 2000; Jenuwein and Allis, 2001; Strahl and Allis, 2000). Recently, NF-κB family members have been shown to be directly targeted by acetylation (reviewed in Quivy and Van Lint, 2004). It has been shown that p65 also interacts with distinct HDAC (histone deacetylase) isoforms to negatively regulate gene expression

(Ashburner *et al.*, 2001; Chen *et al.*, 2001; Ito *et al.*, 2000). HDACs counteract HAT activity. It has been suggested that shifting the balance between acetylation and deacetylation contributes to the regulation of NF-κB-dependent gene expression. Indeed, in a defined subset of genes, p50 homodimers, associated with HDAC-1, are bound to DNA in unstimulated cells. Following stimulation, p50/p65 heterodimers enter the nucleus and displace DNA-bound p50/p50/HDAC-1 complexes. Phosphorylation of nuclear NF-κB determines whether it is associated with CBP/p300 (HATs) or HDAC-1, ensuring that only signal-induced NF-κB entering the nucleus can activate transcription (Zhong *et al.*, 2002).

Recently, it was observed that HATs can also target non-histone proteins. To date, five acetylation sites have been detected in p65. Chen *et al.* identified lysines 218, 221 and 310 as target for acetylation by p300 (Chen *et al.*, 2002). Mutation of K218 did not result in a significant difference in activation of the NF-κB-dependent E-selectin promoter compared to wt p65. In contrast, activation by K221R or K310R mutant p65 was clearly impaired. Acetylation of K221 enhances the binding affinity of the NF-κB complex for the κB consensus sequence. It was suggested that Ac-K221, alone or in combination with Ac-K218, plays a key role in impairing the assembly of p65 with IκBα, thereby preventing nuclear export (Chen *et al.*, 2002). Alternatively, cotreatment of cells with deacetylase inhibitors was suggested to prolong induced NF-κB/DNA-binding activity by delaying the replenishment of the cytoplasmic pool of IκBα by newly synthesized protein (Adam *et al.*, 2003). As DNA-binding was not altered when K310 was mutated, acetylation of K310 seems to enhance p65 transactivation potential (Chen *et al.*, 2002). SIRT1, a nicotinamde adenosine dinucleotide-dependent histone deacetylase, regulates the transcriptional activity of NF-κB through deacetylation of p65 K310 (Yeung *et al.*, 2004).

*In vitro* acetylation assays using p300 or p/CAF identified K122 and K123 as acetyl-acceptor sites (Kiernan *et al.*, 2003). Acetylation of these sites, however, lowers the affinity of NF-κB for the κB-concensus sequence, which facilitates the removal of the transcription factor from enhancer elements by newly synthesized IκBα. In this case, p65 acetylation inhibits the overall transcriptional activity of the NF-κB complex. Deacetylation of these lysine residues can be accomplished by HDAC3.

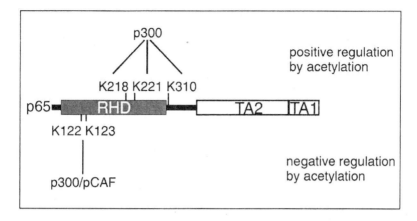

*Figure 2.* p65 acetylation

Similar to p65, acetylation of p50 increases its DNA-binding properties, which coincides with an increased rate of transcription (Deng *et al.*, 2003; Furia *et al.*, 2002). *In vitro* assays revealed 3 acetylation sites: K431, K440 and K441 (Furia *et al.*, 2002).

## 2.3 Pinning and SUMOylation

Pin1 is a peptidyl-prolyl isomerase that binds and isomerizes specific phosphorylated serine or threonine residues that precede proline (pSer/Thr-Pro) in certain proteins. This process induces conformational changes that can effect transcriptional regulation, cell cycle progression, RNA processing, cell proliferation and differentiation (Lu, 2003 and 2004). Recently, Pin1 has been shown to interfere with NF-κB signaling. Upon cytokine treatment, Pin1 binds to the pThr254-Pro motif in p65 and inhibits p65 binding to IκBα, which leads to increased nuclear accumulation and enhanced NF-κB activity. Additionally, association of Pin1 with p65 was shown to stabilize wild type p65 but not a Thr254-mutant. In Pin1-deficient cells, steady-state levels of p65 were found to be much lower when compared to wild type cells. This resulted in reduced NF-κB signaling in response to cytokine treatment (Ryo *et al.*, 2003). Thr254 phosphorylation, as suggested by these authors, has not been observed earlier, nor has the kinase been identified.

Small ubiquitin-related modifier (SUMO) proteins function by covalent binding to other proteins (Johnson, 2004). Next to a large variety of cellular processes, SUMO is also involved in the regulation of NF-κB activity. SUMO-1 conjugation to IκBα is able to inhibit proteasome-mediated degradation of IκBα since it targets the same lysine residue (K21) that is normally ubiquitinated in response to cytokine treatment. Consistently, SUMO-1 overexpression inhibits NF-κB-dependent transcription (Desterro *et al.*, 1998). SUMOylation of IKKγ has also been observed in response to DNA damage, where it is an essential step in the activation of the IKK complex (Hay, 2004; Huang *et al.*, 2003).

## 2.4    p65, a potential target for future therapies?

Small molecule NF-κB inhibitors are being developed by many pharmaceutical companies to be tested as anticancer drugs either alone or in combination with classical chemotherapeutics and/or radiation to counteract activated NF-κB-dependent anti-apoptotic properties. Most of these target IKKβ (reviewed in Haefner, 2002; Karin *et al.*, 2004). Several natural compounds have been proposed to have a role in the treatment or prevention of cancer. Among these are resveratrol, curcumin and green tea extracts. All of these agents have been described to inhibit IKK/NF-κB activation (Surh, 2003). Although NF-κB appears as a logical target for anti-cancer therapeutics, it is not desirable to block NF-κB signaling for prolonged periods of time since the transcription factor also plays an important role in the maintenance of host defense responses. Therefore, intervening selectively with p65 transcriptional activity without completely blocking NF-κB activation, might be a superior strategy.

Despite numerous studies, researchers have not yet reached a consensus as to the extent by which the various p65 residues are phosphorylated/acetylated within a particular cell line, nor as to the contribution and dynamics of each modification to the transcriptional control of the different classes of NF-κB-regulated genes. Indeed, although many genes contain NF-κB-responsive elements, their expression pattern may vary from both a kinetic and quantitative point of view. In addition, post-translational regulation of p65 transcriptional activity appears to be time-dependent and cell type-specific. Further studies directing attention to these intriguing aspects of gene regulation are needed. One might speculate that a specific phosphorylation event is needed for the full expression of certain subclasses of NF-κB-regulated genes but not for that of others. Therefore, it would be interesting to make a list of genes which need specific p65 kinases or phosphorylation at specific sites for full transcriptional activation. This information could be very useful in the search for more specific NF-κB inhibitors as therapeutic agents. Indeed, when a certain kinase is involved in the transcriptional regulation of anti-apoptotic genes but is not essential for the expression of pro-inflammatory genes, inhibition of such kinases might lead to safer drugs for cancer treatment. Alternatively, specific inhibitors of pro-inflammatory genes could be desirable in inflammatory disease therapy.

# 3. ACKNOWLEDGEMENTS

Our research was supported by Interuniversitaire Attractiepolen (IUAP), geconcerteerde onderzoeksacties (GOA) and the Belgian Federation Against Cancer. W.V.B. is a post-doctoral fellow with the Fonds voor Wetenschappelijk Onderzoek-Vlaanderen (FWO-Vlaanderen).

# 4. REFERENCES

Adam, E. *et al.* (2003). Potentiation of tumor necrosis factor-induced NF-κB activation by deacetylase inhibitors is associated with a delayed cytoplasmic reappearance of IκBα. *Mol. Cell. Biol.* **23**: 6200-6209.

Anrather, J. *et al.* (1999). Regulation of NF-κB RelA phosphorylation and transcriptional activity by p21$^{ras}$ and protein kinase Cζ in primary endothelial cells. *J. Biol. Chem.* **274**: 13594-13603.

Ashburner, B.P. *et al.* (2001). The p65 (RelA) subunit of NF-κB interacts with the histone deacetylase (HDAC) corepressors HDAC1 and HDAC2 to negatively regulate gene expression. *Mol. Cell. Biol.* **21**: 7065-7077.

Bird, T.A. *et al.* (1997). Activation of nuclear transcription factor NF-κB by interleukin-1 is accompanied by casein kinase II-mediated phosphorylation of the p65 subunit. *J. Biol. Chem.* **272**: 32606-32612.

Biswas, D.K. *et al.* (2004). NF-κB activation in human breast cancer specimens and its role in cell proliferation and apoptosis. *Proc. Natl. Acad. Sci. USA.* **101**: 10137-10142.

Bohuslav, J. *et al.* (2004). p53 Induces NF-κB activation by an IκB kinase-independent mechanism involving phosphorylation of p65 by ribosomal S6 kinase 1. *J. Biol. Chem.* **279**: 26115-26125.

Buss, H. *et al.* (2004a). Phosphorylation of serine 468 by GSK-3β negatively regulates basal p65 NF-κB activity. *J. Biol. Chem.* **279**: 49571-49574.

Buss, H. *et al.* (2004b). Constitutive and interleukin-1 inducible phosphorylation of p65 NF-κB at serine 536 is mediated by multiple kinases including IKKα, IKKβ, IKKε, TBK1, and an unknown kinase and couples p65 to TAFII31-mediated interleukin-8 transcription. *J. Biol. Chem.* **279**: 55633-55643.

Chantome, A. *et al.* (2004). Casein kinase II-mediated phosphorylation of NF-κB p65 subunit enhances inducible nitric-oxide synthase gene transcription *in vivo*. *J. Biol. Chem.* **279**: 23953-23960.

Chen, L. *et al.* (2001). Duration of nuclear NF-κB action regulated by reversible acetylation. *Science* **293**: 1653-1657.

Chen, L.F. and Greene, W.C. (2004). Shaping the nuclear action of NF-κB. *Nat. Rev. Mol. Cell Biol.* **5**: 392-401.

Chen, L.F. *et al.* (2002). Acetylation of RelA at discrete sites regulates distinct nuclear functions of NF-κB. *EMBO J.* **21**: 6539-6548.

Cheung, P. *et al.* (2000). Signaling to chromatin through histone modifications. *Cell* **103**: 263-271.

De Ketelaere, A. *et al.* (2004). Involvement of GSK-3β in TWEAK-mediated NF-κB activation. *FEBS Lett.* **566**: 60-64.

Deng, W.G. *et al.* (2003). Up-regulation of p300 binding and p50 acetylation in tumor necrosis factor-α-induced cyclooxygenase-2 promoter activation. *J. Biol. Chem.* **278**: 4770-4777.

Desterro, J.M. *et al.* (1998). SUMO-1 modification of IκBα inhibits NF-κB activation. *Mol.Cell* **2**: 233-239.

Duran, A. *et al.* (2003). Essential role of RelA Ser311 phosphorylation by ζPKC in NF-κB transcriptional activation. *EMBO J.* **22**: 3910-3918.

Farrow, B. *et al.* (2004). Inflammatory mechanisms contributing to pancreatic cancer development. *Ann. Surg.* **239**: 763-769: discussion 769-771.

Fognani, C. *et al.* (2000). cRel-TD kinase: a serine/threonine kinase binding *in vivo* and *in vitro* c-Rel and phosphorylating its transactivation domain. *Oncogene* **19**: 2224-2232.

Fujita, F. *et al.* (2003). Identification of NAP1, a regulatory subunit of IκB kinase-related kinases that potentiates NF-κB signaling. *Mol. Cell. Biol.* **23**: 7780-7793.

Furia, B. *et al.* (2002). Enhancement of NF-κB acetylation by coactivator p300 and HIV-1 Tat proteins. *J. Biol. Chem.* **277**: 4973-4980.

Greten, F.R. *et al.* (2004). IKKβ links inflammation and tumorigenesis in a mouse model of colitis-associated cancer. *Cell* **118**: 285-296.

Haefner, B. (2002). NF-κB: arresting a major culprit in cancer. *Drug Discov. Today* **7**: 653-663.

Hay, R.T. (2004). Modifying NEMO. *Nat. Cell Biol.* **6**: 89-91.

Hiscott, J. *et al.* (2001) Hostile takeovers: viral appropriation of the NF-κB pathway. *J. Clin. Invest.* **107**: 143-151.

Hoeflich, K.P. *et al.* (2000). Requirement for glycogen synthase kinase-3β in cell survival and NF-κB activation. *Nature* **406**: 86-90.

Huang, T.T. *et al.* (2003). Sequential modification of NEMO/IKKγ by SUMO-1 and ubiquitin mediates NF-κB activation by genotoxic stress. *Cell* **115**: 565-576.

Israel A. (2000). The IKK complex: an integrator of all signals that activate NF-κB? *Trends Cell Biol.* **10**: 129-133.

Ito, K. *et al.* (2000). Glucocorticoid receptor recruitment of histone deacetylase 2 inhibits interleukin-1β-induced histone H4 acetylation on lysines 8 and 12. *Mol. Cell. Biol.* **20**: 6891-6903.

Jang, M.K. *et al.* (2001). Ca2+/calmodulin-dependent protein kinase IV stimulates nuclear factor-κB transactivation via phosphorylation of the p65 subunit. *J. Biol. Chem.* **276**: 20005-20010.

Jenuwein, T. and Allis, C.D. (2001). Translating the histone code. *Science* **293**: 1074-1080.

Jiang, X. *et al.* (2003). The NF-κB activation in lymphotoxin β receptor signaling depends on the phosphorylation of p65 at serine 536. *J. Biol. Chem.* **278**: 919-926.

Johnson, E.S. (2004). Protein modification by SUMO. *Annu. Rev. Biochem.* **73**: 355-382.

Karin, M. *et al.* (2002). NF-κB in cancer: from innocent bystander to major culprit. *Nat. Rev. Cancer* **2**: 301-310.

Karin, M. *et al.* (2004). The IKK NF-κB system: a treasure trove for drug development. *Nat. Rev. Drug Discov.* **3**: 17-26.

Kiernan, R. *et al.* (2003). Post-activation turn-off of NF-κB-dependent transcription is regulated by acetylation of p65. *J. Biol. Chem.* **278**: 2758-2766.

Leitges, M. *et al.* (2001). Targeted Disruption of the ζPKC Gene Results in the Impairment of the NF-κB Pathway. *Mol. Cell.* **8**: 771-780.

Lu, K.P. (2003). Prolyl isomerase Pin1 as a molecular target for cancer diagnostics and therapeutics. *Cancer Cell* **4**: 175-180.

Lu, K.P. (2004). Pinning down cell signaling, cancer and Alzheimer's disease. *Trends Biochem. Sci.* **29**: 200-209.

Madrid, L.V. *et al.* (2001). Akt stimulates the transactivation potential of the RelA/p65 subunit of NF-κB through utilization of the IκB kinase and activation of the mitogen-activated protein kinase p38. *J. Biol. Chem.* **276**: 18934-18940.

Madrid, L.V. *et al.* (2000). Akt suppresses apoptosis by stimulating the transactivation potential of the RelA/p65 subunit of NF-κB. *Mol. Cell. Biol.* **20**: 1626-1638.

Maier, H.J. *et al.* (2003). Critical Role of RelB Serine 368 for Dimerization and p100 Stabilization. *J. Biol. Chem.* **278**: 39242-39250.

Marienfeld, R. *et al.* (2001). Signal-specific and phosphorylation-dependent RelB degradation: a potential mechanism of NF-κB control. *Oncogene* **20**: 8142-8147.

Mattioli, I. *et al.* (2004a). Transient and selective NF-κB p65 serine 536 phosphorylation induced by T cell costimulation is mediated by IκB kinase β and controls the kinetics of p65 nuclear import. *J. Immunol.* **172**: 6336-6344.

Mattioli, I. *et al.* (2004b). Comparative analysis of T-cell costimulation and CD43 activation reveals novel signaling pathways and target genes. *Blood* **104**: 3302-3304.

Quivy, V. and Van Lint, C. (2004). Regulation at multiple levels of NF-κB-mediated transactivation by protein acetylation. *Biochem. Pharmacol.* **68**: 1221-1229.

Rocha, S. *et al.* (2003). p53- and Mdm2-independent repression of NF-κB transactivation by the ARF tumor suppressor. *Mol. Cell* **12**: 15-25.

Ryo, A. *et al.* (2003). Regulation of NF-κB signaling by Pin1-dependent prolyl isomerization and ubiquitin-mediated proteolysis of p65/RelA. *Mol. Cell* 12: 1413-1426.

Sakurai, H. *et al.* (1999). IκB kinases phosphorylate NF-κB p65 subunit on serine 536 in the transactivation domain. *J. Biol. Chem.* **274**: 30353-30356.

Sakurai, H. *et al.* (2003). Tumor necrosis factor-α-induced IKK phosphorylation of NF-κB p65 on serine 536 is mediated through the TRAF2, TRAF5, and TAK1 signaling pathway. *J. Biol. Chem.* **278**: 36916-36923.

Schmitz, M.L. *et al.* (2001). IκB-independent control of NF-κB activity by modulatory phosphorylations. *Trends Biochem. Sci.* **26**: 186-190.

Schmitz, M.L. *et al.* (1995). Interaction of the COOH-terminal transactivation domain of p65 NF-κB with TATA-binding protein, transcription factor IIB, and coactivators. *J.Biol.Chem.* **270**: 7219-7226.

Schwabe, R.F. and Brenner, D.A. (2002). Role of glycogen synthase kinase-3 in TNF-α-induced NF-κB activation and apoptosis in hepatocytes. *Am. J. Physiol. Gastrointest. Liver Physiol.* **283**: G204-211.

Sizemore, N. *et al.* (2002). Distinct roles of the IκB kinase α and β subunits in liberating NF-κB from IκB and in phosphorylating the p65 subunit of NF-κB. *J. Biol. Chem.* **277**: 3863-3869.

Sizemore, N. *et al.* (1999). Activation of phosphatidylinositol 3-kinase in response to interleukin-1 leads to phosphorylation and activation of the NF-κB p65/RelA subunit. *Mol. Cell. Biol.* **19**: 4798-4805.

Strahl, B.D. and Allis, C.D. (2000). The language of covalent histone modifications. *Nature* **403**: 41-45.

Surh, Y.J. (2003). Cancer chemoprevention with dietary phytochemicals. *Nat. Rev. Cancer* **3**: 768-780.

Takada, Y. *et al.* (2003). Hydrogen peroxide activates NF-κB through tyrosine phosphorylation of IκBα and serine phosphorylation of p65: evidence for the involvement of IκBα kinase and Syk protein-tyrosine kinase. *J. Biol. Chem.* **278**: 24233-24241.

Vermeulen, L. *et al.* (2002). Regulation of the transcriptional activity of the nuclear factor-κB p65 subunit. *Biochem. Pharmacol.* **64**: 963-970.

Vermeulen, L. *et al.* (2003). Transcriptional activation of the NF-κB subunit by mitogen- and stress-activated protein kinase-1 (MSK1). *EMBO J.* **22**: 1313-1324.

Wang, D. and Baldwin, A.S., Jr. (1998). Activation of nuclear factor-κB-dependent transcription by tumor necrosis factor-α is mediated through phosphorylation of RelA/p65 on serine 529. *J. Biol. Chem.* **273**: 29411-29416.

Wang, D. *et al.* (2000). Tumor necrosis factor α-induced phosphorylation of RelA/p65 on Ser529 is controlled by casein kinase II. *J. Biol. Chem.* **275**: 32592-32597.

Wolffe, A.P. and Hayes, J.J. (1999). Chromatin disruption and modification. *Nucleic Acids Res.* **27**: 711-720.

Yang, F. *et al.* (2003). IKKβ plays an essential role in the phosphorylation of RelA/p65 on serine 536 induced by lipopolysaccharide. *J. Immunol.* **170**: 5630-5635.

Yang, J. *et al.* (2001). Protein phosphatase 2A interacts with and directly dephosphorylates RelA. *J. Biol. Chem.* **276**: 47828-47833.

Yeh, P.Y. (2004). Suppression of MEK/ERK signaling pathway enhances cisplatin-induced NF-κB activation by protein phosphatase 4-mediated NF-κB p65 Thr dephosphorylation. *J. Biol. Chem.* **279**: 26143-26148.

Yeung, F. *et al.* (2004). Modulation of NF-κB-dependent transcription and cell survival by the SIRT1 deacetylase. *EMBO J.* **23**: 2369-2380.

Zhong, H. *et al.* (2002). The phosphorylation status of nuclear NF-κB determines its association with CBP/p300 or HDAC-1. *Mol. Cell* **9**: 625-636.

Zhong, H. *et al.* (1997). The transcriptional activity of NF-κB is regulated by the IκB-associated PKAc subunit through a cyclic AMP-independent mechanism. *Cell* **89**: 413-424.

Zhong, H. *et al.* (1998). Phosphorylation of NF-κB p65 by PKA stimulates transcriptional activity by promoting a novel bivalent interaction with the coactivator CBP/p300. *Mol. Cell* **1**: 661-671.

# Chapter 5

# THE ROLE OF IMMUNE CELLS IN THE TUMOR MICROENVIRONMENT

Theresa L. Whiteside
*University of Pittsburgh Cancer Institute,* 5117 Centre Avenue, Pittsburgh, PA 15213

Abstract:     Interactions between tumor infiltrating leukocytes and tumor cells have been of great interest because of the possibility that immune cells either interfere with tumor progression or actively promote tumor growth. The tumor microenvironment is shaped by cells entering it, and their functions reflect the local conditions. Successive changes occurring at the tumor site during tumor progression resemble chronic inflammation. This chronic inflammatory reaction seems to be largely orchestrated by the tumor, and it seems to promote tumor survival. Molecular and cellular mechanisms linking the inflammatory reaction and cancer are emerging, and this review summarizes the current understanding of interactions between inflammatory and cancer cells in the tumor microenvironment.

Keywords:     TIL; immune evasion; immune surveillance; inflammation; cancer

# 1.    INTRODUCTION

Tumor development involves multiple genetic changes, which occur in the progeny of the transformed cell over many years, accumulate and result in the establishment of a malignant phenotype characterized by uncontrolled growth (Zhang *et al.*, 1997). In parallel, a variety of alterations occur in surrounding normal tissues, leading to establishment of the tumor microenvironment. These changes are necessary to assure survival of the tumor at the expense of surrounding normal tissue cells. To meet tumor requirements and sustain its growth, several successive stages of changes have to occur in the tumor microenvironment. In many respects, the tissue changes arising in response to tumor formation resemble the unfolding process of chronic inflammation. Inflammation is a normal component of wound healing or tissue repair. In fact, tumors have been described as wounds that do not heal (Dworak, 1986). Inflammation, when it occurs, generally consists of the initial ischemia, resulting in the interstitial and cellular edema (an immune reaction associated with appearance in tissue of immune cells) and, finally, the appearance of blood capillaries and lymphatics necessary for feeding of the repaired tissues (Ribatti *et al.*, 2003; Aller *et al.*, 2004). These phases of inflammatory response progress from an anerobic tissue environment (ischemia) to the development of oxidative metabolism, which uses oxygen to produce energy in the form of ATP (Mareel and Leroy, 2003; Balkwill and Mantovani, 2001). Inflammation appears to be a ubiquitous tissue response common to many normal conditions, including embryonic development, as well as disease states. Its involvement in shaping the tumor microenvironment has been recognized, and it has been referred to as the "host reaction" to the tumor.

The tumor appears to be able to induce an inflammatory response in the host early on, because the presence of immune cells has been noted even in pre-cancerous or benign lesions (Kornstein *et al.*, 1983; von Kleist *et al.*, 1987; Vacarello *et al.*, 1993). This has been interpreted as an attempt of the host immune system to interfere with tumor growth, otherwise referred to as "immune surveillance". However, the developing tumor is not a passive participant in this interplay. On the contrary, it takes advantage of the host response in order to: (a) use immune cells for elimination of sensitive tumor cells and their gradual replacement by those resistant to immune intervention ("immune selection") and (b) use the host as a participant in creating the microenvironment favorable to tumor progression ("immune evasion"). To this end, lymphocytes, macrophages and dendritic cells (DC) infiltrating the tumor, together with fibroblasts and extracellular matrix forming a scaffold supporting its expansion, contribute to establishing an inflammatory milieu that nourishes the tumor. Thus, the host becomes a participant in the establishment of the tumor by providing structural and trophic elements required for cancer progression.

In this chapter, the role of immune cells in the tumor-host interactions will be considered, with the emphasis placed on capabilities of these cells to modify the tumor microenvironment. To date, the role of tumor cells in shaping their microenvironment has been widely discussed (Bogenrieder and Herlyn, 2003). Yet, it is clear that as a component of the inflammatory reaction, immune cells accumulating at the tumor periphery or those infiltrating the tumor stroma or nest of tumor cells are also involved in modulating tumor progression.

## 1.1 Immune cells in the tumor microenvironment

Immune responses to malignant cells can be categorized as locoregional or systemic. *In situ* or local responses refer mainly to tumor infiltrating lymphocytes (TIL), which accumulate in many human solid tumors and whose role in tumor progression remains controversial. TIL isolated from various human tumors are functionally compromised as compared to normal circulating or tissue-infiltrating lymphocytes. Systemic immunity to tumors, as measured in the peripheral circulation or by delayed-type hypersensitivity (DTH) responses in patients with cancer, is difficult to demonstrate, and tumor-specific responses are particularly elusive. Non-specific proliferative or cytotoxic responses of peripheral lymphocytes in cancer patients are variably impaired (Whiteside, 1993). More recent data indicate that the same functional impairments seen in TIL are found in circulating as well lymph node lymphocytes of patients with cancer (Reichert *et al.*, 2002). In aggregate, the available evidence suggests that in the presence of tumors, both local and systemic antitumor immunity is compromised in patients with cancer. This does not mean that patients with cancer are immunodeficient. Their responses to bacterial and viral antigens remain unimpaired, and only tumor-specific immunity is deficient.

## 1.2 T cells

Among various cells present at the tumor site, T cells ($CD3^+TCR^+$) have received the most attention. They are by far the largest component of mononuclear tumor infiltrates in all human tumors (Mihm *et al.*, 1996), although some tumors may be also generously infiltrated by macrophages (Lin *et al.*, 2001). The hypothesis that TIL-T represent autotumor-specific cytolytic T cells (CTL) has been promoted; however, early limiting dilution studies performed with TIL-T from various human tumors indicated that the frequency of such CTL was low as compared to peripheral blood T lymphocytes (PBL-T) (Miescher *et al.*, 1987). Nevertheless, evidence exists that Vβ-restricted clones of T cells are present in some freshly isolated TIL, and that TIL can selectively recognize and kill autologous tumor cells in some cases (Weidmann *et al.*, 1992). Using tetramers and multi-parameter flow cytometry, it has recently been possible to determine the frequency of tumor-peptide-specific (tetramer$^+$) T cells among TIL with greater accuracy in various human tumors. We reported, for example, that TIL obtained from patients with head and neck cancer (HNC) were significantly enriched in wildtype (wt) p53 epitope-specific T cells, as compared to autologous peripheral blood mononuclear cells (PBMC) (Albers *et al.*, 2005a). The frequency of these tetramer$^+$ TIL was highly variable and ranged from 1/800 to 1/5,000 of CD3$^+$CD8$^+$ TIL, which recognized the wt p53$_{264-272}$ peptide, compared to the mean frequency of 1/6,000 such cells among autologous PBMC (Albers *et al.*, 2005a). Furthermore, our recent analysis of TcR Vβ restrictions in paired TIL and PBMC of patients with HNC indicated the presence of the same Vβ restrictions in both. These oligoclonal expansions of T cells in TIL and PBMC cells were observed in 8/10 patients with HNC and in 0/10 PBMC samples obtained from normal donors. Binding of an HLA-A2.1/p53 tetramer to a high percentage of a Vβ-restricted CD8+ T cell population suggested that the restrictions were tumor related (Albers *et al.*, 2005b). This type of evidence is also available for melanoma (Weidmann *et al.*, 1992 and 1993), and it indicates that TIL may indeed be enriched in tumor-specific T cells.

The phenotypic analysis of T cells in human tumors shows that TIL-T are memory lymphocytes, expressing either CD8 or CD4 markers, although the CD4/CD8 ratio may be highly variable from one tumor to another (Whiteside, 1993). In several studies, the CD4/CD8 ratio was found to be reduced as a result of enrichment in CD8$^+$ T cell, in contrast with nonmalignant inflammatory infiltrates, which consist largely of CD4$^+$ T cells (Whiteside, 1992; Whitford *et al.*, 1990). Some reports have linked a high tumor content of CD8$^+$ T cells with a better prognosis (Baxevanis *et al.*, 1994; Naito *et al.*, 1998), although no consistent data supporting this finding has been obtained. In cervical cancer or in renal cell carcinoma, TIL enrichment in CD8+ T cells seems to be associated with disease progression and a poor prognosis (Sheu *et al.*, 1999; Nakano *et al.*, 2001). When functional attributes of freshly-isolated TIL-T were examined in conventional *ex vivo* assays, their proliferative and anti-tumor functions were found to be significantly depressed compared with equivalent functions of normal T cells. It appears that TIL obtained from advanced or metastatic lesions are more functionally impaired than those from early lesions, suggesting that tumor burden or the potential of more aggressive tumors to suppress immune cells might determine the functional status of TIL-T. The cytokine profile of these cells was also different from that of normal activated T cells, as either no or little type 1 cytokines (IL-2, IFN-γ) were produced by TIL-T and, instead, these cells preferentially secreted down-regulatory cytokines, IL-10 and TGF-β (Vitolo *et al.*, 1993). These functional characteristics of TIL-T were inconsistent with respect to their phenotype, which identified them as predominantly HLA-DR$^+$CD25$^+$ activated T lymphocytes (Whiteside, 1993). More recently, this inconsistency was addressed by examining the hypothesis that TIL-T were enriched in CD4$^+$CD25$^+$ regulatory T cells. Recent reports confirmed the accumulation of regulatory CD4$^+$CD25$^+$ T cells (T$_{reg}$) at the tumor site in several human malignancies (Liyanage *et al.*, 2002; Woo *et al.*, 2001). This enrichment in T$_{reg}$, which are in principle responsible for down-regulation of TIL functions in the tumor microenvironment, could explain the discrepancy between the observed "activation" phenotype (HLA-DR$^+$CD25$^+$) of TIL and their functional impairments. Until recently, however, it was not possible to make a firm distinction between activated CD4$^+$ T cells and T$_{reg}$ due to the lack of specific phenotypic markers for the T$_{reg}$ population. T$_{reg}$ were identified based on the ability to suppress activity of other immune cells in *ex vivo* mixing experiments (Shevach, 2000). We have observed a significant increase in the proportion of CD4$^+$CD25$^+$ T cells in TIL isolated from HNC (a mean of 30 % in TIL vs. 11 % in autologous PBMC; n=17) (Albers *et al.*, 2005a). When the newly available antibodies to FOXp3, a transcription factor expressed in T$_{reg}$ (Ramsdell, 2003), and antibodies to glucocorticoid-induced TNF receptor (GITR) or to CTLA-4 antigen (Stephens *et al.*, 2004; Lee *et al.*, 1998) were used for staining and flow cytometry of permeabilized TIL obtained from patients with HNC, we observed that nearly all CD4$^+$CD25$^+$ TIL were positive for these markers. In contrast, only 1-2% of CD4$^+$CD25$^+$ T cells in PBMC were stained with the antibodies recognizing T$_{reg}$. These preliminary data indicate that tumors indeed "beckon regulatory T cells" (Shevach, 2004). However, these results have to be confirmed by functional studies demonstrating suppressive capabilities of CD4$^+$CD25$^+$ T cells isolated from TIL and PBMC of patients with HNC, similar to those recently performed by Curiel and colleagues with TIL obtained from tumor tissues and ascites of patients with ovarian carcinoma (Curiel *et al.*, 2004). A tentative conclusion that can be drawn from the data available so far is that TIL are enriched in tumor-specific effector cells as well as T$_{reg}$, and that functional paralysis of TIL may, in part, be attributed to suppressive effects mediated by T$_{reg}$, which accumulate in the tumor microenvironment.

Functional impairments observed with TIL isolated from solid tumors can be confirmed by *in situ* studies of signaling molecules in TIL-T. Such studies show that expression of the TcR-associated ζ chain as well as that of NF-κB, the transcription factor regulating expression of a number of immune and inflammatory genes, is significantly decreased in TIL-T compared to their expression in T cells obtained from the peripheral circulation of normal donors (Reichert *et al.*, 1998a; Li *et al.*, 1994). This is particularly evident for TIL evaluated *in situ* or isolated from advanced or metastatic lesions. In a study comprising 132 cases of human oral cell carcinomas, expression of ζ in TIL-T was found to be an independent and highly statistically significant biomarker of prognosis and survival in patients with stage III and IV disease (Reichert *et al.*, 1998b). The patients with tumors infiltrated by T cells with low or absent ζ expression had significantly shorter 5-year survival compared to the patients with tumors infiltrated by T cells with normal ζ expression (Reichert *et al.*, 1998b). Stimulus-dependent activation of NF-κB was found to be impaired in T cells of patients with renal cell carcinoma (RCC). In some patients, the primary defect was the failure of the transactivating complex RelA/NF-κB1 (p50) to accumulate in the nucleus following T-cell activation due to impaired phosphorylation and degradation of the inhibitor IκBα (Uzzo *et al.*, 1999a; Ling *et al.*, 1998). In other patients, NF-κB activation was defective despite normal stimulus-dependent degradation of IκBα (Uzzo *et al.*, 1999b). In both situations, this defective state could be induced by exposure of normal T cells to supernatants of RCC, and the soluble product responsible was identified as an RCC-derived ganglioside (Uzzo *et al.*, 1999b). Impaired NF-κB activity may contribute to reduced T-cell function seen in TIL-T present in RCC, since this transcription factor controls expression of a number of genes encoding cytokines, their receptors and other membrane regulatory molecules essential for T-cell activation (Baeuerle and Baltimore, 1996; May and Ghosh, 1998). It is important to note that defects in function of the ζ chain and activation of NF-κB are observed in TIL-T as well as circulating T cells of patients with cancer (Kuss *et al.*, 1999; Whiteside, 2004). Thus, these signaling defects in T cells are both local and systemic and seem to be related to the tumor burden.

Taken together, functional studies of TIL-T obtained from a variety of human solid tumors in many different laboratories indicate that these cells are functionally incompetent, possibly because of the inhibitory effects mediated by activated $T_{reg}$ in the tumor microenvironment or by factors produced and released by the tumor itself. In addition, it appears that the loss of functions in TIL-T rather than the number or phenotype of T cells infiltrating the tumor may be the important factor for predicting patient survival.

## 1.3    Macrophages

CD45$^+$CD14$^+$ cells are commonly found in human tumors and are referred to as tumor-associated macrophages (TAM). Normal macrophages are phagocytic and antigen-presenting cells, which play an important role in the control of infections. In contrast, TAM are re-programmed to inhibit lymphocyte functions through release of specific cytokines, prostaglandins or reactive oxygen species (ROS). It is hypothesized that re-programming of macrophages occurs in the tumor microenvironment as a result of tumor-driven activation (Al-Sarireh and Eremin, 2000). Possibly, macrophages are the main contributors to removal of dying tumor cells, and the more rapidly proliferating tumors are especially attractive to these scavengers. Evidence has accumulated indicating that invasiveness of tumors, e.g., human primary colon carcinomas, is directly related to the number of TAM detected in the tumor (Al-Sarireh and Eremin, 2000). In invasive breast cancer, an increased TAM count is an independent predictor of reduced relapse-free survival as well as reduced overall survival (Leck *et al.*, 1996). The available data support the active role of TAM in tumor-induced immunosuppression, on the one hand, and in the promotion of tumor growth on the other. The mechanisms that contribute to TAM-mediated inhibition of immune cells are probably numerous, but much attention has been recently devoted to the role of NADPH-dependent ROS, such as superoxide anion or hydrogen peroxide as potential inhibitors of TIL (Kiessling *et al.*, 1996; Hansson *et al.*, 1996). T-cell proliferation and NK-mediated antitumor cytotoxicity are profoundly inhibited by macrophage-derived ROS *in vitro* (Hansson *et al.*, 1996). T and NK cells isolated from human tumors have a decreased expression of CD3ζ and FcγRIII-associated ζ, respectively, and this down-modulation of ζ, a critical signal-transducing molecule for TCR can be induced by ROS produced by TAM (Malmberg *et al.*, 2001). The changes observed in TIL: a loss of normal ζ expression accompanied by a decreased ability to proliferate and subsequent apoptotic cell death, correspond to similar changes induced in T and NK cells co-cultured with activated macrophages (Hansson *et al.*, 1996). Removal of macrophages from these cultures restores T and NK cell functions (Hansson *et al.*, 1996). The overall conclusion from these studies is that immuno-inhibitory activities of TAM, whether due to oxidative stress or to release of inhibitory cytokines, such as IL-10, contribute to making the tumor microenvironment a particularly unfriendly milieu for immune cells. In this, TAM appear to reinforce effects mediated by tumor cells, which also produce ROS, PGE2 and a variety of immuno-inhibitory cytokines (Whiteside *et al.*, 2005). Also, TAM were reported to be associated with angiogenesis and prognosis in breast carcinomas (Leek *et al.*, 1996).

## 1.4      Dendritic cells

Dendritic cells (DC; *Lin*-CD80+CD86+HLA-DR+ cells) are the most potent antigen presenting cells (APC). They are a heterogenous population of highly motile cells that originate from the precursors in the bone marrow and migrate through the blood stream to peripheral non-lymphoid tissues, capturing antigens (Banchereau *et al.*, 2000). They then travel to the lymphoid tissues, where antigen presentation to T cells takes place. The DC compartment is comprised of subpopulations of morphologically and functionally distinct cells, depending on their hematopoietic origin, maturation stage or tissue localization (Banchereau and Steinman, 1998). The two main subpopulations are myeloid-derived DC (DC1) and lymphoid-derived DC (DC2). While in man, this distinction is somewhat blurred, phenotypic and functional differences exist between monocyte-derived CD11c$^+$ DC (MDC) and CD11c$^-$CD123$^+$ (IL-3R$\alpha^{high}$) lymphoid-derived DC (Banchereau and Steinman, 1998; Liu, 2001). The proportion of lymphoid DC is substantially lower than that of myeloid DC, and most of these cells belong to a relatively rare subset of DC known as plasmacytoid DC (pDC), which produce IFN-$\alpha$ in response to viruses (Liu, 2001). Human tumors are frequently infiltrated by MDC but rarely by pDC, although the presence of the latter is associated with poor prognosis (Treilleux *et al.*, 2004). The DC maturation stage determines their functionality: immature DC are primarily responsible for antigen uptake, while mature CD83+ DC primarily serve as antigen-presenting cells (Liu, 2001).

In tumor-bearing hosts, DC are responsible for the uptake, processing and cross-presentation of TAA to naïve or memory T cells, thus playing a crucial role in the generation of tumor-specific effector T cells. Antigen presentation by DC leads to T cell proliferation, which results in either immunity or tolerance, depending on the stage of maturation of the presenting DC. In human solid tumors, DC are often present in substantial numbers, and they express attributes of immature DC (Gabrilovich, 2004). Because antitumor immune responses are inefficient in tumor-bearing individuals, it has been suggested that DC, like T cells, are subverted by the tumor (Gabrilovich, 2004). Phenotypic and functional alterations in DC infiltrating human tumors as well as DC recovered from the peripheral circulation of patients with cancer have been reported (Almand *et al.*, 2000; Hoffmann *et al.*, 2002). Tumor-associated DC (TADC) appear to be immature (lack of expression of CD80 and CD86) and have reduced allostimulatory activity (Troy *et al.*, 1998). TADC are at a particular disadvantage, because tumors or tumor-derived factors have been shown to induce DC apoptosis or impair their maturation (Esche *et al.*, 2001; Gabrilovich *et al.*, 1996a). Co-culture of murine or human DC (obtained from isolated CD34$^+$ precursors or plastic-adherent PBMC, respectively) with a variety of tumor cell lines for 4-48h resulted in apoptotic death of DC, as verified by morphology, TUNEL assays, annexin binding, caspase activation, and DNA laddering (Esche *et al.*, 1999; Shurin *et al.*, 1999). Tumor cells induced DC apoptosis by direct contact or through release of soluble factors. Furthermore, TADC isolated from human tumors contain a high proportion of apoptotic cells (Shurin *et al.*, 1999). Tumor-induced apoptosis of DC was inhibited in the presence of IL-12 and IL-15, an indication that cytokines might regulate DC generation and survival. In fact, these cytokines were shown to stimulate expression of Bcl-2 and Bcl-XL in DC and to protect them from tumor–induced apoptosis (Shurin *et al.*, 1999 and 2001). Experiments performed by Shurin and colleagues further demonstrated that tumor-derived factors, e.g., gangliosides, inhibited DC generation and their function *in vitro* (Shurin *et al.*, 2001). This suppressive effect of gangliosides on DC was found to be mediated by tumor-derived VEGF, a known anti-dendropoietic factor (Gabrilovich *et al.*, 1999). Importantly, cytokines (IL-12, IL-15 and FLT3L) were found to promote DC generation and their functions by exerting a protective anti-apoptotic effect, while tumor-derived factors caused apoptosis in mature DC and inhibited differentiation of hematopoietic precursors into DC. Very recent studies indicate that tumors and tumor supernatants can down-regulate expression of antigen presenting machinery (APM) components in DC, thus interfering with the capacity of these cells to process antigens and present the processed epitopes to T cells (Whiteside *et al.*, 2004; Tourkova *et al.*, 2004). Again, tumor-derived gangliosides were identified as a factor responsible for down-modulation of APM components in DC co-incubated with the tumor (Tourkova *et al.*, 2004). These studies underscore the role of the microenvironment in shaping the functional potential of DC and perhaps other tumor-infiltrating immune cells.

Numerous reports in the literature suggest that despite functional impairments of TADC, their presence in tumors is associated with improved prognosis (Becker, 1993; Reichert *et al.*, 2001). DC infiltrations into tumors have been correlated to significantly prolonged patient survival and reduced incidence of recurrent or metastatic disease in patients with bladder, lung, laryngeal, oral, gastric and nasopharyngeal carcinomas (Reichert *et al.*, 2001; Tsujitani *et al.*, 1987; Lespagnard *et al.*, 1999; Furukawa *et al.*, 1985; Goldman *et al.*, 1998; Giannini *et al.*, 1991). In contrast, patients with lesions reported to be scarcely infiltrated with DC had a relatively poor prognosis (Tsujitani *et al.*, 1990). Fewer DC were observed in metastatic than primary lesions (Murphy *et al.*, 1993). In a recent study, we demonstrated that the number of S-100[+] DC present in the tumor was by far the strongest independent predictor of overall survival as well as disease-free survival and time to recurrence in 132 patients with oral carcinoma, compared with such well established prognostic factors as disease stage or lymph node involvement (Reichert *et al.*, 2001). Another striking observation we made concerns the relationship between the number of DC in the tumor and expression of the TcR-associated ζ chain in TIL. The paucity of DC in the tumor was significantly related to the loss of ζ expression in TIL, and these two factors had a highly significant effect on patient overall survival. The poorest survival and the greatest risk was observed in patients with tumors that had small number of DC and little or no ζ expression in TIL ($p=2.4 \times 10^{-8}$). Our data suggest that both the number of DC and the presence of functionally unimpaired T cells in the tumor microenvironment are important for overall survival of patients with cancer. Interactions of DC and T cells in the tumor appear to sustain TcR-mediated, and presumably tumor-directed, functions of the T cells infiltrating the same area. It is possible that DC protect T cells from tumor-induced immune suppression, although the mechanism responsible for such protection remains unknown and is being actively investigated.

The correlation between TADC presence in the tumor and patient overall survival or relapse free survival has not been confirmed in other more recent studies, in which immunostaining for MDC and pDC subsets was performed. Thus, in primary breast cancer, a strong association of mature DC with CD3$^+$ T cells was observed but did not correlate with prognosis (Treilleux *et al.*, 2004). Rather, it was the infiltration by pDC that predicted a poor survival in the same series. While this and all other reports based on immunostaining of tumor sections may suffer from a bias related to selection of patients, tissues, antibodies used for staining, and methods for cell enumeration, it appears that similar to T-cell infiltrates, the biologic significance of DC presence in the tumor remains undefined.

## 1.5    B cells

B lymphocytes (CD19$^+$, CD20$^+$) are uncommon components of human solid tumors. While anti-tumor antibodies (Abs) are frequently detected in the circulation of cancer patients, it has been assumed that these Abs are made and secreted by plasma cells situated in the tumor draining lymph nodes, spleen or other lymphoid tissues. However, in some carcinomas, plasma cells may be present and, occasionally, represent a substantial infiltrating element (Kornstein *et al.*, 1983). More recent reports indicate that lymphoplasmacytic infiltrates are relatively common in pre-malignant cervical lesions as well as cervical carcinomas (O'Brien *et al.*, 2001) and in medullary ductal breast carcinomas (Coronella *et al.*, 2001). In cervical carcinomas, using antibody phage display, it was possible to show that infiltrating B cells and plasma cells represent an antigen-induced response to human papillomavirus (HPV) infection or transformation (O'Brien *et al.*, 2001). In medullary ductal breast carcinoma, the presence of B and plasma cells is associated with improved prognosis (Fisher *et al.*, 1990), and this has generated considerable interest in the role of these B cells and their products in tumor progression. Several independent studies examined the hypothesis that lymphoplasmacytic infiltrates represented a host humoral response driven by tumor-derived neo-antigens (Coronella *et al.*, 2002; Hansen *et al.*, 2001; Nzula *et al.*, 2003). The data based on patterns and levels of TIL-B IgG H chain hypermutation suggested that tumor-infiltrating B cells are undergoing antigen-driven proliferation and affinity maturation *in situ*. Abs produced by TIL-B may be tumor-specific or may specifically bind an intracellular protein, such as β-actin, translocated and presented to the cell surface upon tumor cell apoptosis (Hansen *et al.*, 2001). It has been suggested that dissection of the intratumoral Ab response using Ig variable region analysis might identify those that bind with high affinity to TAA for the purpose of their isolation (Kotlan *et al.*, 2003). The implication of the presence of ectopic germinal centers in breast cancer and perhaps other solid tumors is that Ab production can occur in the tumor microenvironment under certain circumstances. The biologic significance or the prognostic importance of this is unknown, although it might be that the ability to make Abs *in situ* may be an important aspect of host defense.

## 1.6    Other leukocytes

Human tumors are sometimes infiltrated by granulocytes, and nests of eosinophils may be seen in association with tumor cells in various squamous cell carcinomas, for example. By far the most frequent cell in tumors has characteristics of the immature myeloid cell (iMC). It expresses CD33, a common myeloid marker, but lacks markers of mature myeloid or lymphoid cells and HLA-DR (Almand *et al.*, 2001). The iMC are equivalent to murine Gr-1$^+$CD11b$^+$ cells, which have been shown to inhibit IFN-$\gamma$ production by CD8$^+$ T cells in response to epitopes presented by MHC class I molecules on the surface of these cells (Almand *et al.*, 2001). This inhibition is apparently mediated by ROS produced by iMC, such as $H_2O_2$, which suppress CD3$\zeta$ expression by T cells (Otsuji *et al.*, 1996). Indeed, granulocyte-derived $H_2O_2$ has been shown to be involved in the inhibition of IFN-$\gamma$ production and the suppression of CD3$\zeta$ expression in circulating T cells of patients with advanced malignancy (Schmielau and Finn, 2001). In tumors, where the hypoxic environment prevails, $H_2O_2$-generating iMC might contribute to creating conditions favoring T-cell suppression.

## 2.    INTERACTIONS BETWEEN THE TUMOR AND INFILTRATING LEUKOCYTES

In aggregate, recent phenotypic and functional assessments of tumor-associated leukocytes have provided a broad cross-sectional view of the types of cellular infiltrates present in human solid tumors. While the nature and cellular composition of these infiltrates vary from one tumor type to another or even among individual tumors of the same histologic type, their presence in human solid tumors is a consistent feature. Furthermore, the phenotype, numbers and location in the tumor (i.e., stroma vs. intraepithelial) of infiltrating leukocytes have been in many instances correlated to prognosis and patient survival (see, e.g., Phillips *et al.*, 2004). However, no unified conclusions have emerged to date in this respect, because for every report linking ample leukocyte infiltration to a better prognosis, a report can be found claiming the opposite. It is clear that the presence of leukocytic infiltrates in the tumor is either good or bad but not neutral. There are several aspects of this dilemma that are particularly intriguing, as discussed below.

It is possible to consider leukocytic infiltrates as a component of the inflammatory process representing a "host reaction" to the tumor. In fact, establishing parallels or links between inflammation and cancer has become a popular quest (Balkwill and Coussens, 2004). The initial goal of inflammation is the destruction of the invader, which in this case is the tumor. Hence, the "immune phase" of tumor-driven inflammation involves an influx of anti-tumor effector cells to the affected tissue. In comparison to vigorous cellular and antibody responses that are generated in tissues during the infection by an exogenous pathogen, however, inflammatory responses to tumors are weak. At least one reason for the lack of robust immune responses to the tumor is the absence of a "danger signal" in the tumor microenvironment (Gallucci and Matzinger, 2001; Matzinger, 1998). The immune system perceives infections with bacteria or viruses as "danger" and the tumor as "self." It responds vigorously to contain the external danger introduced by pathogens and only weakly, if at all, to tumor-associated antigens (TAA), which are largely self antigens or altered self antigens. It may be that the attraction of $T_{reg}$ to the tumor is related to an attempt by the host to ill advisedly (in this case) regulate host response to self. Interestingly, inflammatory infiltrates in tumors generally contain few, if any, NK cells which mediate innate immunity and are rich in perforin- or granzyme-containing granules (Whiteside *et al.*, 1998). NK cells are exquisitely attuned to distinguish self from non-self by virtue of a complex system of inhibitory and activating receptors expressed on their surface (Lanier, 2003). They represent "the first line" of defense against pathogens, and their conspicuous absence from tumor infiltrates or even pre-cancerous lesions (Lanier, 2003) suggests that the host's response to the tumor is indeed different in strength and quality from that initiated by exogenous pathogens.

Tolerance to self that needs to be overcome before a full-scale immune response to the tumor can develop is one reason for ineffective anti-tumor host defense (Janeway 1992). But there are others as well. The nature of the tumor microenvironment appears to be quite unique. On the one hand, the tumor creates stress signals, which mobilize the host to initiate an inflammatory cascade. On the other, the tumor microenvironment is characterized by the presence of multiple immuno-suppressive factors and by the excess of antigens produced and released from proliferating or dying tumor cells (Whiteside and Rabinowich, 1998). Thus, inflammatory cells arrive into this environment to be faced by conflicting signals, which orchestrate the local response. Consequently, a somewhat precarious balance is established between the host and the tumor, which clearly favors the tumor, and which has at least two aims: a) to cripple the host immune system so that the tumor can survive, and b) to utilize infiltrating cells and their products for supporting tumor survival. Ample evidence exists to support the existence of both these mechanisms (Whiteside *et al.*, 2005). While tumor escape from the host-mediated surveillance in its various forms has been recently in the limelight (reviewed in Whiteside *et al.*, 2005), those elements of the local inflammatory response that mediate trophic functions and thus support tumor growth have to be recognized as well. Thus, once recruited to the tumor microenvironment, various leukocytes are subjected to non-specific or tumor-specific signals and in response may produce a variety of soluble products, including cytokines and antibodies. In theory, antitumor effects of these products combined with direct cytolytic activity of infiltrating effector cells against tumor targets should result in tumor demise. In most cases, however, the tumor also releases soluble factors, including cytokines, lipids, polyamines and TAA that suppress immune cells and at the same time stimulate tumor growth and survival.

## 3. CHARACTERISTICS OF THE TUMOR MICROENVIRONMENT

Among the factors that may determine the nature of inflammatory infiltrates found in the tumor is the hypoxic environment. It is created early in tumor development through activation of hypoxia responsive genes in tumor cells (Denko *et al.*, 2003), and it obviously favors influx of those inflammatory cells that depend on the glycolytic pathway for survival, namely, phagocytic macrophages and granulocytes (Sitkovsky *et al.*, 2004).

These cells can not only survive in the hypoxic environment but contribute to it by hyperproduction of ROS upon their activation. The tumor milieu, in which apoptosis of rapidly expanding tumor cells is a common feature, provides ample activating signals for phagocytic cells and leads to the generation of ROS. In most inflammatory responses, activities of ROS are mediated by the NF-κB pathway, which in turn is regulated by hypoxia and/or re-oxygenation (Hanada and Yoshimura, 2002). It has been recently proposed that NF-κB activates signaling pathways in both cancer cells and tumor-associated inflammatory cells, thus promoting malignancy (Pikarsky *et al.*, 2004). If progression to malignancy is indeed regulated at the level of NF-κB and a pro-inflammatory mediator TNF-α or other pro-inflammatory cytokines, as some of the animal models of cancer seem to indicate, the missing link between inflammation and cancer may have been identified (Pikarsky *et al.*, 2004; Greten *et al.*, 2004). These cancer models also underscore the importance of the tumor microenvironment, and its interactions with infiltrating inflammatory cells, in cancer progression. The data suggest that the NF-κB pathway is regulated differently in normal vs. malignant tissues. NF-κB is present as an inactive complex in the cytoplasm of many cells, including inflammatory and tissue cells. During inflammation, activation of NF-κB initiated by, e.g., binding of TNF-α to its receptor (TNFR1) expressed on inflammatory cells in the microenvironment initiates regulated expression of cytokine genes which control cell proliferation and cell death. Tumor cells depend on these cytokines for proliferation, and leukocytes activated in the tumor microenvironment are re-programmed to continually release these cytokines. Responding to this cytokine cascade, tumor and stromal cells produce a panoply of soluble factors with biologic effects ranging from enhancement of cell proliferation, matrix remodeling, vessel growth, inhibition of cellular differentiation to sustained release of pro-inflammatory mediators. Inhibition of NF-κB activation in tumor cells favors cell death and arrests tumor progression. This model is consistent with observed correlations between the numbers and maturation stages of inflammatory cells in the tumor, levels of cytokines produced and tumor prognosis (Balkwill, 2004). The role of TNF-α in driving tumor progression has been emphasized by Balkwill and colleagues (Malik *et al.*, 1998), and it offers an interesting example of the efficiency of tumors in their ability to usurp the normal biologic process of inflammation to promote tumor progression.

As tumor cells successively modify their microenvironment, they often adopt the phenotypic characteristics of immune cells. They co-opt signaling molecules, chemokines, selectins and their receptors normally expressed by leukocytes to serve for tumor migration, invasion and metastasis. It is likely that soluble factors produced during the immune phase, such as colony-stimulating factor (CSF-1), could contribute to this adoption by tumor cells of a myeloid-like phenotype. The plasticity of tumor cells allows them to express chemokines and chemokine receptors, which usually function as chemoattractants and activating factors in leukocytes. Functions associated with neutrophils, such as the production of extracellular proteases, including matrix metalloproteinases (MMPs) that modify the extracellular matrix and fit it into the tumor scaffolding, are also adopted by tumor cells (Engbring and Kleinman, 2003). The use of a leukocyte-like metabolism by tumor cells, i.e., their ability to metabolize glucose via the glycolytic pathway and to synthesize ROS, is another example of how the properties of leukocytes are co-opted to maintain the hypoxic state in the tumor microenvironment (Borregaard and Herlin, 1982). Masquerading as inflammatory cells, tumor cells acquire the ability to further alter the microenvironment, migrate by responding to signals and pathways normally reserved for the cells of the immune system and establish metastases to organs rich in resident macrophages, where conditions are favorable for proliferation (i.e., lung, liver and bone). Thus, the leukocytes infiltrating the tumor contribute to the maintenance of the cytokine-rich microenvironment, which facilitates adoption of the leukocyte-like phenotype by tumor cells.

In inflammation, the immune phase is followed by the appearance of blood vessels and lymphatics in the repaired tissue. The process of angiogenesis is a prominent component of the tumor microenvironment (Bamias and Dimipoulos, 2003). Vascular endothelial growth factor (VEGF) is produced by most tumors and plays a crucial role in the development of tumor vasculature (Gabrilovich *et al.*, 1996b). Increased levels of VEGF in the plasma of patients with cancer were shown to correlate with a poor prognosis (Ellis and Fidler, 1996). Evidence points to VEGF as one of the factors responsible for inducing defects in DC differentiation in the tumor. As TAM play an important role in angiogenesis, it is not surprising that the tumor re-programs the myeloid precursors to express the secretory phenotype, which serves to promote vessel development, rather than their maturation to DC capable of priming T cells for antitumor responses. The appearance of blood vessels in the tumors signals another major change in the tumor microenvironment, namely a switch from hypoxic to oxidative metabolism. Oxidative phosphorylation with an increase in ATP synthesis is necessary to drive tumor cell proliferation, and it is enabled by angiogenesis promoted by combined activities of tumor-infiltrating leukocytes and tumor cells.

Once established, the tumor microenvironment is not a friendly place for infiltrating leukocytes. While they are clearly conscripted by the host to interfere with abnormal tissue growth, once in the tumor, they come in contact with a variety of soluble factors that impede their maturation, inhibit their functions or simply induce their apoptosis (reviewed in Whiteside *et al.*, 2005). Cytokines are known to be present in tumors and are known to affect maturation, differentiation or functions and survival of immune cells (Toi, 2002). They include M-CSF, GM-CSF, IL-6, IL-10, TGFβ and other tumor-derived soluble factors (Whiteside *et al.*, 2005). The degree of impairment of immune cells in the tumor microenvironment differs widely in individual tumors. While the inhibitory effects are the strongest in the tumor, they are not confined locally but are systemic, especially in patients with advanced disease (Whiteside, 2002). Functional abnormalities and apoptosis of T lymphocytes are seen not only at the tumor site but are common in the circulation of patients with cancer. However, it is important to note that these patients generally have normal immune responses to recall antigens and can mount normal primary responses, except for those with terminal cancers. The mechanisms involved in selective and persistent inhibition of antitumor immune responses in patients with cancer are numerous and have been reviewed (Whiteside *et al.*, 2005). Tumors grow progressively and metastasize despite prominent leukocyte infiltrations, largely because they evolve strategies for escape from immune intervention (Whiteside *et al.*, 2005). Consequently, the fate of immune cells infiltrating the tumor is to be corrupted by the tumor into helping its progression, to lose their functional attributes or to die. Tumor aggressiveness depends on the efficiency with which this can be accomplished.

Successive changes that take place during chronic inflammation in the tumor imply that the nature and composition of the inflammatory infiltrates change as well. The characteristic feature of the tumor microenvironment is that it undergoes alterations in concert with tumor progression. It is for this reason that snapshots of the tumor microenvironment obtained by immunohistology of tumor sections or studies of TIL isolated from tumors at one stage of their progression provide an incomplete picture of cellular interactions *in situ*. Therefore, correlations of the numbers or phenotype of inflammatory cells in the tumor with clinical data or with patient prognosis may not be informative. Indeed, conflicting reports available in the literature regarding the significance of immune cells in the tumor microenvironment reflect the difficulties in interpretation of events that unfold and change in the context of host-tumor interactions.

## 4. CONCLUSIONS

New developments in molecular immunology in conjunction with newly developed animal models, as discussed above, have altered our perception of *in situ* interactions between infiltrating leukocytes and tumor cells. More recent evidence favors the view of the developing tumor as a site of chronic inflammatory reaction that is orchestrated not by the host but by the tumor. Its success in co-opting functions of leukocytes toward promoting tumor survival depends on a variety of molecular mechanisms, and these are beginning to be elucidated. At least one link between inflammation and cancer in the form of the NF-κB pathway, which can either promote survival of cells with the malignant phenotype or sustain the production of pro-inflammatory cytokines in inflammatory cells within the tumor, has been identified. This discovery dramatically emphasizes the fact that the same molecular pathway can be harnessed to mediate opposite effects, depending on the context in which they operate. It also reminds us that dysregulated production of pro-inflammatory cytokines and chemokines can and does lead to tissue pathology. An understanding of the complex role of inflammatory infiltrates in the tumor progression is essential for devising novel and more effective anticancer therapies of the future.

# 5. REFERENCES

Albers, A.E. *et al.* (2005). Immune response to p53 in patients with cancer: enrichment in tetramer+p53 peptide-specific T cells and regulatory T cells at tumor sites. *Cancer Immunol, Immunother.* in press.

Albers, A.E. *et al.* (2005). T-cell receptor variable gene β-restricted T lymphocytes are sensitive to apoptosis in patients with squamous cell carcinoma of the head and neck. Submitted.

Aller, M.A. *et al.* (2004). Posttraumatic inflammation is a complex response based on the pathological expression of the nervous, immune and endocrine function systems. *Exp. Biol. Med.* **229**: 170-181.

Almand, B. *et al.* (2000). Clinical significance of defective dendritic cell differentiation in cancer. *Clin. Cancer Res.* **6**: 1755-1766.

Almand, B. *et al.* (2001). Increased production of immature myeloid cells in cancer patients: a mechanism of immunosuppression in cancer. *J. Immunol.* **166**: 678-689.

Al-Sarireh, B. and Eremin, O. (2000). Tumour-associated macrophages (TAMS): disordered function, immune suppression and progressive tumour growth. *J. R. Coll. Surg. Edinb.* **45**: 1-16.

Baeuerle, P.A. and Baltimore, D. (1996). NF-kappaB: ten years after. *Cell* **87**: 13-20.

Balkwill, F. and Mantovani, A. (2001). Inflammation and cancer: back to Virchow? *Lancet* **357**: 539-545.

Balkwill, F. (2004). Cancer and the chemokine network. *Nat. Rev.Cancer* **4**: 540-550.

Balkwill, F. and Coussens, L.M. (2004). Cancer: An inflammatory link. *Nature* **431**: 405-406.

Bamias, A. and Dimipoulos, M.A. (2003). Angiogenesis in human cancer: implications in cancer therapy. *Eur. J. Intern. Med.* **14**: 459-469.

Banchereau, J. and Steinman, R.M. (1998). Dendritic cells and the control of immunity. *Nature* **392**: 245-252.

Banchereau, J. *et al.* (2000). Immunobiology of dendritic cells. *Annu. Rev. Immunol.* **18**: 767-811.

Baxevanis, C.N. *et al.* (1994). Tumor specific cytolysis by tumor infiltrating lymphocytes in breast cancer. *Cancer* **74**: 1275-1282.

Becker, Y. (1993). Dendritic cell activity against primary tumors: an overview. *In Vivo* **7**: 187-191.

Bogenrieder, T. and Herlyn, M. (2003). Axis of evil: molecular mechanisms of cancer metastasis. *Oncogene* **22**: 6524-6536.

Borregaard, N. and Herlin T. (1982). Energy metabolism of human neutrophils during phagocytosis. *J. Clin. Invest.* **70**: 550-557.

Coronella, J.A. *et al.* (2001). Evidence for an antigen-driven humoral immune response in medullary ductal breast cancer. *Cancer Res.* **61**: 7889-7899.

Coronella, J.A. *et al.* (2002). Antigen-driven oligoclonal expansion of tumor-infiltrating B cells in infiltrating ductal carcinoma of the breast. *J. Immunol.* **169**: 1829-1836.

Curiel, T.J. *et al.* (2004). Specific recruitment of regulatory T cells in ovarian carcinoma fosters immune privilege and predicts reduced survival. *Nature Med.* **10**: 942-949.

Dworak, H.F. (1986). Tumors: Wounds that do not heal. Similarities between tumor stroma generation and wound healing. *N. Engl. J. Med.* **315**: 1650-1659.

Denko, N.C. *et al.* (2003). Investigating hypoxic tumor physiology through gene expression patterns. *Oncogene* **22**: 5907-5914.

Engbring, J.A. and Kleinman, H.K. (2003). The basement membrane matrix in malignancy. *J. Pathol.* **200**: 465-470.

Ellis, L.M. and Fidler, I.J. (1996). Angiogenesis and metastasis. *Eur. J. Cancer* **32A**: 2451-2460.

Esche, C. *et al.* (1999). Tumor's other immune targets: dendritic cells. *J. Leukocyte Biol.* **66**: 336-344.

Esche, C. *et al.* (2001). Tumor necrosis factor-alpha-promoted expression of Bcl-2 and inhibition of mitochondrial cytochrome C release mediated resistance of mature dendritic cells to melanoma-induced apoptosis. *Clin. Cancer Res.* **7**: 974s-979s.

Fisher, E.R. *et al.* (1990). Medullary cancer of the breast revisited. *Breast Cancer Res. Treat.* **16**: 215-229.

Furukawa, T. *et al.* (1985). T-zone histiocytes in adenocarcinoma of the lung in relation to postoperative prognosis. *Cancer* **56**: 2651-2656.

Gabrilovich, D.I. *et al.* (1996a). Decrease in antigen presentation by dendritic cells in patients with breast cancer. *Nat. Med.* **2**: 1096-1103.

Gabrilovich, D.I. *et al.* (1996b). Vascular endothelial growth factor produced by human tumors inhibits the functional maturation of dendritic cells. *Nature Med.* **2**: 1096-1103.

Gabrilovich, D. *et al.* (1999). Antibodies to vascular endothelial growth factor enhance the efficacy of cancer immunotherapy by improving endogenous dendritic cell functions. *Clin. Cancer Res.* **5**: 2963-2970.

Gabrilovich, D. (2004). Mechanisms and functional significance of tumor-induced dendritic cell defects. *Nature Med.* **4**: 941-952.

Gallucci, S. and Matzinger, P. (2001). Danger signals: SOS to the immune system. *Curr. Opin. Immunol.* **13**: 114-119.

Giannini, A. *et al.* (1991). Prognostic significance of accessory cells and lymphocytes in nasopharygeal carcinoma. *Pathol. Res. Pract.* **187**: 496-502.

Goldman, S.A. *et al.* (1998). Peritumoral CD1a-positive dendritic cells are associated with improved survival in patients with tongue carcinoma. *Arch. Otolaryngol. Head Neck Surg.* **124**: 641-646.

Greten, F.R. *et al.* (2004). IKKbeta links inflammation and tumorigenesis in a mouse model of colitis-associated cancer. *Cell* **118**: 285-296.

Hanada, T. and Yoshimura, A. (2002). Regulation of cytokine signaling and inflammation. *Cytokine Growth Factor Rev.* **13**: 413-421.

Hansen, M.H. *et al.* (2001). The tumor-infiltrating B cell response in medullary breast cancer is oligoclonal and directed against the autoantigen actin exposed on the surface of apoptotic tumor cells. *Proc. Natl Acad. Sci. U.S.A.* **98**: 12659-12664.

Hansson, M. *et al.* (1996). Induction of apoptosis in NK cells by monocyte-derived reactive oxygen metabolites. *J. Immunol.* **156**: 42-47.

Hoffmann, T.K. *et al.* (2002). Spontaneous apoptosis of circulating T lymphocytes in patients with head and neck cancer and its clinical importance. *Clin. Cancer Res.* **8**: 2553-2562.

Janeway Jr., C.A. (1992). The immune system evolved to discriminate infectious nonself from noninfectious self. *Immunol. Today* **13**: 11-16.

Kiessling, R. *et al.* (1996). Immunosuppression in human tumor-host interaction: role of cytokines and alterations in signal-transducing molecules. *Springer Sem .Immunopathol.* **18**: 227-242.

Kornstein, M.J. *et al.* (1983). Immunoperoxidase localization of lymphocyte subsets in the host responses to melanoma and nevi. *Cancer Res,* **43**: 2749-2753.

Kotlan, B. *et al.* (2003). Immunoglobulin reprtoire of B lymphocytes infiltrating breast medullary carcinoma. *Hum. Antibodies* **12**: 113-121.

Kuss, I. *et al.* (1999). Clinical significance of decreased $\zeta$ chain expression in peripheral blood lymphocytes of patients with head and neck cancer. *Clin.Cancer Res.* **5**: 329-334.

Lanier, L.L. (2003). Natural killer cell receptor signaling. *Curr. Opin. Immunol.* **15**: 308-314.

Lee, K.M. *et al.* (1998). Molecular basis of T-cell inactivation by CTLA-4. *Science* **282**: 2263-2266.

Leek, R.D. *et al.* (1996). Association of macrophage infiltration with angiogenesis and prognosis in invasive breast carcinoma. *Cancer Res.* **56**: 4625-4629.

Lespagnard, L. *et al.*, (1999) Tumor-infiltrating dendritic cells in adenocarcinomas of the breast: a study of 143 neoplasms with a correlation to usual prognostic factors and to clinical outcome. *Int. J. Cancer* **84**: 309-314.

Li, X. *et al.* (1994). T cells from renal cell carcinoma patients exhibit an abnormal pattern of kappa B-specific DNA-binding activity: a preliminary report. *Cancer Res.* **54**: 5424 5429.

Lin, E.Y. *et al.* (2001). Colony-stimulating factor 1 promotes progression of mamary tumors to malignancy. *J. Exp. Med.* **193**: 727-740.

Ling, W. *et al.* (1998). Impaired activation of NFκB in T cells from a subset of renal cell carcinoma patients is mediated by inhibition of phosphorylation and degradation of the inhibitor, IκBα. *Blood* **92**: 1334-1341.

Liu, Y.J. (2001). Dendritic cell subsets and lineages and their functions in innate and adoptive immunity. *Cell* **106**: 259-262.

Liyanage, U.K. *et al.* (2002). Prevalence of regulatory T cells is increased in peripheral blood and tumor microenvironment of patients with pancreas or breast adenocarcinoma. *J. Immunol.* **169**: 2756-2761.

Malik, S.T.A. *et al.* (1989). Paradoxical effects of tumor necrosis factor in experimental ovarian cancer. *Int. J. Cancer* **44**: 918-925.

Malmberg, K.J. *et al.* (2001). Inhibition of activated/memory (CD45RO(+)) T cells by oxidative stress associated with block of NK-kappaB activation. *J. Immunol.* **167**: 2595-2601.

Mareel, M. and Leroy, A. (2003). Clinical cellular, and molecular aspects of cancer invasion. *Physiol. Rev.* **83**: 337-376.

Matzinger, P. (1998). An innate sense of danger. *Semin. Immunol.* **10**: 399-415.

May, M.J. and Ghosh, S. (1998). Signal transduction through NF-κB. *Immunol. Today* **19**: 80-88.

Miescher, S. *et al.* (1987). Clonal and frequency analyses of tumor-infiltrating T lymphocytes from human solid tumors. *J. Immunol.* **138**: 4004-4011.

Mihm, M.C. *et al.* (1996). Tumor infiltrating lymphocytes in lymph node melanoma metastases – a histopathologic prognostic indicator and an expression of local immune response. *Lab. Invest.* **74**: 43-47.

Murphy, G.F. *et al.* (1993). Autologous melanoma vaccine induces inflammatory responses in melanoma metastases: relevance to immunologic regression and immunotherapy. *J. Invest. Dermatol.* **100**: 335s-341s.

Naito, Y. *et al.* (1998). CD8+ T cells infiltrated within cancer cell nests as a prognostic factor in human colorectal cancer. *Cancer Res.* **58**: 3491-3494.

Nakano, O. *et al.* (2001). Proliferative activity of intratumoral CD8+ T lymphocytes as aprognostic factor in human renal cell carcinoma: Clinicopathologic demonstration of antitumor immunity. *Cancer Res.* **61**: 5132-5136.

Nzula, S. *et al.* (2003). Antigen-driven clonal proliferation, somatic hypermutation and selection of B lymphocytes infiltrating human ductal breast carcinomas. *Cancer Res.* **63**: 3275-3280.

O'Brien, P.M. *et al.* (2001). Immunoglobin genes expressed by B-lymphocytes infiltrating cervical carcinomas show evidence of antigen-driven selection. *Cancer Immunol. Immunother.* **50**: 523-532.

Otsuji, M. *et al.* (1996). Oxidative stress by tumor-derived macrophagessuppresses the expression of CD3 ζ chain of T-cell receptor complex and antigen-specific cell responses. *Proc. Natl Acad. Sci.U.S.A.* **93**: 13119-13124.

Phillips, S.M. *et al.* (2004). Tumour-infiltrating lymphocytes in colorectal cancer with microsatellite instability are activated and cytotoxic. *Br. J. Cancer* **91**: 469-475.

Pikarsky, E. *et al.* (2004). NF-kappaB functions as a tumor promoter in inflammation-associated cancer. *Nature* **431**: 461-466.

Ramsdell, F. (2003). Foxp3 and natural regulatory T cells: key to a cell lineage? *Immunity* **19**: 165-168.

Reichert, T.E. *et al.* (1998a). Human immune cells in the tumor microenvironment: mechanisms responsible for signaling and functional defects. *J. Immunother.* **21**: 295-306.

Reichert, T.E. *et al.* (1998b). Absent of low expression of the ζ chain in T cells at the tumor site correlates with poor survival in patients with oral carcinoma. *Cancer Res.* **58**: 5344-5347.

Reichert, T.E. *et al.* (2001). The number of intratumoral dendritic cells and ζ-chain expression in T cells as prognostic and survival biomarkers in patients with oral carcinoma. *Cancer* **91**: 2136-2147.

Reichert, T.E. *et al.* (2002). Signaling abnormalities and reduced proliferation of circulating and tumor-infiltrating lymphocytes in patients with oral carcinoma. *Clin. Cancer Res.* **8**: 3137-3145.

Ribatti, D. *et al.* (2003). New non-angiogenesis dependent pathways for tumor growth. *Eur. J. Cancer* **39**: 1835-1841.

Schmielau, J. and Finn, O.J. (2001). Activated granulocytes and granulocyte-derived hydrogen peroxide are the underlying mechanism of suppression of T-cell function in advanced cancer patients. *Cancer Res.* **61**: 4756-4760.

Sheu, B.C. *et al.* (1999). Reversed CD4/CD8 percentages of tumor-infiltrating lymphocytes correlate with disease progression in human cervical cancer. *Cancer* **86**: 1537-1543.

Shevach, E.M. (2000). Regulatory T cells in autoimmunity. *Annu. Rev. Immunol.* **18**: 423-449.

Shevach, E.M. (2004). Fatal attraction: tumors becon regulatory T cells. *Nature Med.* **10**: 900-901.

Shurin, M.R. *et al.* (1999). 'Apoptosis in dendritic cells' in Dendritic Cells: Biology and Clinical Applications. M.T. Lotze and A.W. Thomson (eds), Academic Press, New York, 673-692.

Shurin, G.V. *et al.* (2001). Neuroblastoma-derived gangliosides inhibit dendritic cell generation and function. *Cancer Res.* **61**: 363-369.

Sitkovsky, M.V. *et al.* (2004). Physiological control of immune response and inflammatory tissue damage by hypoxia-inducible factors and adenosine $A_{2A}$ receptors. *Annu. Rev. Immunol.* **22**: 657-682.

Stephens, G.L. *et al.* (2004). Engagement of glucocorticoid induced TNFR family-related receptor on effector T cells by its ligand mediates resistance to suppression by CD4+CD25+ T cells. *J. Immunol.* **173**: 5008-5020.

Toi, M. (2002). Proinflammation in human tumor microenvironment: its status and implication. *Med. Sci. Monit.* **8**: 25-26.

Tourkova, I.L. *et al.* (2004). IL-15 restores MHC class I antigen processing machinery in human dendritic cells inhibited by tumor-derived gangliosides. Submitted.

Tsujitani, S. *et al.* (1987). Langerhans cells and prognosis in patients with gastric carcinoma. *Cancer* **59**: 501-505.

Tsujitani, S. *et al.* (1990). Infiltration of dendritic cells in relation to tumor invasion and lymph node metastasis in human gastric cancer. *Cancer* **66**: 2012-2016.

Treilleux, I. *et al.* (2004). Dendritic cell infiltration and prognosis of early stage breast cancer. *Clin. Cancer Res.* **10**: 7466-7474.

Troy, A.J. *et al.* (1998). Minimal recruitment and activation of dendritic cells in within renal cell carcinoma. *Clin. Cancer Res.* **4**: 585-593.

Uzzo, R.G. *et al.* (1999a). Renal cell carcinoma-derived gangliosides suppress NFκB activation in T cells. *J. Clin. Invest.* **104**: 769-776.

Uzzo, R.G. *et al.* (1999b). Alterations in NFκB activation in T lymphocytes of patients with renal cell carcinoma. *J. Nat. Cancer Inst.* **91**: 718-721.

Vacarello, L. *et al.* (1993). Tumor-infiltrating lymphocytes from ovarian tumors of low malignant potential. *Int. J. Gynecol. Path.* **12**: 41-50.

Vitolo, D. *et al.* (1993). *In situ* hybridization for cytokine gene transcripts in the solid tumor microenvironment. *Eur. J. Cancer* **3**: 371-377.

Von Kleist, S. *et al.* (1987). Immunohistochemical analysis of lymphocyte subpopulations infiltrating breast carcinomas and benign lesions. *Int. J. Cancer* **40**: 18-23.

Weidmann, E. *et al.* (1992). The T-cell receptor V beta gene usage in tumor-infiltrating lymphocytes and blood of patients with hepatocellular carcinoma. *Cancer Res.* **52**: 5913-5920.

Weidmann, E. *et al.* (1993). Usage of T-cell receptor V beta chain genes in fresh and cultured tumor-infiltrating lymphocytes from human melanoma. *Int. J. Cancer* **54**: 383-390.

Whiteside, T.L. (1992). Tumor Infiltrating Lymphocytes as antitumor effector cells. *Biotherapy* **5**: 47-61.

Whiteside, T.L. (1993). Tumor Infiltrating Lymphocytes in Human Malignancies. Medical Intelligence Unit, R.G. Landes Co., Austin, TX.

Whiteside, T.L. *et al.* (1998). Natural killer cells and tumor therapy. *Curr. Topics Microbiol. Immunol.* **230**: 221-244.

Whiteside, T.L. and Rabinowich, H. (1998). The role of Fas/FasL in immunosuppression induced by human tumors. *Cancer Immunol. Immunother.* **46**: 175-184.

Whiteside, T.L. (2002). Tumor-induced death of immune cells: its mechanisms and consequences. *Sem. Cancer Biol.* **12**: 43-50.

Whiteside, T.L. (2004). Down-regulation of ζ chain expression in T cells: A biomarker of prognosis in cancer? *Cancer Immunol. Immunother.* **53**: 865-876.

Whiteside, T.L. *et al.* (2004). Antigen processing machinery (APM) in human dendritic cells: up-regulation by maturation and down regulation by tumor cells. *J. Immunol.* **173**: 1526-1534.

Whiteside, T.L. *et al.* (2005). 'Tumor induced immune suppression and immune escape: Mechanisms and possible solutions' in: Monitoring T cell Directed Vaccine Trials in Cancer Patients. D. Nagorsen and F. Manincola (eds) in press.

Whitford, P. *et al.* (1990). Flow cytometric analysis of tumour infiltrating lymphocytes in breast cancer. *Br. J. Cancer* **62**: 971-975.

Woo, E.Y. *et al.* (2001). Regulatory CD4+ CD25+ T cells in tumors from patients with early-stage non-small cell lung cancer and late stage ovarian cancer. *Cancer Res.* **61**: 4766-4772.

Zhang, L. *et al.* (1997). Gene expression profiles in normal and cancer cells. *Science* **276**: 1268-1272.

# Chapter 6

# TUMOR-MICROENVIRONMENT INTERACTIONS:

## The Selectin-Selectin Ligand Axis in Tumor-Endothelium Cross Talk

Isaac P. Witz

*Department of Cell Research and Immunology, The George S. Wise Faculty of Life Sciences, Tel Aviv University, Tel Aviv. 69978, Israel, ipwitz@post.tau.ac.il*

Abstract:    Interactions of cancer cells with components of their microenvironment are crucial determinants in the decision making process which determines whether the cancer cells will progress towards a highly malignant phenotype or whether they will stay dormant or disappear altogether. The tumor microenvironment is composed of a plethora of soluble and cellular components. Many of these components deliver signals to tumor cells and thus modulate their phenotype thereby driving tumor progression. This chapter focuses on the interaction of tumor cells with endothelial cells through endothelial selectins and their fucosylated ligands expressed by the tumor cells. Comparisons are drawn between the utilization of this interaction axis by inflammatory leukocytes and by tumor cells.

Key words:    tumor microenvironment; metastasis; endothelium; selectins; selectin-ligands; fucose; FX enzyme; transendothelial migration; extravasation

# 1.    THE ROAD TO METASTASIS IS PAVED WITH SEVERAL INVASION EVENTS

Metastasis is the principal cause of treatment failure, poor prognosis, morbidity and mortality in cancer patients. Invasion of surrounding or distant tissues by cancer cells is the critical event in neoplastic diseases. An understanding of the molecular mechanisms involved in this process will aid in the identification of specific therapeutic targets that may allow tailored therapies for patients with metastasis or even the prevention of cancer progression.

There are several distinct events in the metastatic cascade in which cancer cells invade surrounding tissues. Detached cells from the primary tumor lesion equipped with the proper machinery (e.g., proteinases and other lytic enzymes; motility etc.) invade the extra cellular matrix on their way to the blood or lymph vasculature. Some cells invade these vessels and enter the circulation (intravasation). The next invasion event is transendothelial migration of the tumor cells into the surrounding tissue. This event is also termed extravasation. Those cancer cells that survive all the previous steps may form metastases at distant sites.

Intravasation and, in particular extravasation of tumor cells, require a close and intimate cross talk between tumor and endothelial cells. Such interactions are, however not unique to tumor cells. Other extravasating cells, most notably inflammatory leukocytes also interact with vascular endothelium in the inflammatory process. In fact, our comprehension of tumor cell extravasation is based on mechanisms underlying leukocyte-endothelium interactions leading to the extravasation of the leukocytes.

This review will focus on the involvement of the selectin-selectin ligand axis in cancer-endothelium interactions.

# 2.    MICROENVIRONMENT-DRIVEN MOLECULAR EVOLUTION OF CANCER CELLS

The concept that cancer cells are autonomous with respect to growth factor requirements has prevailed for a long time (Haran-Ghera, 1965; Noble and Hoover, 1975; Chigira *et al.*, 1990; Hanahan and Weinberg, 2000). Cancer autonomy has been ascribed to the capacity of cancer cells to produce and respond to their own growth factors delivering autocrine proliferation signals (Herlyn *et al.*, 1990; Berthois and Martin, 1989; Sporn and Roberts, 1985).

Growth factor autonomy may be meaningful at the first stages of carcinogenesis but is certainly much less conspicuous at the later stages of this process. Invasion and metastasis do not seem to be significantly influenced by growth factor autonomy. Moreover, evidence is rapidly accumulating that invasion, metastasis and in some cases even the formation of primary tumors depends on the microenvironment of the cancer cells (Paget, 1889; Witz, 1977; Yeatman and Nicolson, 1993; Fidler, 1995; Witz et al., 1996; Park et al., 2000; Liotta and Kohn, 2001; Witz, 2001; Eshel et al., 2002a; Witz, 2002; Fidler, 2002a and 2002b; Roskelley and Bissel, 2002; Jung et al., 2002; Wilson and Balkwill, 2002; Ghia et al., 2002; Mueller and Fusenig, 2002; Fidler , 2002; Lynch and Matrisian, 2002; Ben-Baruch, 2003; Vincent-Salomon and Thiery, 2003; Hendrix et al., 2003; Cunha et al., 2003; Kenny and Bissel, 2003; Mantovani et al., 2004; Henning et al., 2004; Lin and Pollard, 2004). Experiments performed in our laboratory over 15 years ago (Halachmi and Witz, 1989) convincingly illustrate this point. In our model, BALB/c 3T3 cells transformed in vitro with a temperature-sensitive mutant of polyoma virus were cloned. These cloned cells were passaged once in syngeneic mice. Cells from the resulting tumors were recultured. The in vitro proliferative capacity of the cells that remained in culture and that of the in vivo passaged cells was essentially identical. However, the in vivo tumorigenicity phenotype of the in vivo passaged cells was considerably augmented as compared to that of their clonal ancestors remaining in culture.

Based on these experiments demonstrating that an in vivo passage increased the tumorigenicity phenotype of the tumor cells, the following hypotheses were formulated:

1. An autocrine stimulation of the in vivo passaged tumor cells by a growth factor intrinsic to these cells can be ruled out.
2. Factors operating in the in vivo microenvironment, and not present in tissue culture medium, are involved in the induction of molecules capable of conferring a high tumorigenicity phenotype upon the tumor cells. A subsequent selection of variants expressing such molecules probably ensues, resulting in growth advantage.

One such microenvironment-induced molecule with the capacity to confer a high malignancy phenotype upon mouse tumor cells was identified in our laboratory as an immunoglobulin receptor, the Fc-γ receptor type IIB1 (Ran et al., 1992; Zusman et al., 1996a and 1996b). In an unpublished study, we identified the factor capable of inducing the expression of the Fc receptor to be an interferon-γ, a cytokine known to be present in the microenvironment of several cancer types (Hess *et al.*, 2003; Lebel-Binay *et al.*, 2003).

The studies summarized above as well as many others clearly attest to the fact that tumor cells possess the potential to interact with factors in their microenvironment. Such interactions may modify gene expression in the cancer cells thereby driving their molecular evolution. The molecular evolution of cancer cells may lead to a modified tumorigenicity phenotype of these cells.

The tumor microenvironment is a highly complex milieu. The recent study of Celis *et al.* (2004) illustrates this point. This group carried out a proteomic analysis of the interstitial fluid of breast cancer. They identified in this microenvironment over two hundred proteins involved in various cellular functions such as proliferation, invasion, angiogenesis, metastasis, inflammation, protein synthesis, transport and folding, to name but a few.

Basically the tumor microenvironment is composed, in addition to the tumor cells themselves, of resident cells such as stroma and endothelial cells, extracellular matrix, infiltrating cells such as macrophages and lymphocytes, soluble products, namely growth factors, cytokines and antibodies, proteases as well as other types of enzymes (Witz, 2001; Jung *et al.*, 2002; Wilson and Balkwill, 2002; Mueller and Fusenig, 2002; Lynch and Matrisian, 2002; Ben-Baruch, 2003; Cunha *et al.*, 2003; Mantovani, 2004; Lin and Pollard, 2004; Vlodavsky and Friedmann, 2001).

All these microenvironmental components are capable of interacting with cancer cells, thus driving their molecular evolution. The ensuing altered molecular profile of the tumor could promote or alternatively restrain tumor progression (Witz *et al.*, 1996; Witz, 2002; Eshel *et al.*, 2002a).

## 3. THE INTERACTION OF ENDOTHELIAL SELECTINS WITH FUCOSYLATED COUNTER-RECEPTORS (SELECTIN LIGANDS) EXPRESSED BY LEUKOCYTES LEADS TO THEIR EXTRAVASATION

Tissue-specific leukocyte localization is a requirement for immune surveillance and plays a key role in the pathogenesis of various inflammatory diseases. Leukocyte adhesion to endothelial cells is crucial for their extravasation to sites of inflammation. Extravasating leukocytes migrate through the endothelial barrier by first adhering to the endothelial cell surface and then transmigrating through the endothelial cell layer. Adhesion to the endothelium usually requires a cascade of steps mediated by the selectins, leukocyte activating chemotactic factors, and endothelial activating proinflammatory cytokines as well as by integrins. These molecules act in concert and regulate the sequence of distinct steps. The transendothelial migration process requires the active participation of the endothelial cells. Leukocyte binding probably delivers signals to the endothelial cells that promote the opening of endothelial cell junctions thus facilitating the transendothelial passage of the leukocytes (Vestweber, 2002; Middleton *et al.*, 2002; Rosen, 2004).

Selectins are transmembrane C-type lectins that bind carbohydrate moieties expressed by their ligands (Vestweber, 1992; Weis *et al.*, 1998; Vestweber and Blanks, 1999; Ley, 2003; Cambi and Figdor, 2003; Ehrhardt *et al.* 2004). The three known selectins P, E and L are structurally very similar to each other. Each has a carbohydrate-binding domain at the NH$_2$-terminus, an EGF-like domain and various numbers of consensus repeats with homology to complement regulatory proteins. A transmembrane domain anchors the selectins to the membrane. All three selectins contain a cytoplasmatic tail (Vestweber, 1992; Weis *et al.*, 1998; Vestweber and Blanks, 1999; Ley, 2003; Cambi and Figdor, 2003; Ehrhardt *et al.* 2004) that confers the capacity to act as signaling receptors (Yoshida *et al.*, 1998; Simon *et al.*, 1999; Kiely *et al.*, 2003). In addition, soluble forms of selectins were found in serum (Ehrhardt *et al.*, 2004; Ushiyama *et al.*, 1993). These circulating molecules may be generated by proteolysis or may represent splice variants lacking the transmembrane domain (Ushiyama *et al.*, 1993). In the immune system, C-type-lectins may exert a dual function. They may function both as adhesion receptors and as pathogen recognition receptors (Cambi and Figdor, 2003). Such a dual function has, however, not been reported for selectins.

P and E selectins are expressed by endothelial cells. The interaction between these selectins with their ligands expressed by various leukocytes, such as neutrophils, is the initiating event of the extravasation of these leukocytes and their subsequent migration towards inflammatory sites (Ley, 2003). Selectins are also highly important in the adaptive immune system. In this case, L selectin expressed by T lymphocytes and other leukocytes is rather the major player (Ley, 2003).

The first step of leukocyte localization to many tissues involves transient interactions of E and P selectins present on endothelial cells and of L selectin present on T cells and other leukocytes, with carbohydrate ligands displayed, correspondingly, on glycoprotein scaffolds on both leukocytes and endothelial cells (Vestweber, 2002; Middleton *et al.*, 2002; Rosen, 2004; Vestweber, 1992; Weis *et al.*, 1998; Vestweber and Blanks, 1999; Ley, 2003; Cambi and Figdor, 2003; Ehrhardt *et al.* 2004; Varki 1994). These interactions cause tethering and rolling of flowing leukocytes on the endothelial cell surface. The slow velocity of rolling leukocytes on selectins favors encounters with glycosaminoglycan-bound chemokines presented on the endothelial lining to chemokine receptors expressed by leukocytes (Middleton *et al.*, 2002). Short-lived selectin–glycoprotein interactions mediate the rolling of the leukocytes along the endothelial cells. Selectins bind weakly to free sialylated glycans, but with high affinity to specific glycoprotein counter-receptors (Vestweber, 2002; Middleton *et al.*, 2002; Rosen, 2004; Vestweber, 1992; Weis *et al.*, 1998; Vestweber and Banks, 1999; Ley, 2003; Cambi and Figdor, 2003; Ehrhardt, 2004; Varki, 1994). In addition to facilitating leukocyte-endothelium interactions, selectins, being equipped with a cytoplasmic tail, may receive outside-in signals from selectin ligands (Yoshida *et al.*, 1998; Simon *et al.*, 1999; Kiely *et al.*, 2003).

The proper functioning of selectin ligands requires their fucosylation (Varki, 1994; Smith *et al.*, 2002; Becker and Lowe, 2003) mainly by the fucose-generating FX enzyme (Smith *et al.*, 2002; Becker and Lowe; 2003; Eshel *et al.* 2000 and 2001). Fucose is a component of many surface-localized and secreted molecules. It decorates the terminal portions of N-, O-, or lipid-linked glycans and modifies the core of some N-linked glycans (Smith *et al.*, 2002; Becker and Lowe, 2003). Terminal fucosylated glycans in humans constitute several blood group antigens and function as selectin ligands (Smith *et al.*, 2002; Becker and Lowe, 2003). Fucosylation of these ligands determines their ability to bind to the selectin family of cell adhesion molecules and therefore controls pivotal steps of selectin-dependent leukocyte adhesion and trafficking (Smith *et al.*, 2002; Becker and Lowe, 2003; Homeister *et al.*, 2001; Carlow *et al.*, 2001). The final steps of fucose biosynthesis are mediated by the GDP-D-mannose 4, 6 dehydratase (GMD) generating GDP-mannose-4-keto-6-D-deoxymannose. This sugar is converted to GDP-L-fucose by the FX enzyme functioning both as an epimerase and a reductase (Sullivan *et al.*, 1998; Ohyama *et al.*, 1998) . The GDP-L fucose is then transported to the Golgi. Fucosylation of mammalian glycans is catalyzed by distinct fucosyltransferases, with catalytic activities characterized by specificity for certain glycoconjugate substrates and a requirement for GDP-fucose (Lopez-Ferrer *et al.*, 2000).

The generation of FX knock-out mice allowed to conclude that fucosylation events are essential for fertility, early growth and development, as well as for intercellular adhesion (Smith *et al.*, 2002; Becker and Lowe, 2003). FX knockout resulted in massive intrauterine mortality. Live-born FX-null mice exhibited a virtually complete deficiency of cellular fucosylation and a postnatal failure to thrive. FX (-/-) adults suffer from an extreme neutrophilia, myeloproliferation, and absence of leukocyte selectin ligand expression reminiscent of LAD-II/CDG-IIc (Smith *et al.*, 2002; Becker and Lowe, 2003; Etzioni *et al.*, 1999; Becker and Lowe, 1999).

Fucose participates not only in controlling adhesive properties, but also in other functions such as modifying signal transduction events. For example, Fringe, a fucose-specific glycosyltransferase initiates elongation of O-linked fucose residues attached to epidermal growth factor-like sequence repeats of Notch (Moloney *et al.*, 2000) This glycosylation modulates Notch-mediating signaling (Bruckner *et al.*, 2000). Another example is the O-fucose modification of Cripto. This modification is essential for Nodal-dependent signaling (Haltiwanger, 2002).

## 4.  THE INVOLVEMENT OF THE FUCOSE-GENERATING FX ENZYME IN TUMOR-ENDOTHELIUM INTERACTIONS

Studies performed in our laboratory demonstrated that the fucose generating FX enzyme is involved in the biosynthesis of sialyl Lewis–x (sLe-x) in activated T or B cells (Eshel *et al.*, 2001). In head and neck squamous cell carcinomas, the FX enzyme plays a key role and is a limiting factor in the biosynthesis of selectin ligands such as sialyl Lewis–a (sLe-a) and in the interaction of these cancer cells with endothelial cells (Eshel *et al.*, 2000 and 2002b). In lymphocytes. as well as in head and neck squamous cell carcinomas, the FX enzyme is regulated by outside-in signaling (Eshel *et al.*, 2000 and 2001). We also reported that a functional relationship between the expression level of the FX enzyme and that of the selectin ligand sLe-a exists in colorectal cancer (CRC) cells (Zipin *et al.*, 2004). This conclusion was based on a direct and positive correlation between expression levels of FX and those of sLe-a by several CRC cell lines. Furthermore, down-regulating FX expression by FX siRNA transfection decreased sLe-a expression. We also documented a functional axis linking FX and sLe-a expression to the capacity of CRC cells to adhere to E-selectin. It was thus found that the FX enzyme is a limiting factor for the capacity of at least certain CRC cells, to adhere to endothelium. This conclusion is supported both by correlative evidence as well as by direct evidence provided by transfection experiments (Zipin *et al.*, 2004).

It is assumed that highly metastatic tumor variants extravasate more efficiently than cells with a low metastatic phenotype (Voura *et al.*, 1998; Laferriere *et al.*, 2002; Thurin and Kieber-Emmons, 2002). This implies that the former variants would adhere better to endothelial cells than the latter ones. Indeed, highly metastatic CRC variants adhered better to endothelial cells than low metastatic variants originating from the same tumor (Zipin *et al.*, 2004). Additional results led us to tentatively conclude that the degree of malignancy of CRC cells correlates positively with expression of the fucose-generating FX enzyme and of its selectin ligand product sLe-a (Zipin *et al.*, 2004).

Noda *et al.* (2003) confirmed the role of the FX enzyme and fucose synthesis in hepatocellular carcinoma and in hepatoma. They demonstrated that GDP-L-fucose in human hepatocellular carcinoma was significantly higher than in non-involved liver tissue and in normal liver.

Based on the studies summarized above, one may hypothesize that the fucose-generating FX enzyme controls, by regulating selectin ligand biosynthesis, the interaction of at least certain tumor cells with endothelium and thus the capacity to extravasate and form metastases.

The FX enzyme supplies about 90% of the cellular fucose while the rest is supplied by the salvage pathway (Smith *et al.*, 2002; Marquardt *et al.*, 1999; Niittymaki *et al.*, 2004). In this pathway, extra cellular fucose is taken up by the cell, phosphorylated by a fucose-kinase and subsequently converted to GDP L-fucose by GDP-fucose-pyrophosphorylase. The GDP L-fucose generated by the salvage pathway undergoes an identical biosynthetic route as the GDP L-fucose generated by the FX enzyme (Smith *et al.*, 2002; Becker and Lowe, 2003). In order to fully assess the role of the FX enzyme in regulating various fucose-dependent reactions such as adhesion or in Notch or Cripto-mediated signaling, one should determine the relative contribution of the salvage pathway to the fucose supply in various cells.

## 5. DO TUMOR CELLS, SIMILARLY TO LEUKOCYTES, UTILIZE THE SELECTIN-SELECTIN LIGAND AXIS TO INTERACT WITH ENDOTHELIAL CELLS?

Does the extravasation of pre-metastatic tumor cells from blood vessels follow the pathway of leukocyte extravasation? While this question is still not entirely solved, a large body of data suggests that the interaction of selectin ligand-expressing tumor cells with selectin-expressing endothelial cells is an initial and crucial event in the interaction of tumor cells with endothelium resulting in tumor cell transendothelial migration (Voura *et al.*, 1988; Laferriere *et al.*, 2002; Mannori *et al.*, 1995; Kim *et al.*, 1999; Burdick *et al.*, 2003).

Takada *et al.* (1991) demonstrated that the adhesion of cancer cells to vascular endothelium is mediated by the interaction of sLe-a and sLe-x expressed by tumor cells to E-selectin expressed by endothelial cells. Similar findings were subsequently reported for various tumors (Laferriere *et al.*, 2002; Majuri *et al.*, 1992; Wenzel *et al.*, 1995; Ito *et al.*, 2001; Dimitroff *et al.*, 2004). An interesting approach to answer the question if tumor cells utilize the leukocyte extravasation strategy was to modify selectin-selectin ligand interactions by various means and then examine the effects of such modulations on tumor cell adhesion and on metastasis. Among the approaches used were selectin-ligand mimetics (Ohrlein, 2001; Otvos *et al.*, 2002), diversion of the biosynthesis of selectin ligands toward non-adhesive structures (Mathieu *et al.*, 2004), modification or inhibition of the carbohydrate moieties that participate in selectin-selectin-ligand interactions (Hiramatsu *et al.*, 1998; Haroun-Bouhedja *et al.*, 2002) or inhibition of E-selectin expression (Nubel *et al.*, 2004). The excellent reviews by Renkonen *et al.* (1997) and by Kannagi *et al.* (2004) are recommended in order to obtain a comprehensive picture of this field.

Indirect support for the involvement of the selectin-selectin ligand axis in tumor progression was provided by studies demonstrating a correlation between a high expression of selectin ligands by cancer cells, notably epithelial cancer, and a high rate of metastasis and poor prognosis (Thurin and Kieber-Emmons, 2002; Shirahama *et al.*, 1993; Izumi *et al.*, 1995). In fact, sLe-a and sLe-x are tumor markers detected by monoclonal antibodies (Magnani, 2004). The CA19-9 antibody is probably one of the better known ones used in the diagnostics of gastrointestinal and pancreatic cancer (Magnani, 2004).

# 6.     THE ROLE OF SELECTINS IN DISEASE AND IN TUMOR PROGRESSION

In view of the fact that trafficking of leukocytes is controlled to a large extend by interactions between selectins and their ligands, it is logical to expect that such interactions constitute a double-edged sword. Whereas selectin-selectin ligand mediated leukocyte adhesion to endothelial cells and their subsequent transendothelial migration is an important component of host defense, these interactions may be involved in various pathological states such as inflammatory disorders including adult respiratory distress syndrome, acute lung injury, acute ischemic stroke and rheumatoid arthritis (for reviews see Ley, 2003 and Ehrhardt *et al.*, 2004).

Patients with a variety of diseases have elevated plasma levels of soluble selectins. Among them are connective tissue diseases, malaria, systemic sclerosis, acute lung injury, acute stroke, bronchial asthma and Graves' disease (Ehrhardt *et al.*, 2004). In view of the fact that the level of soluble selectins often correlates with disease severity, one may conclude that the soluble selectins contribute to pathogenesis.

An absence of selectins or of their ligands may also have severe consequences. For example patients with leukocyte adhesion deficiency type II (LAD-II) have a mutation in the gene encoding a fucose transporter thus rendering selectin ligands on the neutrophils of these patients incapable of interacting with selectins. This leads to a diminished ability to interact with endothelium and to extravasate. These patients suffer from recurrent infections and persistent leukocytosis (Etzioni *et al.*, 1999; Becker and Lowe, 1999; Marquardt *et al.*, 1999). For further details on the consequences of selectin deficiencies see Ley, 2003.

As mentioned above, tumor progression may be associated with an elevated expression of selectin ligands on the tumor cells, which facilitates their interactions with E and P selectins. These interactions seem to promote metastatic spread as documented by the following examples. Laferriere reported that E-selectin expressed on the membrane of endothelial cells plays an important role in extravasation of cancer cells (Laferriere *et al.*, 2002). Hematogenous metastasis is significantly facilitated by interactions between platelets and tumor cells (Honn *et al.*, 1992). The molecules involved in this interaction are P-selectin expressed by the platelets and selectin ligands expressed by the tumor cells (Varki and Varki, 2002).

A number of clinical studies suggested that elevated levels of E-selectin in the serum of patients with various types of cancer reflect tumor progression (Wittig *et al.*, 1996; Alexiou *et al.*, 2001 and 2003; Zhang and Adachi, 1999; Hebbar and Peyrat, 2000; Ito *et al.*, 2001; Uner *et al.*, 2004). This suggestion is however, not supported by other clinical studies (Velikova *et al.*, 1998; Hebbar *et al.*, 1998; Cervello *et al.*, 2000) and by results demonstrating that the local growth of human colon carcinoma or melanoma in selectin-deficient mice was significantly enhanced (Taverna *et al.*, 2004). The authors explained these results by the deficient monocyte/macrophage infiltration into tumors propagated in the selectin null mice.

Taken together, the studies cited above do not allow a definitive conclusion regarding the role of selectins in tumor progression.

## 7.    SELECTIN-SELECTIN LIGAND MEDIATED INTERACTIONS BETWEEN EXTRAVASATING AND ENDOTHELIAL CELLS AS POSSIBLE TARGETS FOR NOVEL THERAPEUTIC MODALITIES

As mentioned earlier, selectin-selectin ligand interactions play multifaceted and crucial roles in various pathological states such as inflammatory disorders, metastasis formation and possibly autoimmunity.

These interactions have, therefore, become targets for development of new anti-inflammatory and anti-cancer therapy. Various strategies have been employed in the development of drugs that interfere with selectin-selectin ligand interactions (for detailed reviews on this subject please refer to Ley, 2003; Ehrhardt *et al.*, 2004; Magnani, 2004; Boehnke and Schon, 2003). Among the approaches used are: targeting selectins by anti-selectin antibodies, by liposomes or by polymer-based particles, modulation or blocking of selectin expression (Nubel *et al.*, 2004), glycomimetic drugs, selectin ligand competitors, cell surface fucose ablation (Listinsky *et al.*, 2001), inhibition of the synthesis of fucosyltransferases or modulation of their activities.

All these approaches are still in the research and development stage and await efficacy testing in a clinical setting.

## ACKNOWLEDGEMENTS

This chapter was written while spending a sabbatical period at the Department of Cancer Biology, The University of Texas, MD Anderson Cancer Center, Houston, Texas. I thank Dr. Menashe Bar Eli for useful suggestions concerning this review.

The research performed by the group of IPW is supported by: The Jacqueline Seroussi Memorial Foundation for Cancer Research, The Ela Kodesz Institute for Research on Cancer Development and Prevention, Tel Aviv University, The Israel Cancer Association, The Fainbarg Family Fund (Orange County, CA), The Fred August and Adele Wolpers Charitable Fund (Clifton, NJ), Arnold and Ruth Feuerstein (Orange County, CA), and the Pikovsky Fund (Jerusalem, Israel) and by Natan Blutinger (West Orange, NJ). I. Witz is the incumbent of the David Furman Chair in Immunobiology of Cancer.

## REFERENCES

Alexiou, D. *et al.* (2001). Serum levels of E-selectin, ICAM-1 and VCAM-1 in colorectal cancer patients: correlations with clinicopathological features, patient survival and tumour surgery. *Eur. J. Cancer* **37**: 2392-2397.

Alexiou, D. *et al.* (2003). Clinical significance of serum levels of E-selectin, intercellular adhesion molecule-1, and vascular cell adhesion molecule-1 in gastric cancer patients. *Am. J. Gastroenterol.* **98**: 478-485.

Becker, D.J. and Lowe, J.B. (1999). Leukocyte adhesion deficiency type II. *Biochim. Biophys. Acta* **1455**: 193-204.

Becker, D.J. and Lowe, J.B. (2003). Fucose: biosynthesis and biological function in mammals. *Glycobiology* **13**: 41R-53R.

Ben-Baruch, A. (2003). Host microenvironment in breast cancer development: inflammatory cells, cytokines and chemokines in breast cancer progression: reciprocal tumor-microenvironment interactions. *Breast Cancer Res.* **5**: 31-36.

Berthois, Y. and Martin, P. M. (1989). Growth factors and oncogenes. *Biomed. Pharmacother.* **43**: 635-639.

Boehncke, W.H. and Schon, M.P. (2003). Interfering with leukocyte rolling - a promising therapeutic approach in inflammatory skin disorders? *Trends Pharmacol. Sci.* **24**: 49-52.

Bruckner, K. *et al.* (2000). Glycosyltransferase activity of Fringe modulates Notch-Delta interactions. *Nature* **406**: 411-415.

Burdick, M.M. *et al.* (2003). Colon carcinoma cell glycolipids, integrins, and other glycoproteins mediate adhesion to HUVECs under flow. *Am. J. Physiol. Cell Physiol.* **284**: C977-C987.

Cambi, A. and Figdor, C.G. (2003). Dual function of C-type lectin-like receptors in the immune system. *Curr. Opin. Cell Biol.* **15**: 539-546.

Carlow, D.A. *et al.* (2001). IL-2, -4, and -15 differentially regulate O-glycan branching and P-selectin ligand formation in activated CD8 T cells. *J. Immunol.* **167**: 6841-6848.

Celis, J.E. *et al.* (2004). Proteomic characterization of the interstitial fluid perfusing the breast tumor microenvironment: a novel resource for biomarker and therapeutic target discovery. *Mol. Cell Proteomics* **3**: 327-344.

Cervello, M. *et al.* (2000). Serum concentration of E-selectin in patients with chronic hepatitis, liver cirrhosis and hepatocellular carcinoma. *J. Cancer Res. Clin. Oncol.* **126**: 345-351.

Chigira, M. *et al.* (1990). Autonomy in tumor cell proliferation. *Med. Hypotheses* **32**: 249-254.

Cunha, G.R. *et al.* (2003). Role of the stromal microenvironment in carcinogenesis of the prostate. *Int. J. Cancer* **107**: 1-10.

Dimitroff, C.J. *et al.* (2004). Rolling of human bone-metastatic prostate tumor cells on human bone marrow endothelium under shear flow is mediated by E-selectin. *Cancer Res.* **64**: 5261-5269.

Ehrhardt, C. *et al.* (2004). Selectins-an emerging target for drug delivery. *Adv. Drug Deliv. Rev.* **56**: 527-549.

Eshel, R. *et al.* (2000). The GPI-linked Ly-6 antigen E48 regulates expression levels of the FX enzyme and of E-selectin ligands on head and neck squamous carcinoma cells. *J. Biol. Chem.* **275**: 12833-12840.

Eshel, R. *et al.* (2001). The FX enzyme is a functional component of lymphocyte activation. *Cell. Immunol.* **213**: 141-148.

Eshel, R. *et al.* (2002a). Receptors involved in microenvironment-driven molecular evolution of cancer cells. *Semin. Cancer Biol.* **12**: 139-147.

Eshel, R. *et al.* (2002b). Human Ly-6 antigen E48 (Ly-6D) regulates important interaction parameters between endothelial cells and head-and-neck squamous carcinoma cells. *Int. J. Cancer* **98**: 803-810.

Etzioni, A. *et al.* (1999). Of man and mouse: leukocyte and endothelial adhesion molecule deficiencies. *Blood* **94**: 3281-3288.

Fidler, I.J. (1995). Modulation of the organ microenvironment for the treatment of cancer metastasis (editorial). *J. Natl Cancer Inst.* **84**: 1588–1592.

Fidler, I.J. (2002a). Critical determinants of metastasis. *Semin. Cancer Biol.* **12**: 89-96.

Fidler, I.J. (2002b). The organ microenvironment and cancer metastasis. *Differentiation* **70**: 498-505.

Ghia, P. *et al.* (2002). Chronic B cell malignancies and bone marrow microenvironment. *Semin. Cancer Biol.* **12**: 149-155.

Halachmi, E. and Witz, I.P. (1989). Differential tumorigenicity of 3T3 cells transformed *in vitro* with polyoma virus and *in vivo* selection for high tumorigenicity. *Cancer Res.* **49**: 2383-2389.

Haltiwanger, R.S. (2002). Regulation of signal transduction pathways in development by glycosylation. *Curr. Opin. Struct. Biol.* **12**: 593-598.

Hanahan, D. and Weinberg, R.A. (2000). The hallmarks of cancer. *Cell* **100**: 57-70.

Haran-Ghera, N. (1965). Autonomy and dependence of preneoplastic mammary nodules in mice. *Br. J. Cancer* **19**: 816-823.

Haroun-Bouhedja, F. *et al.* (2002). *In vitro* effects of fucans on MDA-MB231 tumor cell adhesion and invasion. *Anticancer Res.* **22**: 2285-2292.

Hebbar, M. *et al.* (1998). The relationship between concentrations of circulating soluble E-selectin and clinical, pathological, and biological features in patients with breast cancer. *Clin. Cancer Res.* **4**: 373-380.

Hebbar, M. and Peyrat, J.P. (2000). Significance of soluble endothelial molecule E-selectin in patients with breast cancer. *Int. J. Biol. Markers* **15**: 15-21.

Hendrix, M.J. *et al.* (2003). Remodeling of the microenvironment by aggressive melanoma tumor cells. *Ann. N. Y. Acad. Sci.* **995**: 151-161.

Henning, T. *et al.* (2004). Relevance of tumor microenvironment for progression, therapy and drug development. *Anticancer Drugs* **15**: 7-14.

Herlyn, M. *et al.* (1990) Growth-regulatory factors for normal, premalignant, and malignant human cells in vitro. *Adv. Cancer Res.* **54**: 213-234.

Hess, S.D. *et al.* (2003). Human CD4+ T cells present within the microenvironment of human lung tumors are mobilized by the local and sustained release of IL-12 to kill tumors in situ by indirect effects of IFN-gamma. *J. Immunol.* **170**: 400-412.

Hiramatsu, Y. *et al.* (1998). Studies on selectin blockers. 6. Discovery of homologous fucose sugar unit necessary for E-selectin binding. *J. Med. Chem.* **41**: 2302-2307.

Homeister, J. W. *et al.* (2001). The alpha(1,3)fucosyltransferases FucT-IV and FucT-VII exert collaborative control over selectin-dependent leukocyte recruitment and lymphocyte homing. *Immunity* **15**: 115-126.

Honn, K.V. *et al.* (1992). Platelets and cancer metastasis: a causal relationship? *Cancer Metastasis Rev.* **11**: 325-351.

Ito, K. *et al.* (2001). Paired tumor marker of soluble E-selectin and its ligand sialyl Lewis A in colorectal cancer. *J. Gastroenterol.* **36**: 823-829.

Izumi, Y. *et al.* (1995). Characterization of human colon carcinoma variant cells selected for sialyl Lex carbohydrate antigen: liver colonization and adhesion to vascular endothelial cells. *Exp. Cell Res.* **216**: 215-221.

Jung, Y.D. *et al.* (2002). The role of the microenvironment and intercellular cross-talk in tumor angiogenesis. *Semin. Cancer Biol.* **12**: 105-112.

Kannagi, R. *et al.* (2004). Carbohydrate-mediated cell adhesion in cancer metastasis and angiogenesis. *Cancer Sci.* **95**: 377-384.

Kenny, P.A. and Bissell, M.J. (2003). Tumor reversion: correction of malignant behavior by microenvironmental cues. *Int. J. Cancer* **107**: 688-695.

Kiely, J.M. *et al.* (2003). Lipid raft localization of cell surface E-selectin is required for ligation-induced activation of phospholipase C gamma. *J. Immunol.* **171**: 3216-3224.

Kim, Y.J. *et al.* (1999). Distinct selectin ligands on colon carcinoma mucins can mediate pathological interactions among platelets, leukocytes, and endothelium. *Am. J. Pathol.* **155**: 461-472.

Laferriere, J. *et al.* (2002). Regulation of the metastatic process by E-selectin and stress-activated protein kinase-2/p38. *Ann. N. Y. Acad. Sci.* **973**: 562-572.

Lebel-Binay, S. *et al.* (2003). IL-18 is produced by prostate cancer cells and secreted in response to interferons. *Int. J. Cancer* **106**: 827-835.

Ley, K. (2003). The role of selectins in inflammation and disease. *Trends Mol. Med.* **9**: 263-268.

Lin, E.Y. and Pollard, J.W. (2004). Role of infiltrated leucocytes in tumour growth and spread. *Br. J. Cancer* **90**: 2053-2058.

Liotta, L.A. and Kohn, E.C. (2001). The microenvironment of the tumour–host interface. *Nature* **411**: 375–379.

Listinsky, J.J. *et al.* (2001). Cell surface fucose ablation as a therapeutic strategy for malignant neoplasms. *Adv. Anat. Pathol.* **8**: 330-337.

Lopez-Ferrer, A. *et al.* (2000). Role of fucosyltransferases in the association between apomucin and Lewis antigen expression in normal and malignant gastric epithelium. *Gut* **47**: 349-356.

Lynch, C.C. and Matrisian, L.M. (2002). Matrix metalloproteinases in tumor-host cell communication. *Differentiation* **70**: 561-573.

Majuri, M.L. *et al.* (1992). Recombinant E-selectin-protein mediates tumor cell adhesion via sialyl-Le(a) and sialyl-Le(x). *Biochem. Biophys. Res. Commun.* **182**: 1376-1382.

Magnani, J.L. (2004). The discovery, biology, and drug development of sialyl Lea and sialyl Lex. *Arch. Biochem. Biophys.* **426**: 122-131.

Mannori, G. *et al.* (1995). Differential colon cancer cell adhesion to E-, P-, and L-selectin: role of mucin-type glycoproteins. *Cancer Res.* **55**: 4425-4431.

Mantovani, A. *et al.* (2004). Tumour-associated macrophages as a prototypic type II polarised phagocyte population: role in tumour progression. *Eur. J. Cancer* **40**: 1660-1667.

Marquardt, T. *et al.* (1999). Correction of leukocyte adhesion deficiency type II with oral fucose. *Blood,* **94**: 3976-3985.

Mathieu, S. *et al.* (2004). Transgene expression of alpha(1,2)-fucosyltransferase-I (FUT1) in tumor cells selectively inhibits sialyl-Lewis x expression and binding to E-selectin without affecting synthesis of sialyl-Lewis a or binding to P-selectin. *Am. J. Pathol.* **164**: 371-383.

Middleton, J. *et al.* (2002). Leukocyte extravasation: chemokine transport and presentation by the endothelium. *Blood* **100**: 3853-3860.

Moloney, D.J. *et al.* (2000). Fringe is a glycosyltransferase that modifies Notch. *Nature* **406**: 369-375.

Mueller, M.M. and Fusenig, N.E. (2002). Tumor-stroma interactions directing phenotype and progression of epithelial skin tumor cells. *Differentiation* **70**: 486-497.

Niittymaki, J. *et al.* (2004). Cloning and expression of murine enzymes involved in the salvage pathway of GDP-L-fucose. *Eur. J. Biochem.* **271**: 78-86.

Noble, R.L. and Hoover, L. (1975). A classification of transplantable tumors in Nb rats controlled by estrogen from dormancy to autonomy. *Cancer Res.* **35**: 2935-2941.

Noda, K. *et al.* (2003). Relationship between elevated FX expression and increased production of GDP-L-fucose, a common donor substrate for fucosylation in human hepatocellular carcinoma and hepatoma cell lines. *Cancer Res.* **63**: 6282-6289.

Nubel, T. *et al.* (2004). Lovastatin inhibits Rho-regulated expression of E-selectin by TNFalpha and attenuates tumor cell adhesion. *FASEB J.* **18**: 140-142.

O, I. *et al.* (2002). Role of SA-Le(a) and E-selectin in metastasis assessed with peptide antagonist. *Peptides* **23**: 999-1010.

Ohyama, C. *et al.* (1998). Molecular cloning and expression of GDP-D-mannose-4,6-dehydratase, a key enzyme for fucose metabolism defective in Lec13 cells. *J. Biol. Chem.* **273**: 14582-14587.

Ohrlein, R. (2001). Carbohydrates and derivatives as potential drug candidates with emphasis on the selectin and linear-B area. *Mini Rev. Med. Chem.* **1**: 349-361.

Paget, S. (1889). The distribution of secondary growth in cancer of the breast, *Lancet* **1**: 571–573.

Park, C.C. *et al.* (2000). The influence of the microenvironment on the malignant phenotype. *Mol. Med. Today* **6**: 324–329.

Ran, M. *et al.* (1992). Possibilities of interference with the immune system of tumor bearers by non-lymphoid Fc gamma RII expressing tumor cells. *Immunobiology* **185**: 415-425.

Renkonen, R. *et al.* (1997). In vitro experimental studies of sialyl Lewis x and sialyl Lewis a on endothelial and carcinoma cells: crucial glycans on selectin ligands. *Glycoconj J.* **14**: 593-600.

Rosen, S.D. (2004). Ligands for L-selectin: homing, inflammation, and beyond. *Annu. Rev. Immunol.* **22**: 129-156.

Roskelley, C.D. and Bissell, M.J. (2002). The dominance of the microenvironment in breast and ovarian cancer. *Semin. Cancer Biol.* **12**: 97-104.

Shirahama, T. *et al.* (1993). The binding site for fucose-binding proteins of Lotus tetragonolobus is a prognostic marker for transitional cell carcinoma of the human urinary bladder. *Cancer* **72**: 1329-1334.

Simon, S.I. *et al.* (1999). Signaling functions of L-selectin in neutrophils: alterations in the cytoskeleton and colocalization with CD18. *J. Immunol.* **163**: 2891-2901.

Smith, P.L. *et al.* (2002). Conditional control of selectin ligand expression and global fucosylation events in mice with a targeted mutation at the FX locus. *J. Cell Biol.* **158**: 801-815.

Sporn, M.B. and Roberts, A.B. (1985). Autocrine growth factors and cancer. *Nature* **313**: 745-747.

Sullivan, F.X. *et al.* (1998). Molecular cloning of human GDP-mannose 4,6-dehydratase and reconstitution of GDP-fucose biosynthesis in vitro. *J. Biol. Chem.* **273**: 8193-8202.

Takada, A. *et al.* (1991). Adhesion of human cancer cells to vascular endothelium mediated by a carbohydrate antigen, sialyl Lewis A. *Biochem. Biophys. Res. Commun.* **179**: 713-719.

Taverna, D. *et al.* (2004). Increased primary tumor growth in mice null for beta3- or beta3/beta5-integrins or selectins. *Proc. Natl. Acad. Sci. U.S.A.* **101**: 763-768.

Thurin, M. and Kieber-Emmons, T. (2002). SA-Lea and tumor metastasis: the old prediction and recent findings. *Hybrid. Hybridomics,* **21**: 111-116.

Uner, A. *et al.* (2004). Serum levels of soluble E-selectin in colorectal cancer, *Neoplasma* **51**: 269-274.

Ushiyama, S. *et al.* (1993). Structural and functional characterization of monomeric soluble P-selectin and comparison with membrane P-selectin. *J. Biol. Chem.* **268**: 15229-15237.

Varki, A. (1994). Selectin ligands. *Proc. Natl Acad. Sci. U.S.A.* **91**: 7390-7397.

Varki, N.M. and Varki, A. (2002). Heparin inhibition of selectin-mediated interactions during the hematogenous phase of carcinoma metastasis: rationale for clinical studies in humans. *Semin. Thromb. Hemost.* **28**: 53-66.

Velikova, G. *et al.* (1998). Serum concentrations of soluble adhesion molecules in patients with colorectal cancer. *Br. J. Cancer* **77**: 1857-1863.

Vestweber, D. (1992). Selectins: cell surface lectins which mediate the binding of leukocytes to endothelial cells. *Semin. Cell Biol.* **3**: 211-220.

Vestweber, D. and Blanks, J.E. (1999). Mechanisms that regulate the function of the selectins and their ligands. *Physiol. Rev.* **79**: 181-213.

Vestweber, D. (2002). Regulation of endothelial cell contacts during leukocyte extravasation. *Curr. Opin. Cell Biol.* **14**: 587-593.

Vincent-Salomon, A. and Thiery, J.P. (2003). Host microenvironment in breast cancer development: epithelial-mesenchymal transition in breast cancer development. *Breast Cancer Res.* **5**: 101-106.

Vlodavsky, I. and Friedmann, Y. (2001). Molecular properties and involvement of heparanase in cancer metastasis and angiogenesis. *J. Clin. Invest.* **108**: 341-347.

Voura, E.B. *et al.* (1998). Cell-cell interactions during transendothelial migration of tumor cells. *Microsc. Res. Tech.* **43**: 265-275.

Weis, W.I. *et al.* (1998). The C-type lectin superfamily in the immune system. *Immunol. Rev.* **163**: 19-34.

Wenzel, C.T. *et al.* (1995). Adhesion of head and neck squamous cell carcinoma to endothelial cells. The missing links. *Arch. Otolaryngol. Head Neck Surg.* **121**: 1279-1286.

Wilson, J. and Balkwill, F. (2002). The role of cytokines in the epithelial cancer microenvironment. *Semin. Cancer Biol.* **12**: 113-120.

Wittig, B.M. *et al.* (1996). Elevated serum E-selectin in patients with liver metastases of colorectal cancer. *Eur. J. Cancer* **32A**: 1215-1218.

Witz, I.P. (1977). Tumor-bound immunoglobulins: in situ expression of humoral immunity. *Adv. Cancer Res.* **25**: 95–148.

Witz, I.P. *et al.* (1996) in *Premalignancy and Tumor Dormancy*, edited by Yefenof, E. and Scheuermann, R.H. (R.G. Landes Company/Springer-Verlag, Heidelberg), 147–160.

Witz, I.P. (2001). Presence and functions of immune components in the tumor microenvironment. *Adv. Exp. Med. Biol.* **495**: 317-324.

Witz, I.P. (2002). The tumour microenvironment-introduction, *Semin. Cancer Biol.* **12**: 87-88.

Yeatman, T.J. and Nicolson, G.L. (1993). Molecular basis of tumor progression: mechanisms of organ-specific tumor metastasis. *Semin. Surg. Oncol.* **9**: 256–263.

Yoshida, M. *et al.* (1998). Phosphorylation of the cytoplasmic domain of E-selectin is regulated during leukocyte-endothelial adhesion. *J. Immunol.* **161**: 933-941.

Zhang, G.J. and Adachi, I. (1999). Serum levels of soluble intercellular adhesion molecule-1 and E-selectin in metastatic breast carcinoma: correlations with clinicopathological features and prognosis. *Int. J. Oncol.* **14**: 71-77.

Zipin, A. *et al.* (2004). Tumor-microenvironment interactions: the fucose-generating FX enzyme controls adhesive properties of colorectal cancer cells. *Cancer Res.* **64**: 6571-6578.

Zusman, T. *et al.* (1996a). The murine Fc-gamma (Fc gamma) receptor type II B1 is a tumorigenicity-enhancing factor in polyoma-virus-transformed 3T3 cells. *Int. J. Cancer* **65**: 221-229.

Zusman, T. *et al.* (1996b). Contribution of the intracellular domain of murine Fc-gamma receptor type IIB1 to its tumor-enhancing potential. *Int. J. Cancer* **68**: 219-227.

Chapter 7

# CD95L/FASL AND TRAIL IN TUMOUR SURVEILLANCE AND CANCER THERAPY

Harald Wajant

*Department of Molecular Internal Medicine, Medical Polyclinic, University of Wuerzburg, Roentgenring 11, 97070 Wuerzburg, Germany*

Abstract: The membrane-bound death ligands CD95L/FasL and TRAIL, which activate the corresponding death receptors CD95/Fas, TRAILR1 and TRAILR2, induce apoptosis in many tumour cells, but can also elicit an inflammatory response. This chapter focuses on the relevance of CD95L/FasL and TRAIL for the tumour surveillance function of natural killer cells and cytotoxic T-cells and discuss current concepts of utilizing these ligands in tumour therapy.


Key words: apoptosis; CD95L; FasL; TRAIL; tumour

# 1.     INTRODUCTION

Several lines of evidence obtained during the last three decades indicated that a network of immune cells responds to tumour cells (Smyth *et al.*, 2002; Dunn *et al.*, 2004). Innate and adaptive immunity have both been implicated in immune surveillance. This is especially evident from gene-targeted mice deficient in the expression of recombinase activating genes RAG1 and RAG2. These mice are unable to rearrange antigen receptors and have therefore neither functional T-cells or B-cells nor NKT-cells and have been shown to develop tumours faster than strain-matched wild-type mice (Shankaran *et al.*, 2001; Smyth *et al.*, 2001b). The most relevant cells in anti-tumour immunity are natural killer (NK) cells and cytotoxic T-cells (CTLs) which can both be directly responsible for killing malignant cells (Figure 1). Noteworthy, these cells do not act independently, but rather in an integrated manner since NK-cells prepare the ground for a subsequent CTL response. NK-cell mediated destruction of tumour cells delivers tumour antigens to dendritic cells. Furthermore, cytokines secreted by activated NK-cells, especially IFNγ, in addition, establish a CTL and helper T-cell activating microenvironment. NK-cell activity is mainly regulated by receptors of the immunoglobulin superfamily (e.g., killer inhibitory factor, KIR) and the C-type lectin family (e.g., lymphocyte antigen 49, Ly49). These receptors receive activating and inhibitory signals from MHC class I or related molecules and still unknown ligands expressed on tumour cells or virus-infected cells (Smyth *et al.*, 2002). By means of their inhibitory receptors, NK-cells sense the normal expression of their cognate MHC class I ligands resulting in the blockage of their effector functions. Thus, inhibition of the expression of MHC class I molecules, which is often the consequence of tumorigenesis or viral infection, helps cells escape an adaptive immune response and leads to NK-cell activation, especially when activating or costimulatory ligands such as CD27L, CD80 or CD86 are available (Smyth *et al.*, 2002). In fact, it has been shown that blockage of the interaction between inhibitory receptors and tumour expressed MHC class I molecules increased the anti-tumoral activity of NK-cells. (Bakker *et al.*, 1998; Smith *et al.*, 1998; Idris *et al.*, 1998, Idris *et al.*, 1999; Koh *et al.*, 2001). Tumour cells expressing sufficient MHC class I molecules to stimulate the inhibitory NK-cell receptors efficiently can also be destroyed by NK-cells when they are triggered via their activating receptors. For example, the NK-cell activating receptor NKG2D is triggered by the MHC class I chain-related molecules A and B (MICA/B), the UL16 binding protein (ULBP), and by lymphocyte effector cell toxicity-activating ligand (Letal) (Cosman *et al.*, 2001, Pende *et al.*, 2002, Conejo-Garcia *et al.*, 2003). Expression of these ligands is very rare in normal tissue but occurs frequently in primary carcinomas of the colon, prostate, ovary, lung, liver and kidney and in melanomas (Groh *et al.*, 1999; Vetter *et al.*, 2002; Pende *et al.*, 2002; Jinushi *et al.*, 2003; Conejo-Garcia *et al.*, 2003) allowing a discrimination of malignantly transformed cells from healthy cells by NK-cells. Although the activating NK-cell receptor ligands are often described as stress-induced, the reasons why their expression is causally linked to cancer and their relevance for tumour biology are poorly understood. NK-cell activation can also be facilitated by stimulating cytokines such as IFNα, interleukin (IL)-2, IL-12, IL-15 (Smyth *et al.*, 2002). NK-cells destroy target cells mainly by three effector systems (Figure 1). Firstly, by expression of the death ligands CD95L/FasL, TRAIL and TNF that may induce apoptosis in target cells by the mechanisms described in detail below. Secondly, by releasing perforin and granzyme containing granules. The importance of the latter effector system for NK-cell-mediated elimination of transformed cells is evident from studies of gene-targeted mice lacking perforin that showed a reduced capacity to inhibit the growth of MHC class I deficient syngenic tumours (van de Broek *et al.*, 1995; van de Broek *et al.*, 1996; Smyth *et al.*, 1999). Thirdly, by production of effector cytokines, especially IFNγ, which among other functions interferes with tumour angiogenesis, stimulates adaptive immunity, e.g., by upregulation of MHC molecules, and sensitizes for death receptor-induced apoptosis. Indeed, several studies have demonstrated that IFNγ deficiency enhanced the development of chemically-induced and spontaneous tumours (Dighe *et al.*, 1994; Kaplan *et al.*, 1998; Shankaran *et al.*, 2001; Street *et al.*, 2001; Street *et al.*, 2002).

Figure 1

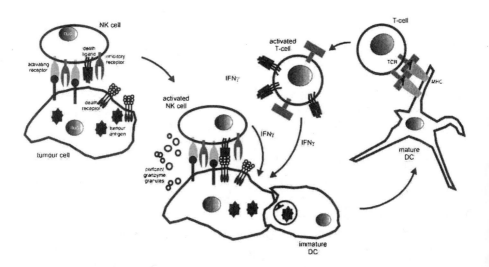

*Figure 1.* Effector functions of NK-cells and CTLs. Tumour-expressed NK-cells activating ligands and/or lack of MHC I class molecule expression on tumour cells activate NK-cells leading, among other things, to perforin/granzyme release, TRAIL upregulation and IFNγ secretion. Apoptotic debris is phagocytosed by dendritic cells allowing activation of tumour-specific CTLs.

## 2.    MECHANISMS OF DEATH RECEPTOR-INDUCED APOPTOSIS

Death receptors form a subgroup of the tumour necrosis factor (TNF) receptor superfamily and are characterized by a protein-protein interaction domain in their cytoplasmic tail called the death domain (Fesik, 2000). By means of their death domain some (CD95, TRAILR1, TRAILR2, TNFR1, DR3), but not all death receptors engage the apoptotic machinery of the cell (Wajant, 2003). This relies on interaction with the death domain-containing adapter protein FADD and the FADD interacting procaspase-8 and is best studied for CD95/Fas. The death receptor CD95/Fas, as other members of the TNFR family, assembles at the cell surface into signalling incompetent complexes (Siegel *et al.*, 2000). CD95/Fas signalling is initiated by binding of CD95L/FasL. Together with the ligands of the other TNFR family members CD95L/FasL forms a family of structurally related trimeric proteins – the TNF ligand family (Locksley *et al.*, 2001). The ligands of this family are normally expressed as type II membrane proteins but soluble variants can be generated by proteolysis or alternative splicing. Trimeric membrane CD95L/FasL interacts with three CD95/Fas molecules which after secondary clustering by yet poorly understood mechanisms become signalling competent and recruit FADD (Chinnaiyan *et al.*, 1995; Boldin *et al.*, 1995). CD95/Fas-bound FADD in turn mediates recruitment of procaspase-8 (Muzio *et al.*, 1996). In the context of the clusters formed by CD95L/FasL, CD95/Fas, FADD and procaspase-8, the latter assembles in enzymatically active dimers, which subsequently undergo autoproteolytical processing in two steps (Donepudi *et al.*, 2003: Boatright *et al.*; 2003), (Figure 2). First, the C-terminal p12 subunit of the caspase homology domain is cleaved off the FADD-bound procaspase-8 molecules, but remains in the complex by non-covalent interaction with the remaining p43/41 fragment of caspase-8. In the second cleavage step, the caspase-8 p43/41 fragment is cleaved between the prodomain, which interacts with CD95/Fas-bound FADD, and the p20 subunit of the caspase homology domain. As a consequence, the mature caspase-8 heterotetramer ($p20_2p12_2$) is formed and released from the CD95/Fas signalling complex. Then the CD95/Fas-bound prodomain of FADD can be replaced by a novel procaspase-8 molecule and a new cycle of caspase-8 activation and processing can begin. Thus, the CD95L/FasL-CD95/Fas-FADD-caspase-8 clusters act as a caspase-8 converting complex, which has been named death-inducing signalling complex (DISC; Kischkel *et al.*, 1995). Several lines of evidence suggest that TRAILR1 and TRAILR2 activate procaspase-8 in a similar manner by forming a corresponding TRAILR1 and TRAILR2 DISC (Kischkel *et al.*, 2000; Sprick *et al.*, 2000; Bodmer *et al.* 2000). TNFR1-induced apoptosis is also mediated by caspase-8 and FADD, but in this case, no TNFR1 DISC is formed (Harper *et al.*, 2003). Instead stimulation of TNFR1 triggers, by yet poorly defined mechanisms, the formation of a cytoplasmic complex containing FADD and procaspase-8 and, in addition, TRAF2, RIP and TRADD (Micheau and Tschopp, 2003). While TRAF2 and RIP have been implicated in non-apoptotic TNFR1 signalling and are dispensable for apoptosis induction, TRADD seems to play a crucial role in TNFR1-mediated activation of the FADD-procaspase-8 axis (Hsu *et al.*, 1995). Due to its high degree of homology to TNFR1, the death receptor DR3 most likely signals apoptosis via the cytoplasmic FADD-procaspase-8 complex, too. The crucial role of FADD and caspase-8 for death receptor induced apoptosis is especially evident in FADD or caspase-8 deficient cells, which are fully resistant to death receptor-induced apoptosis (Juo *et al.*, 1998;

1999; Zhang *et al.*, 1998; Yeh *et al.*, 1998, Varfolomeev *et al.*, 1998; Kuang *et al.*, 2000). Mature active caspase-8 heterotetramers that are released from the DISC or the TNFR1-induced cytoplasmic FADD-caspase-8 complexes can cleave a narrow range of substrates, especially effector caspases such as caspase-3 and caspase-7, which become activated in this way. Active caspase-3 and caspase-7 in turn cleave a growing number of cellular proteins and thereby orchestrate the execution phase of apoptosis. In some cells death receptor-induced caspase-8 activation is too weak to activate directly effector caspases to an extent sufficient for robust apoptosis induction. In such cells, called type II cells, death receptor-induced apoptosis, in addition, depends on caspase-8 mediated cleavage of BID (Peter and Krammer, 2003). This pro-apoptotic protein belongs to the Bcl2 family as it contains a Bcl2 homology-3 domain (Cory *et al.*, 2003). Cleavage of BID results in a truncated fragment (tBID) which translocates to mitochodria where it triggers a conformational change in BAX and BAK (Cory *et al.*, 2003). As a consequence these proteins form pores in the outer membrane of the mitochondria allowing the release of a variety of apoptogenic proteins from the mitochondrial intermembrane space, such as apoptosis-inducing factor (AIF), endonuclease G, cytochrome c, second mitochondria-derived activator of caspase/direct IAP-binding protein with low pI (SMAC/Diablo), and high-temperature requirement protein A2 (HtrA2/OMI) (Saelens *et al.*, 2004). Especially the latter three proteins enforce caspase-3 activation and therefore enhance indirectly caspase-3 activation via caspase-8. SMAC/Diablo and HtrA2/OMI facilitate caspase-3 activation by depletion and degradation of the inhibitor of apoptosis proteins that block effector caspases (Vaux and Silke, 2003). Cytosolic cytochrome c together with ATP, Apaf1 and caspase-9 forms a complex, called the apoptosome, in which caspase-9 becomes active and is therefore able to cleave and activate caspase-3 (Shi 2002). In type II cells the mitochondrial branch of apoptotic events measurably contributes to death receptor-induced apoptosis. In such cells overexpression of Bcl2 or Bcl-XL therefore delays and attenuates CD95/Fas-induced apoptosis. *Vice versa*, cells are called type I cells when the direct caspase-8 mediated activation of effector caspases is so rapid and robust that Bcl2 overexpression has no effect (Peter and Krammer, 2003).

Figure 2

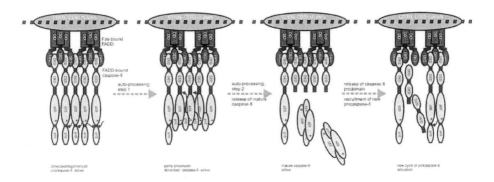

*Figure 2.* Mechanisms of CD95L-induced caspase-8 activation. Interaction of membrane CD95L/FasL and CD95/Fas leads to the formation of supramolecular clusters of CD95L/FasL and CD95/Fas. These clusters bind FADD, which in turn mediates recruitment of several pro-caspase 8 molecules into CD95L/CD95 signalling aggregates. In the environment of this death-inducing signaling complex (DISC), pro-caspase-8 becomes activated by dimerization and subsequently undergoes maturation to its heterotetrameric active form in two-steps by trans-autoprocessing.

## 3. TRAIL AND CD95L/FASL IN TUMOUR SURVEILLANCE

TRAIL is expressed on NK-cells after stimulation with IL-2, IL-12, IL-15 or interferons and contributes to NK-cell induced apoptosis *in vitro* (Zamai *et al.*, 1998; Kayagaki *et al.*, 1999; Smyth *et al.*, 2001a). While freshly isolated liver NK-cells express constitutively low levels of TRAIL on the cell surface, NK-cells from spleen, lung or blood exert no significant TRAIL expression without stimulation (Smyth *et al.*, 2001a). The constitutive expression of TRAIL in liver NK-cells seems to be at least partly caused by IFNγ production of the liver NK-cells themselves for the following reasons: Firstly, liver NK-cells isolated from gene targeted mice deficient in the expression of IFNγ or the IFNγ receptor display no TRAIL expression. Secondly, IFNγ rapidly induces TRAIL in liver NK-cells of IFNγ deficient mice. Thirdly, a significant portion of liver NK-cells, but not of spleen NK-cells, produces IFNγ (Smyth *et al.*, 2001a). Protection against death receptor-induced apoptosis promotes metastasis (Djerbi *et al.* 1999; Medema *et al.*, 1999; Lee *et al.*, 2000; Schroter *et al.*, 2000) and NK-cells have implicated in the control of metastasis (Talmadge *et al.*, 1980; Kärre *et al.*, 1986). This points to the possibility that NK-cell-expressed death ligands, especially TRAIL, contribute to surveillance of metastasis. In agreement with this idea, NK-cell depletion and neutralizing TRAIL and CD95L/FasL specific antibodies enhance liver metastasis of L929, CB27.4 and Renca cells. Especially TRAIL neutralization had no effect in NK depleted mice (Takeda *et al.*, 2001). Perforin deficiency also lead to an increase in liver metastasis, which was further enhanced by TRAIL-blocking antibodies, suggesting that TRAIL and perforin act independently of each other (Takeda *et al.*, 2001). IL-12 and α-galactosylceramide induce IFNγ production and stimulate cytotoxic NK-cell action (Gately *et al.*, 1994; Kawamura *et al.*, 1998; Burdin *et al.* 1998; Eberl *et al.*, 2000). In some mouse models these reagents show strong anti-metastatic activity, which relies on NK-cells and the NK effector molecules IFNγ, perforin and TRAIL. Again, the TRAIL-dependent, but not the perforin-dependent anti-metastatic effect was abrogated in IFNγ-deficient mice suggesting a model, in which IL-12 or α-galactosylceramide induce IFNγ in NK-cells, which in turn upregulates TRAIL. The latter acts then in concert with the perforin/granzyme system to suppress metastasis (Smyth *et al.*, 2001a). Remarkably, the relative contribution of perforin and TRAIL to the anti-metastatic effect of NK-cells is dependent on the organ investigated (Smyth *et al.*, 2001a).

Recent studies have implicated TRAIL also in host surveillance against primary tumour development. In a model where development of primary sarcoma was induced by the carcinogen methylcholanthrene (MCA), TRAIL-neutralizing antibodies accelerated the onset of fibrosarcoma development (Takeda *et al.*, 2002). In particular, tumour cell lines derived from mice that had been treated with TRAIL-specific antibodies, were more sensitive to TRAIL stimulation than corresponding cell lines derived from Ig-treated mice suggesting that TRAIL-sensitive tumour cells were eliminated *in vivo* (Takeda *et al.*, 2002). The outgrowth of subcutaneously inoculated TRAIL-sensitive fibrosarcoma cell lines was enhanced by anti-TRAIL treatment whereas TRAIL resistant cell lines remained unaffected by this regime. Moreover, MCA-cell lines established from mice, in which NK-cells has been depleted by anti-ASGM1, are often more sensitive to TRAIL-induced apoptosis than similar cells derived from control mice, arguing for a role for NK-cell expressed TRAIL in inhibition of MCA-induced tumours (Takeda *et al.*, 2002). It is noteworthy that in the cited study, depletion of NK-cells did not abrogate the tumour-promoting effect of anti-TRAIL antibody administration indicating a tumour-suppressive, NK-cell independent source of TRAIL (Takedea *et al.*, 2002). The inhibitory effect of TRAIL on the development of primary tumours is also evident from mice with a defective p53 allele. Anti-TRAIL treatment of such $p53^{+/-}$ mice resulted in earlier and more aggressive development of spontaneous tumours (Takeda *et al.*, 2002). Cell lines derived from the anti-TRAIL-treated mice were again more sensitive to TRAIL, whereas TRAIL showed no proapoptotic effect on cell lines established from Ig-treated mice. The natural tumour inhibitory potential of TRAIL is also reflected by its importance in graft versus tumour (GVT) activity of allogeneic T-cells in allogeneic hematopoietic cell transplantation. GVT activity relies on the recognition of allo- and tumour-antigens and is therefore inevitably accompanied by graft versus host disease (GVDH). Remarkably, it has been found in different models of bone marrow transplantation that TRAIL is more relevant for GVT than for GVHD, while, *vice versa*, CD95L/FasL seemed to be more important in GVT than in GVHD. Perforin, finally, contributes to both GVT and GVHD. The different importance of TRAIL and CD95L/FasL for GVT and GVHD could prompt novel strategies in allogeneic hematopoietic cell transplantation in which harmful CD95/Fas activation is blocked and TRAIL activity is pushed (Schmaltz *et al.*, 2002).

Although TRAIL seems to be more relevant than CD95L/FasL to tumour surveillance, a crucial role of the latter has been deduced form several lines of experimental evidence. Lpr and gld mice, which have severe genetic defects in CD95/Fas and CD95L/FasL, respectively, develop plasmacytoid tumours at older age. Furthermore, cross-breading of lpr or gld mice with mice that are predisposed to tumours such as E mu L-MYC transgenic mice, leads to offspring that has a significantly increase in tumour incidence (Zornig *et al.*, 1995; Peng *et al.*, 1996; Traver *et al.*, 1998; Davidson *et al.*, 1998). In gld mice, melanoma metastasis was found to be enhanced (Owen-Schaub *et al.*, 1998; Owen-Schaub *et al.*, 2000). The anti-tumoral effect of IL-12, which has been reported in some murine models, relies in part on CD95/Fas signalling, too (Wigginton *et al.*, 2001 and 2002).

## 4.     CD95L/FASL AND THE TUMOUR COUNTERATTACK

Death receptor-, in particular CD95/Fas-induced apoptosis, is not only used by the immune system to suppress metastasis and primary tumour development, but it can also be utilized by tumours to escape immune responses by expressing CD95L/FasL and inducing apoptosis in infiltrating immune cells. In agreement with this concept, named tumour counterattack, apoptosis of tumour infiltrating lymphocytes has been shown in CD95L/FasL-expressing tumours. Moreover, some CD95/Fas-resistant tumours express CD95L/FasL and are able to kill CD95/Fas sensitive cells (O'Connell *et al.*, 1996; Hahne *et al.*, 1996; Strand *et al.*, 1996; Niehans *et al.*, 1997; Villunger *et al.*, 1997; Bennett *et al.*, 1998). Furthermore, better growth of some CD95L/FasL expressing tumours compared to their corresponding CD95L/FasL deficient counterparts has been found in wild type mice, whereas in lpr mice, no effect or even a reduction was observed (Hahne *et al.*, 1996; Arai *et al.*, 1997; Nishimatsu *et al.*, 1999). Interestingly, the opposite effect of CD95L/FasL expression, namely accelerated rapid destruction of CD95L/FasL positive grafts and tumours, has also been found in several cases (Yagita *et al.*, 1996; Seino *et al.*, 1997; Okamoto *et al.*, 1999; Shimizu *et al.*, 1999; Behrens *et al.*, 2001). Thus, secondary, yet poorly characterized events have to determine the *in vivo* effects of CD95L/FasL expression on tumours. CD95L/FasL expression can drive the destruction of CD95/Fas-resistant tumour cells *in vivo* and infiltrating neutrophils have been regularly observed in CD95L/FasL positive tumours (Yagita *et al.*, 1996; Seino *et al.*, 1997; Okamoto *et al.*, 1999; Shimizu *et al.*, 1999; Behrens *et al.*, 2001). Thus, it is unlikely that the anti-tumoral effect of CD95L/FasL expression is due to apoptosis induction in the tumour cells. Instead, destruction by neutrophils seems possible. In accordance with such a role for neutrophils in CD95L/FasL-dependent tumour suppression, the development of CD95L/FasL-expressing tumour cells was increased in gene-targeted mice deficient for the neutrophil chemoattractant MIP1 (Simon *et al.*, 2002). The early events by which CD95L/FasL triggers neutrophil recruitment are complex and poorly understood. While some early *in vitro* studies demonstrated direct chemotactic action of soluble CD95L/FasL for neutrophils (Seino *et al.*, 1998; Ottonello *et al.*, 1999), other studies failed to confirm this result *in vivo* and instead reported that a non-cleavable deletion mutant of membrane CD95L/FasL is sufficient to induce neutrophil recruitment (Shudo *et al.*, 2001; Hohlbaum *et al.*, 2000; Kang *et al.*, 2000; Simon *et al.*, 2002). Especially tumours only expressing soluble CD95L/ FasL failed to mount a neutrophilic response. Thus, direct chemotactic action of CD95L/FasL seems to be secondary or even irrelevant to CD95L/FasL-induced neutrophil recruitment *in vivo*. An obvious explanation for the CD95L/FasL-induced neutrophil attraction is that CD95L/FasL expressed on tumour cells induces chemoattractant proteins in the surrounding cells. Indeed, it has been found that CD95L/FasL can induce IL-8 and other chemokines in peritoneal macrophages, fibroblasts and various cell lines (Miwa *et al.*, 1998). Moreover, several studies have shown *in vitro* that TRAIL induces chemokines, too (Wajant 2004). This death ligand could therefore have CD95L/FasL-related proinflammatory effects *in vivo*. The tumour suppressive effect of CD95L/FasL and TRAIL is not only due to induction of apoptosis in sensitive cells by CD95L/FasL and/or TRAIL bearing NK- and T-cells, but seems to rely also on secondary local immune responses triggered by non-apoptotic CD95/Fas and TRAIL receptor signalling in tumour or tumour-associated cells. Thus, the proinflammatory potential of CD95L/FasL and TRAIL, which is independent of apoptosis, could restrict the deleterious effect of CD95L/FasL in the tumour counterattack.

## 5.     ANTI-TUMORAL POTENTIAL OF RECOMBINANT CD95L/FASL VARIANTS AND AGONISTIC CD95/FAS ANTIBODIES

*In vivo*, CD95L/FasL occurs as a transmembrane protein (membrane CD95L/FasL) and in a soluble form which is derived from membrane CD95L/FasL by proteolytic processing or, in mice, in addition by alternative splicing. While membrane CD95L/FasL induces CD95/Fas signalling, soluble CD95L/FasL does normally not activate CD95/Fas and can even act as competitive inhibitor of membrane CD95L/FasL (Suda *et al.*, 1997; Schneider *et al.*, 1998). Remarkably, soluble CD95L/FasL trimers can be converted into active ligands by immobilization on the extracellular matrix or by secondary crosslinking (Schneider *et al.*, 1998; Aoki *et al.*, 2001). For example, aggregates of recombinant soluble Flag-tagged CD95L/FasL trimers crosslinked by anti-Flag antibodies or a hexameric fusion protein of CD95L/FasL are able to activate CD95/Fas (Schneider *et al.*, 1998; Holler *et al.*, 2003). The requirement of crosslinking reflects most likely a need for secondary aggregation of trimeric CD95L/FasL-CD95/Fas (CD95L/FasL$_3$-CD95/Fas$_3$) complexes into supramolecular clusters to gain signalling competence. In accordance with this idea, it has been noted that agonistic CD95/Fas-specific antibodies belong to the multimeric IgM or IgG3 subclass (Kischkel *et al.*, 1995). Moreover, non-agonistic CD95/Fas antibodies, e.g., of the IgG2b subtype, can act as potent CD95/Fas agonists after crosslinking with protein A (Kischkel *et al.*, 1995; Huang *et al.*, 1999).

Activation of CD95/Fas in the liver leads to deadly liver damage. Systemic activation of CD95/Fas, e.g., with crosslinked soluble CD95L/FasL, is therefore certainly no option for tumour therapy. Instead, tumour treatment concepts that allow selective activation of CD95/Fas are necessary to make this death receptor a useful target. One development in this direction is based on the unexpected observation that agonistic anti-

CD95/Fas antibodies differ in the quality of CD95/Fas activation. While the hamster anti-mouse CD95/Fas monoclonal antibody Jo2 kills cultured primary hepatocytes and thymocytes, the hamster anti-mouse CD95/Fas mAb RK8 only triggers apoptosis in the latter cells (Nishimura *et al.*, 1997a). The qualitatively different bioactivities of Jo2 and RK8 are also evident *in vivo*. While systemic treatment with Jo2 leads to rapid liver failure (Ogasawara *et al.*, 1993), treatment with RK8 has no toxic effects on the liver, but induces thymocyte apoptosis and thymic atrophy with comparable efficiency as Jo2 (Nishimura *et al.*, 1997 a and b). The different quality of Jo2 and RK8 becomes particular obvious when gld mice are treated with these antibodies. Jo2 kills the mice due to its toxic effects on the liver whereas RK8 inhibits the lymphoadenopathy and splenomegaly of gld mice as the consequence of a defect in the CD95L/FasL gene (Nishimura *et al.*, 1997 a and b). Gene-targeted mice deficient in Bid or in Bax and Bak are less sensitive to CD95/Fas-mediated liver damage than wild-type mice indicating a contribution of mitochondria-associated apoptogenic proteins to CD95/Fas-mediated apoptosis (for a review see Cory *et al.*, 2003). Hepatocytes have therefore been classified as type II cells. Thymocytes from wild-type, Bid-deficient and Bak/Bax double deficient mice, on the other hand are equally sensitive and are therefore type I cells. It is tempting to speculate that, for unknown reasons, RK8 is able to trigger CD95/Fas on type I cells, but fails to activate this receptor on type II cells, whereas Jo2 stimulates CD95/Fas on both type I and type II cells. To obtain anti-human CD95/Fas antibodies with a similar cell type restricted activity as RK8, CD95/Fas deficient mice have been immunized with human CD95/Fas (Ichikawa *et al.*, 2000). Indeed, one antibody recognizing CD95/Fas from various species including men and mice has been isolated this way and named HEF7A. This antibody exerted no hepatotoxicity in mice, marmosets and crab-eating monkey but significantly attenuated the phenotype of gld mice. However, broader studies concerning safety and therapeutic potential are still necessary (Ichikawa *et al.*, 2000).

The latent CD95/Fas-stimulating capability of soluble CD95L/FasL, which becomes apparent after secondary crosslinking, indicates that soluble CD95L/FasL bears, in principle, all structural information necessary for CD95/Fas activation. This is also in agreement with the observation that soluble CD95L/FasL, bound to the extracellular matrix, is bioactive (Aoki *et al.*, 2001). It has therefore been speculated, that artificial immobilization of soluble CD95L/FasL on the cell surface of tumour cells restrict CD95/Fas activation to these tumour cells or to cells adjacent to the targeted cells. This idea was experimentally proven using a trimeric fusion protein of soluble CD95L/FasL and a N-terminal single-chain antibody domain recognizing the fibroblast activation protein (FAP) (Samel *et al.*, 2003). FAP is a transmembrane protein normally only expressed during embryonal development and wound healing, but is also abundantly expressed on activated fibroblasts that surround a variety of solid tumours (Scanlan *et al.*, 1994). The scFAP-CD95L/FasL fusion protein was as inactive as soluble CD95L/FasL on FAP-negative cells. However, on FAP expressing cells it was as active, or even more so, as crosslinked sCD95L/FasL. Using FAP-specific antibodies that block the scFAP-FAP interaction, a crucial role for FAP-binding in the activation of CD95/Fas by scFAP-CD95L/FasL (Samel *et al.*, 2003) was demonstrated. The scFAP-CD95L/FasL fusion protein showed no toxic effects in mice, even after administration of 100 µg per mouse, but it interfered with the development of FAP expressing, xenotransplants (Samel *et al.*, 2003). Further studies will show whether the principle of cell surface immobilization-mediated activation of soluble CD95L/FasL fusion proteins (Figure 3) can be widely used to develop CD95L/FasL variants with no or reduced side effects. Higher activity of single chain fusion proteins containing TNF and TRAIL as effector domains on cells expressing the appropriate cell surface antigen have also been demonstrated (Wajant *et al.*, 2001; Wuest *et al.*, 2002). TNF and TRAIL interact with two (TNFR1, TNFR2), respectively three (TRAILR1, TRAILR2, TRAILR4), distinct transmembrane receptors that have different activation requirements with respect to the nature of their ligand. While soluble TNF predominantly activates TNFR1, its corresponding transmembrane form also stimulates TNFR2 (Grell *et al.*, 1995). Likewise, membrane TRAIL activates TRAILR1 and TRAILR2 whereas soluble TRAIL acts mainly via TRAILR1 (Wajant *et al.*, 2001). The activation requirements of TRAILR4 are unknown. Thus, the cell surface antigen dependent activities of the TNF and TRAIL fusion proteins rely on activation of TNFR2 and TRAILR2 and are therefore highly dependent on the expression patterns of the corresponding receptors. It is noteworthy that cell surface immobilization also enables bispecific antibodies containing a non-agonistic CD95/Fas-specific antibody fragment to activate CD95/Fas (Jung *et al.*, 2001).

Figure 3

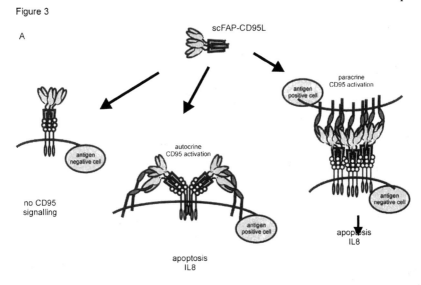

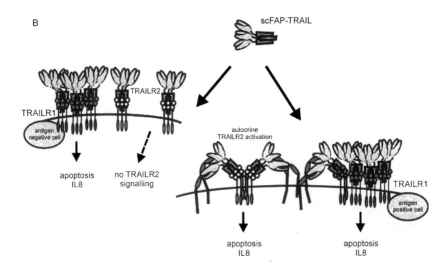

*Figure 3*. Cell surface antigen dependent activation of CD95/Fas. Fusion proteins of the extracellular receptor-binding domain of CD95L/FasL and a single chain antibody fragment recognizing a cell surface antigen convert to an entity with membrane CD95L/FasL-like activity after antigen binding (A). Similarly, in contrast to soluble TRAIL, predominantly stimulating TRAILR1, a corresponding single chain fusion protein of TRAIL, in addition, activates TRAILR2, gaining membrane TRAIL activity (B).

## 6. ANTI-TUMORAL POTENTIAL OF RECOMBINANT TRAIL VARIANTS AND AGONISTIC TRAIL RECEPTOR ANTIBODIES

Although one or both TRAIL death receptors are expressed in most tissue, administration of recombinant soluble TRAIL variants showed no toxic effects in mice, cynomolgus monkey, and chimpanzees (Ashkenazi *et al.*, 1999; Walczak *et al.*, 1999). Moreover, with very few exceptions, primary human cells were TRAIL insensitive. In contrast, many tumour cells were TRAIL sensitive or become so after treatment with chemotherapeutic drugs. It appeared therefore that in most normal cells, TRAIL-induced apoptosis is prevented by yet only poorly understood mechanisms that, for unknown reasons, are less active in tumour cells. However, this promising "tumour"-selective action was seen with soluble recombinant TRAIL variants that homogenously form trimers and these results were challenged when secondary aggregated complexes of soluble TRAIL trimers were used. For example, in contrast to soluble TRAIL trimers, bacterial produced His-tagged soluble TRAIL, which forms higher aggregates, strongly induces apoptosis in hepatocytes (Jo *et al.*, 2000; Lawrence *et al.*, 2001). Moreover, liver toxicity has been observed with membrane TRAIL encoding adenoviral vectors (see below for details). Likewise, primary cultures of normal prostate epithelial cells and keratinocytes are resistant against soluble TRAIL but are killed by membrane TRAIL (Voelkel-Johnson *et al.*, 2002) or aggregated TRAIL (Jo *et al.*, 2000). It has been speculated that aggregated preparations of trimeric soluble TRAIL or antibody-crosslinked TRAIL trimers, but not soluble TRAIL trimers, over-multimerize the TRAIL death receptors leading to the generation of apoptotic signals surpassing the apoptotic threshold of normal cells (Almasan and Ashkenazi, 2003). In this regard, the obvious question arises whether such an over-multimerization of TRAILR1 and/or TRAILR2 reflects a non-natural artificial capability of aggregated soluble TRAIL to activate TRAIL receptors or whether this is due to reduced limited activity of recombinant soluble TRAIL compared to the naturally occurring membrane TRAIL. In fact, as already discussed above, it has been shown for some other ligands of the TNF family (e.g., TNF, CD95L/FasL, CD40L) that the membrane-bound form is more active as the corresponding soluble trimer. A similar differential activity of soluble trimeric TRAIL, on the one hand, and membrane TRAIL, or aggregated trimers of soluble TRAIL, on the other hand, in the activation of TRAILR1 and TRAILR2 has recently been described (Wajant *et al.*, 2001). Thus, the severe toxic effects of aggregated TRAIL preparations on normal cells, such as hepatocytes, could therefore be mainly caused by TRAILR2 activation and have no significance upon predominant activation of TRAILR1 with "safe" trimeric preparations of recombinant soluble TRAIL. If this scenario is correct, trimeric TRAIL may be a promising treatment for TRAILR1 sensitive cancers, but would fail to have a significant effect on tumours that predominantly signal via TRAILR2. Superior activity of cross-linked soluble TRAIL has been observed in several tumour cell lines (Gong and Almasan 2000; Chen *et al.*, 2001; Muhlenbeck *et al.*, 1999; Leverkus *et al.*, 2003). It therefore seems possible that TRAIL variants activating both TRAIL death receptors could be used for the treatment of a broader range of tumours. However, the use of reagents systemically activating TRAILR1 and TRAILR2 is most likely limited by severe side effects. Thus, similar to CD95L/FasL, the development of strategies that ensure local action of such reagents is necessary. Cell surface antigen-dependent activation of trimeric soluble ligand fusion proteins, as discussed above for CD95L/FasL, could be a possibility. Indeed, two independent studies have already shown that trimeric single chain-TRAIL fusion proteins activate TRAILR2 mainly after binding to the corresponding cell surface antigen while TRAILR1 signalling is triggered by theses fusion proteins independent of their interaction with the antigen (Wajant *et al.*, 2001; Bremer *et al.*, 2004). Cell surface immobilization of TRAIL fusion proteins may also partly compensate for the poor pharmacokinetic properties of soluble TRAIL (Walczak *et al.*, 1999; Kelley *et al.*, 2001). The avoidance of systemic toxicity, which is required for a potential use of aggregated TRAIL variants and membrane TRAIL, could also be of considerable relevance to *per se* safe trimeric TRAIL preparations in situations of co-treatment with chemotherapeutic drugs. In fact, TRAIL, especially trimeric TRAIL, alone has often only minor apoptotic effects on tumour cells and requires their prior sensitization with chemotherapeutic drugs. However, experiments with primary keratinocytes have shown that such treatments can also reduce the TRAIL resistance of normal cells (Leverkus *et al.*, 2003). In this regard the systemic toxicity of trimeric TRAIL variants in combination with chemotherapeutic drugs has, as yet, been only poorly addressed and needs urgent verification.

Only some initial studies using agonistic TRAILR1- or TRAILR2-specific monoclonal antibodies have been published, yet. Strong anti-tumoral activities were described with anti-human TRAILR1 and anti-human TRAILR2 mAbs in nude mice or SCID mice with human xenografts (Chuntharapai *et al.*, 2001; Ichikawa *et al.*, 2001). Naturally, these initial studies cannot answer the question for systemic side effects of these antibodies as murine DR5, the homologue of human TRAILR2, was not activated. Intererstingly, the TRAILR2-specific agonistic antibody used in one of these studies induces apoptosis in xenografts but does not kill human liver cells (Ichikawa *et al.*, 2001). At first glance, this is at variance with the concept of TRAILR2-mediated toxic effects in normal cells discussed above. However, it has to be taken into consideration that agonistic receptor antibodies have not necessarily the same signalling capacity as the natural, membrane-bound ligand or its crosslinked soluble counterpart. In fact, agonistic antibodies may not only differentially act on type I and type II cells as discussed above for the anti-CD95/Fas mAbs Jo2 and RK8, but can also show further enhancement of their activity by protein A crosslinking when they are already active on type II cells. The functional importance of *in vivo* crosslinking of TRAIL receptor-specific antibodies became also evident in a recent study with a hamster-derived anti-mouse DR5 antibody. This antibody requires crosslinking by Fc-receptors expressed on macrophages or dendritic cells to acquire agonistic activity *in vivo*, but then gains the capability to suppress metastasis (Takeda *et al.*, 2004). Remarkably, no toxic side effects after systemic administration were observed using this antibody.

# 7.    CD95L/FASL AND TRAIL IN GENE THERAPY

Intravenous injection of adenoviruses carrying a CMV promoter driven CD95L/FasL gene results in hepatocyte apoptosis and liver failure (Ichikawa *et al.*, 2001), the hallmark of systemic CD95/Fas activation. Thus, not unexpectedly, a major requirement for CD95L/FasL based gene therapy strategies is the avoidance of CD95/Fas-mediated systemic toxicity. In some cases, localized activation of CD95/Fas should be possible by physical barriers preventing distribution of CD95L/FasL throughout the body. An example for such a therapeutic strategy is the treatment of rheumatoid arthritis with membrane CD95L/FasL-encoding adenoviral constructs. The inflammatory cells and tissue in arthritic joints are "encapsulated" in a cavity allowing localized adenovirus-mediated CD95L/FasL-gene transfer into inflamed joints. In a collagen-induced murine arthritis model, adenovirus driven CD95L/FasL expression reduced disease by triggering apoptosis in synovial fibroblasts without having systemic side effects (Zhang *et al.*, 1997; Guery *et al.*, 2000; Kim *et al.*, 2002). A more general strategy to circumvent systemic CD95L/FasL toxicity in gene therapy is the use of replication-defective adenovirus with inducible tissue-specific promoters. Indeed, lack of liver damage and localized CD95/Fas activation have been demonstrated in mouse models using adenoviral vectors expressing membrane CD95L/FasL under the control of neuronal-, astrocyte- or smooth muscle cell-specific promoters (Morelli *et al.*, 1999; Ambar *et al.*, 1999; Aoki *et al.*, 2000). Regulated adenoviral expression of membrane CD95L/FasL gene has been demonstrated *in vitro* also with a tetracyclin-regulated promoter (Hyer *et al.*, 2000; Rubinchik *et al.*, 2000 and 2001). However, it remains to be seen whether, *in vivo*, a localized induction of CD95L/FasL can be achieved by this method.

Potent anti-tumoral activity after adenoviral gene transfer of TRAIL, which even overcame impaired responses against aggregated and non-aggregated soluble TRAIL in some reports, has been described in several studies. However, as mentioned above, adenoviral encoded membrane TRAIL, in contrast to soluble trimeric TRAIL, induces severe apoptosis in primary human hepatocytes (Armeanu *et al.*, 2003). Adenovirus infection elicits an immune response in the liver. Although adenoviral transduction does not sensitize hepatocytes to soluble TRAIL (Armeanu *et al.*, 2003), it is still possible that adenoviral infection primes hepatocytes to membrane TRAIL-induced apoptosis. However, the hepatotoxicity of adenoviral-encoded membrane TRAIL could also reflect the higher activity of membrane TRAIL as compared to soluble TRAIL. Administration of adenovector-encoded membrane TRAIL must be therefore either locally restricted or controlled at the transcriptional level to limit its action to tumour tissue. Indeed, both concepts have already been experimentally demonstrated in animal models. For example, the intralesional administration of adenoviral TRAIL suppressed the development of human prostate and breast tumour xenografts in SCID mice and in a rabbit model of arthritis, intra-articular-delivered adenoviral TRAIL induced apoptosis in cells of the activated synovium and reduced infiltration of immune cells (Griffith and Broghammer, 2001; Lin *et al.*, 2002; Yao *et al.*, 2003). Furthermore, aerosolized administration of an adenovector expressing a fusion protein of GFP and TRAIL has been successfully used to suppress metastatic nodules derived from breast cancer cells (Lin *et al.*, 2003). As in this study, TRAIL expression was controlled not only by the way of administration, but also by using the human telomerase reverse transcriptase promoter, the safety of this route of delivery for vectors constitutively expressing TRAIL remains to be demonstrated. For an oncolytic TRAIL-encoding adenovirus, efficient intratumoral spread and metastases suppression have been demonstrated in a colon cancer model after tail vein infusion (Sova *et al.*, 2004).

In recent years much progress has been made in the development of concepts for the use of TRAIL and CD95L/FasL in tumour therapy. Now, the future must show whether some of those can make it to the clinic.

# 8.     REFERENCES

Ambar, B.B. *et al.* (1999). Treatment of experimental glioma by administration of adenoviral vectors expressing Fas ligand. *Hum. Gene Ther.* **10**: 1641-1648.

Almasan, A. and Ashkenazi, A. (2003). Apo2L/TRAIL: apoptosis signaling, biology, and potential for cancer therapy. *Cytokine Growth Factor Rev.* **14**: 337-48.

Aoki, K. *et al.* (2000). Restricted expression of an adenoviral vector encoding Fas ligand (CD95L) enhances safety for cancer gene therapy. *Mol. Ther.* **1**: 555-565.

Aoki, K. *et al.* (2001). Extracellular matrix interacts with soluble CD95L: retention and enhancement of cytotoxicity. *Nat. Immunol.* **2**: 333-337.

Arai H. *et al.* (1997). Inhibition of the alloantibody response by CD95 ligand. *Nat. Med.* **3**: 843-848.

Armeanu, S. *et al.* (2003). Adenoviral gene transfer of tumor necrosis factor-related apoptosis-inducing ligand overcomes an impaired response of hepatoma cells but causes severe apoptosis in primary human hepatocytes. *Cancer Res.* **63**: 2369-2372.

Ashkenazi, A. *et al.* (1999). Safety and antitumor activity of recombinant soluble Apo2 ligand. *J. Clin. Invest.* **104**: 155-162.

Bakker, A.B. *et al.* (1998). Killer cell inhibitory receptors for MHC class I molecules regulate lysis of melanoma cells mediated by NK cells, gamma delta T cells, and antigen-specific CTL. *J. Immunol.* **160**: 5239-5245.

Behrens, C.K. *et al.* (2001). CD95 ligand-expressing tumors are rejected in anti-tumor TCR transgenic perforin knockout mice. *J. Immunol.* **166**: 3240-3247.

Bennett, M.W. *et al.* (1998). The Fas counterattack *in vivo*: apoptotic depletion of tumor-infiltrating lymphocytes associated with Fas ligand expression by human esophageal carcinoma. J. Immunol. **160**: 5669-5675.

Boatright, K.M. *et al.* (2003). A unified model for apical caspase activation. *Mol. Cell.* **11**: 529-541.

Bodmer, J.L. *et al.* (2000). TRAIL receptor-2 signals apoptosis through FADD and caspase-8. *Nat. Cell Biol.* **2**: 241-243.

Boldin, M.P. *et al.* (1995). A novel protein that interacts with the death domain of Fas/APO1 contains a sequence motif related to the death domain. *J. Biol. Chem.* **270**: 7795-7798.

Bremer, E. *et al.* (2004). Target cell-restricted and -enhanced apoptosis induction by a scFv: sTRAIL fusion protein with specificity for the pancarcinoma-associated antigen EGP2. *Int. J. Cancer* **109**: 281-290.

Burdin, N. *et al.* (1998). Selective ability of mouse CD1 to present glycolipids: alpha-galactosylceramide specifically stimulates V alpha 14+ NK T lymphocytes. *J. Immunol.* **161**: 3271-3281.

Chen, Q. *et al.* (2001). Apo2L/TRAIL and Bcl-2-related proteins regulate type I interferon-induced apoptosis in multiple myeloma. *Blood* **98**: 2183-2192.

Chinnaiyan, A.M. *et al.* (1995). FADD, a novel death domain-containing protein, interacts with the death domain of Fas and initiates apoptosis. *Cell* **81**: 505-512.

Chuntharapai, A. *et al.* (2001). Isotype-dependent inhibition of tumor growth *in vivo* by monoclonal antibodies to death receptor 4. *J. Immunol.* **166**: 4891-4898.

Conejo-Garcia, J.R. *et al.* (2003). Letal, A tumor-associated NKG2D immunoreceptor ligand, induces activation and expansion of effector immune cells. *Cancer Biol. Ther.* **2**: 446-451.

Cory, S. *et al.* (2003). The Bcl-2 family: roles in cell survival and oncogenesis. *Oncogene* **22**: 8590-8607.

Cosman, D. *et al.* (2001). ULBPs, novel MHC class I-related molecules, bind to CMV glycoprotein UL16 and stimulate NK cytotoxicity through the NKG2D receptor. *Immunity* **14**: 123-133.

Davidson, W.F. *et al.* (1998). Spontaneous development of plasmacytoid tumors in mice with defective Fas-Fas ligand interactions. *J. Exp. Med.* **187**: 1825-1838.

Dighe, A.S. *et al.* (1994). Enhanced *in vivo* growth and resistance to rejection of tumor cells expressing dominant negative IFN gamma receptors. *Immunity* **1**: 447-456.

Djerbi, M. *et al.* (1999). The inhibitor of death receptor signaling, FLICE-inhibitory protein defines a new class of tumor progression factors. *J. Exp. Med.* **190**: 1025-1032.

Donepudi, M. *et al.* (2003). Insights into the regulatory mechanism for caspase-8 activation. *Mol. Cell* **11**: 543-549.

Dunn, G.P. *et al.* (2004). The immunobiology of cancer immunosurveillance and immunoediting. *Immunity* **21**: 137-148.

Eberl, G. and MacDonald, H.R. (2000). Selective induction of NK cell proliferation and cytotoxicity by activated NKT cells. *Eur. J. Immunol.* **30**: 985-992.

Fesik, S.W. (2000). Insights into programmed cell death through structural biology. *Cell* **103**: 273-282.

Gately, M.K. *et al.* (1994). Interleukin-12: a cytokine with therapeutic potential in oncology and infectious diseases. *Ther. Immunol.* **1**: 187-196.

Gong, B. and Almasan, A. (2000). Apo2 ligand/TNF-related apoptosis-inducing ligand and death receptor 5 mediate the apoptotic signaling induced by ionizing radiation in leukemic cells. *Cancer Res.* **60**: 5754-5760.

Griffith, T.S. and Broghammer, E.L. (2001). Suppression of tumor growth following intralesional therapy with TRAIL recombinant adenovirus. *Mol. Ther.* **4**: 257-266.

Groh, V. *et al.* (1999). Broad tumor-associated expression and recognition by tumor-derived gamma delta T cells of MICA and MICB. *Proc. Natl Acad. Sci. U.S.A.* **96**: 6879-6884.

Guery, L. *et al.* (2000). Expression of Fas ligand improves the effect of IL-4 in collagen-induced arthritis. *Eur. J. Immunol.* **30**: 308-315.

Hahne, M. *et al.* (1996). Melanoma cell expression of Fas(Apo-1/CD95) ligand: implications for tumor immune escape. *Science* **274**: 1363-1366.

Harper, N. *et al.* (2003). Fas-associated death domain protein and caspase-8 are not recruited to the tumor necrosis factor receptor 1 signaling complex during tumor necrosis factor-induced apoptosis. *J. Biol. Chem.* **278**: 25534-25541.

Hohlbaum, A.M. *et al.* (2000). Opposing effects of transmembrane and soluble Fas ligand expression on inflammation and tumor cell survival. *J. Exp. Med.* **191**: 1209-1220.

Holler, N. *et al.* (2003). Two adjacent trimeric Fas ligands are required for Fas signaling and formation of a death-inducing signaling complex. *Mol. Cell Biol.* **23**: 1428-1440.

Hsu, H. *et al.* (1995). The TNF receptor 1-associated protein TRADD signals cell death and NF-kappa B activation. *Cell* **81**: 495-504.

Huang, D.C. *et al.* (1999). Activation of Fas by FasL induces apoptosis by a mechanism that cannot be blocked by Bcl-2 or Bcl-x(L). *Proc. Natl Acad. Sci. U.S.A.* **96**: 14871-14876.

Hyer, M.L. *et al.* (2000). Intracellular Fas ligand expression causes Fas-mediated apoptosis in human prostate cancer cells resistant to monoclonal antibody-induced apoptosis. *Mol. Ther.* **2**: 348-358.

Ichikawa, K. *et al.* (2000). A novel murine anti-human Fas mAb which mitigates lymphadenopathy without hepatotoxicity. *Int. Immunol.* **12**: 555-562.

Idris, A.H. *et al.* (1998). Genetic control of natural killing and *in vivo* tumor elimination by the Chok locus. *J. Exp. Med.* **188**: 2243-2256.

Idris, A.H. *et al.* (1999). The natural killer gene complex genetic locus Chok encodes Ly-49D, a target recognition receptor that activates natural killing. *Proc. Natl Acad. Sci. U.S A.* **96**: 6330-6335.

Jinushi, M. *et al.* (2003). Expression and role of MICA and MICB in human hepatocellular carcinomas and their regulation by retinoic acid. *Int. J. Cancer* **104**: 354-361.

Jo, M. *et al.* (2000). Apoptosis induced in normal human hepatocytes by tumor necrosis factor-related apoptosis-inducing ligand. *Nat. Med.* **6**: 564-567.

Jung, G. *et al.* (2001). Target cell-restricted triggering of the CD95 (APO-1/Fas) death receptor with bispecific antibody fragments. *Cancer Res.* **61**: 1846-1848.

Juo, P. *et al.* (1998). Essential requirement for caspase-8/FLICE in the initiation of the Fas-induced apoptotic cascade. *Curr. Biol.* **8**: 1001-1008.

Juo, P. *et al.* (1999). FADD is required for multiple signaling events downstream of the receptor Fas. *Cell Growth Differ.* **10**: 797-804.

Kang, S.M. *et al.* (2000). A non-cleavable mutant of Fas ligand does not prevent neutrophilic destruction of islet transplants. *Transplantation* **69**: 1813-1817.

Kaplan, D.H. *et al.* (1998). Demonstration of an interferon gamma-dependent tumor surveillance system in immunocompetent mice. *Proc. Natl Acad. Sci. U.S.A.* **95**: 7556-7561.

Karre, K. *et al.* (1986). Selective rejection of H-2-deficient lymphoma variants suggests alternative immune defence strategy. *Nature* **319**: 675-678.

Kawamura, T. *et al.* (1998). Critical role of NK1+ T cells in IL-12-induced immune responses *in vivo*. *J. Immunol.* **160**: 16-19.

Kayagaki, N. *et al.* (1999). Expression and function of TNF-related apoptosis-inducing ligand on murine activated NK cells. *J. Immunol.* **163**: 1906-1913.

Kelley, S.K. *et al.* (2001). Preclinical studies to predict the disposition of Apo2L/tumor necrosis factor-related apoptosis-inducing ligand in humans: characterization of *in vivo* efficacy, pharmacokinetics, and safety. *J. Pharmacol. Exp. Ther.* **299**: 31-38.

Kim, S.H. *et al.* (2002). Effective treatment of established mouse collagen-induced arthritis by systemic administration of dendritic cells genetically modified to express FasL. *Mol. Ther.* **6**: 584-590.

Kischkel, F.C. *et al.* (1995). Cytotoxicity-dependent APO-1 (Fas/CD95)-associated proteins form a death-inducing signaling complex (DISC) with the receptor. *EMBO J.* **14**: 5579-5588.

Kischkel, F.C. *et al.* (2000). Apo2L/TRAIL-dependent recruitment of endogenous FADD and caspase-8 to death receptors 4 and 5. *Immunity* **12**: 611-620.

Koh, C.Y. *et al.* (2001). Augmentation of antitumor effects by NK cell inhibitory receptor blockade *in vitro* and *in vivo*. *Blood* **97**: 3132-3137.

Kuang, A.A. *et al.* (2000). FADD is required for DR4- and DR5-mediated apoptosis: lack of trail-induced apoptosis in FADD-deficient mouse embryonic fibroblasts. *J. Biol. Chem.* **275**: 25065-25068.

Lawrence, D. *et al.* (2001). Differential hepatocyte toxicity of recombinant Apo2L/TRAIL versions. *Nat. Med.* **7**: 383-385.

Lee, J.K. *et al.* (2000). IFN-gamma-dependent delay of *in vivo* tumor progression by Fas overexpression on murine renal cancer cells. *J. Immunol.* **164**: 231-239.

Leverkus, M. et al. (2003). Proteasome inhibition results in TRAIL sensitization of primary keratinocytes by removing the resistance-mediating block of effector caspase maturation. *Mol. Cell Biol.* **23**: 777-790.

Lin, T. *et al.* (2002). Long-term tumor-free survival from treatment with the GFP-TRAIL fusion gene expressed from the hTERT promoter in breast cancer cells. *Oncogene* **21**: 8020-8028.

Lin, T. *et al.* (2003). Combination of TRAIL gene therapy and chemotherapy enhances antitumor and antimetastasis effects in chemosensitive and chemoresistant breast cancers. *Mol. Ther.* **8**: 441-448.

Locksley, R.M. *et al.* (2001). The TNF and TNF receptor superfamilies: integrating mammalian biology. *Cell* **104**: 487-501.

Medema, J.P. *et al.* (1999). Immune escape of tumors *in vivo* by expression of cellular FLICE-inhibitory protein. *J. Exp. Med.* **190**: 1033-1038.

Micheau, O. and Tschopp, J. (2003). Induction of TNF receptor I-mediated apoptosis via two sequential signaling complexes. *Cell* **114**: 181-190.

Miwa, K. *et al.* (1998). Caspase 1-independent IL-1beta release and inflammation induced by the apoptosis inducer Fas ligand. *Nat. Med.* **4**: 1287-1292.

Morelli, A.E. *et al.* (1999). Neuronal and glial cell type-specific promoters within adenovirus recombinants restrict the expression of the apoptosis-inducing molecule Fas ligand to predetermined brain cell types, and abolish peripheral liver toxicity. *J. Gen. Virol.* **80**: 571-583.

Muhlenbeck, F. *et al.* (2000). The tumor necrosis factor-related apoptosis-inducing ligand receptors TRAIL-R1 and TRAIL-R2 have distinct cross-linking requirements for initiation of apoptosis and are non-redundant in JNK activation. *J. Biol. Chem.* **275**: 32208-32213.

Muzio, M. *et al.* (1996). FLICE, a novel FADD-homologous ICE/CED-3-like protease, is recruited to the CD95 (Fas/APO-1) death--inducing signaling complex. *Cell* **85**:817-827.

Niehans, G.A. *et al.* (1997). Human lung carcinomas express Fas ligand. *Cancer Res.* **57**: 1007-1012.

Nishimatsu, H. *et al.* (1999). CD95 ligand expression enhances growth of murine renal cell carcinoma *in vivo*. *Cancer Immunol. Immunother.* **48**: 56-61.

Nishimura, Y. *et al.* (1997a). *In vivo* analysis of Fas antigen-mediated apoptosis: effects of agonistic anti-mouse Fas mAb on thymus, spleen and liver. *Int. Immunol.* **9**: 307-316.

Nishimura-Morita, Y. *et al.* (1997b). Amelioration of systemic autoimmune disease by the stimulation of apoptosis-promoting receptor Fas with anti-Fas mAb. *Int. Immunol.* **9**: 1793-1799.

O'Connell, J. *et al.* (1996). The Fas counterattack: Fas-mediated T cell killing by colon cancer cells expressing Fas ligand. *J. Exp. Med.* **184**: 1075-1082.

Ogasawara, J. *et al.* (1993). Lethal effect of the anti-Fas antibody in mice. *Nature* **364**: 806-809.

Okamoto, S. *et al.* (1999). Overexpression of Fas ligand does not confer immune privilege to a pancreatic beta tumor cell line (betaTC-3). *J. Surg. Res.* **84**: 77-81.

Ottonello, L. *et al.* (1999). Soluble Fas ligand is chemotactic for human neutrophilic polymorphonuclear leukocytes. *J. Immunol.* **162**: 3601-3606.

Owen-Schaub, L.B. *et al.* (1998). Fas and Fas ligand interactions suppress melanoma lung metastasis. *J. Exp. Med.* **188**: 1717-1723.

Owen-Schaub, L. *et al.* (2000). Fas and Fas ligand interactions in malignant disease. *Int. J. Oncol.* **17**: 5-12.

Pende, D. *et al.* (2002). Major histocompatibility complex class I-related chain A and UL16-binding protein expression on tumor cell lines of different histotypes: analysis of tumor susceptibility to NKG2D-dependent natural killer cell cytotoxicity. *Cancer Res.* **62**: 6178-6186.

Peng, S.L. *et al.* (1996). A tumor-suppressor function for Fas (CD95) revealed in T cell-deficient mice. *J. Exp. Med.* **184**: 1149-1154.

Peter, M.E. and Krammer, P.H. (2003). The CD95(APO-1/Fas) DISC and beyond. *Cell Death Differ.* **10**: 26-35.

Rubinchik, S. *et al.* (2000). Adenoviral vector which delivers FasL-GFP fusion protein regulated by the tet-inducible expression system. *Gene Ther.* **7**: 875-885.

Rubinchik, S. *et al.* (2001). A complex adenovirus vector that delivers FASL-GFP with combined prostate-specific and tetracycline-regulated expression. *Mol. Ther.* **4**: 416-426.

Saelens, X. *et al.* (2004). Toxic proteins released from mitochondria in cell death. *Oncogene* **23**: 2861-2874.

Samel, D. *et al.* (2003). Generation of a FasL-based proapoptotic fusion protein devoid of systemic toxicity due to cell-surface antigen-restricted Activation. *J. Biol. Chem.* **278**: 32077-32082.

Scanlan, M.J. *et al.* (1994). Molecular cloning of fibroblast activation protein alpha, a member of the serine protease family selectively expressed in stromal fibroblasts of epithelial cancers. *Proc. Natl Acad. Sci. U.S.A.* **91**: 5657-5661.

Schmaltz, C. *et al.* (2002). T cells require TRAIL for optimal graft-versus-tumor activity. *Nat. Med.* **8**: 1433-1437.

Schneider, P. *et al.* (1998). Conversion of membrane-bound Fas(CD95) ligand to its soluble form is associated with downregulation of its proapoptotic activity and loss of liver toxicity. *J. Exp. Med.* **187**: 1205-1213.

Schroter, M. *et al.* (2000). Fas-dependent tissue turnover is implicated in tumor cell clearance. *Oncogene* **19**: 1794-1800.

Seino, K. *et al.* (1997). Antitumor effect of locally produced CD95 ligand. *Nat. Med.* **3**: 165-170.

Seino, K. *et al.* (1998) Chemotactic activity of soluble Fas ligand against phagocytes. *J. Immunol.* **161**: 4484-4488.

Shankaran, V. *et al.* (2001). IFNgamma and lymphocytes prevent primary tumour development and shape tumour immunogenicity. *Nature* **410**: 1107-1111.

Shi, Y. (2002). Apoptosome: the cellular engine for the activation of caspase-9. *Structure* (Camb.) **10**: 285-288.

Shimizu, M. *et al.* (1999). Induction of antitumor immunity with Fas/APO-1 ligand (CD95L)-transfected neuroblastoma neuro-2a cells. *J. Immunol.* **162**: 7350-7357.

Shudo, K. *et al.* (2001). The membrane-bound but not the soluble form of human Fas ligand is responsible for its inflammatory activity. *Eur. J. Immunol.* **31**: 2504-2511.

Siegel, R.M. *et al.* (2000). Fas preassociation required for apoptosis signaling and dominant inhibition by pathogenic mutations. *Science* **288**: 2354-2357.

Simon, A.K. *et al.* (2002). Fas ligand breaks tolerance to self-antigens and induces tumor immunity mediated by antibodies. *Cancer Cell.* **2**: 315-322.

Smith, K.M. *et al.* (1998). Ly-49D and Ly-49H associate with mouse DAP12 and form activating receptors. *J. Immunol.* **161**: 7-10.

Smyth, M.J. *et al.* (1999). Perforin is a major contributor to NK cell control of tumor metastasis. *J. Immunol.* **162**: 6658-6662.

Smyth, M.J. *et al.* (2001a). Tumor necrosis factor-related apoptosis-inducing ligand (TRAIL) contributes to interferon gamma-dependent natural killer cell protection from tumor metastasis. *J. Exp. Med.* **193**: 661-670.

Smyth, M.J. *et al.* (2001b). NK cells and NKT cells collaborate in host protection from methylcholanthrene-induced fibrosarcoma. *Int. Immunol.* **13**: 459-463.

Smyth, M.J. *et al.* (2002). New aspects of natural-killer-cell surveillance and therapy of cancer. *Nat. Rev. Cancer* **2**: 850-861.

Sordillo, E.M. and Pearse, R.N. (2003). RANK-Fc: a therapeutic antagonist for RANK-L in myeloma. *Cancer* **97**: 802-812.

Sova, P. *et al.* (2004). A tumor-targeted and conditionally replicating oncolytic adenovirus vector expressing TRAIL for treatment of liver metastases. *Mol. Ther.* **9**: 496-509.

Sprick, M.R. *et al.* (2000). FADD/MORT1 and caspase-8 are recruited to TRAIL receptors 1 and 2 and are essential for apoptosis mediated by TRAIL receptor 2. *Immunity* **12**: 599-609.

Strand, S. *et al.* (1996). Lymphocyte apoptosis induced by CD95 (APO-1/Fas) ligand-expressing tumor cells - a mechanism of immune evasion? *Nat. Med.* **2**: 1361-1366.

Street, S.E. *et al.* (2001). Perforin and interferon-gamma activities independently control tumor initiation, growth, and metastasis. *Blood* **97**: 192-197.

Street, S.E. *et al.* (2002). Suppression of lymphoma and epithelial malignancies effected by interferon gamma. *J. Exp. Med.* **196**: 129-134.

Suda, T. *et al.* (1997). Membrane Fas ligand kills human peripheral blood T lymphocytes, and soluble Fas ligand blocks the killing. *J. Exp. Med.* **186**: 2045-2050.

Takeda, K. *et al.* (2001). Involvement of tumor necrosis factor-related apoptosis-inducing ligand in NK cell-mediated and IFN-gamma-dependent suppression of subcutaneous tumor growth. *Cell. Immunol.* **214**: 194-200.

Takeda, K. *et al.* (2002). Critical role for tumor necrosis factor-related apoptosis-inducing ligand in immune surveillance against tumor development. *J. Exp. Med.* **195**: 161-169.

Takeda, K. *et al.* (2004). Induction of tumor-specific T cell immunity by anti-DR5 antibody therapy. *J. Exp. Med.* **199**: 437-448.

Talmadge, J.E. *et al.* (1980a). Role of natural killer cells in tumor growth and metastasis: C57BL/6 normal and beige mice. *J. Natl Cancer Inst.* **65**: 929-935.

Talmadge, J.E. *et al.* (1980b). Role of NK cells in tumour growth and metastasis in beige mice. *Nature* **284**: 622-624.

Traver, D. *et al.* (1998). Mice defective in two apoptosis pathways in the myeloid lineage develop acute myeloblastic leukemia. *Immunity* **9**: 47-57.

van den Broek, M.E. *et al.* (1996). Decreased tumor surveillance in perforin-deficient mice. *J. Exp. Med.* **184**: 1781-1790.

van den Broek M.E. *et al.* (1995) Perforin dependence of natural killer cell-mediated tumor control *in vivo*. *Eur. J. Immunol.* **25**: 3514-3516.

Varfolomeev, E.E. *et al.* (1998). Targeted disruption of the mouse Caspase 8 gene ablates cell death induction by the TNF receptors, Fas/Apo1, and DR3 and is lethal prenatally. *Immunity* **9**: 267-276.

Vaux, D.L. and Silke, J. (2003). Mammalian mitochondrial IAP binding proteins. *Biochem. Biophys. Res. Commun.* **304**: 499-504.

Vetter, C.S. *et al.* (2002). Expression of stress-induced MHC class I related chain molecules on human melanoma. *J. Invest. Dermatol.* **118**: 600-605.

Villunger, A. *et al.* (1997). Constitutive expression of Fas (Apo-1/CD95) ligand on multiple myeloma cells: a potential mechanism of tumor-induced suppression of immune surveillance. *Blood* **90**: 12-20.

Voelkel-Johnson, C. *et al.* (2002). Resistance of prostate cancer cells to soluble TNF-related apoptosis-inducing ligand (TRAIL/Apo2L) can be overcome by doxorubicin or adenoviral delivery of full-length TRAIL. *Cancer Gene Ther.* **9**: 164-172.

Wajant, H. (2003). Death receptors. *Essays Biochem.* **39**: 53-71.

Wajant, H. (2004). TRAIL and NFkappaB signalling -a complex relationship. *Vitam. Horm.* **67**: 101-132.

Wajant, H. *et al.* (2001). Differential activation of TRAIL-R1 and -2 by soluble and membrane TRAIL allows selective surface antigen-directed activation of TRAIL-R2 by a soluble TRAIL derivative. *Oncogene* **20**: 4101-4106.

Walczak, H. *et al.* (1999). Tumoricidal activity of tumor necrosis factor-related apoptosis-inducing ligand *in vivo*. *Nat. Med.* **5**: 157-163.

Wigginton, J.M. *et al.* (2001). IFN-gamma and Fas/FasL are required for the antitumor and antiangiogenic effects of IL-12/pulse IL-2 therapy. *J. Clin. Invest.* **108**: 51-62.

Wigginton, J.M. *et al.* (2002). Synergistic engagement of an ineffective endogenous anti-tumor immune response and induction of IFN-gamma and Fas-ligand-dependent tumor eradication by combined administration of IL-18 and IL-2. *J. Immunol.* **169**: 4467-4474.

Wuest, T. *et al.* (2002). TNF-selectokine: a novel prodrug generated for tumor targeting and site-specific activation of tumor necrosis factor. *Oncogene* **21**: 4257-4265.

Yagita, H. *et al.* (1996). CD95 ligand in graft rejection. *Nature* **379**: 682.

Yao, Q. *et al.* (2003). Intra-articular adenoviral-mediated gene transfer of trail induces apoptosis of arthritic rabbit synovium. *Gene Ther.* **10**: 1055-1060.

Yeh, W.C. *et al.* (1998) FADD: essential for embryo development and signaling from some, but not all, inducers of apoptosis. *Science* **279**: 1954-1958.

Zamai, L. *et al.* (1998). Natural killer (NK) cell-mediated cytotoxicity: differential use of TRAIL and Fas ligand by immature and mature primary human NK cells. *J. Exp. Med.* **188**: 2375-2380.

Zhang, H. *et al.* (1997). Amelioration of collagen-induced arthritis by CD95 (Apo-1/Fas)-ligand gene transfer. *J. Clin. Invest.* **100**: 1951-1957.

Zhang, J. *et al.* (1998). Fas-mediated apoptosis and activation-induced T-cell proliferation are defective in mice lacking FADD/Mort1. *Nature* **392**: 296-300.

Zornig, M. *et al.* (1995). Loss of Fas/Apo-1 receptor accelerates lymphomagenesis in E mu L-MYC transgenic mice but not in animals infected with MoMuLV. *Oncogene* **10**: 2397-2401.

Chapter 8

# INFECTION & NEOPLASTIC GROWTH 101
*The required reading for microbial pathogens aspiring to cause
cancer*

Jessica Bertout & Andrei Thomas-Tikhonenko
*University of Pennsylvania, 3800 Spruce Street, Philadelphia, PA 19104-6051*

Abstract:     The role of infectious agents in the development of cancer is well-established.
              For example, numerous RNA and DNA viruses express dedicated
              oncoproteins that are able to transform cells *in vitro* and induce rapid tumor
              formation in experimental animals. Curiously, these acutely-transforming
              viruses are seldom associated with naturally occurring neoplasms of humans
              or animals. Conversely, the microbial pathogens that are linked to cancers in
              natural hosts rarely encode acutely transforming proteins. Moreover, they tend
              to down-regulate most of their genes except for genes affecting cell survival,
              often via the NF-κB pathway. This allows the pre-neoplastic cell to avoid
              triggering cytotoxic immunity and the ensuing acute inflammation. These host
              responses not only kill tumor cells directly, but also strongly suppress the
              development of new blood vessels (neovascularization), which is absolutely
              essential for neoplastic growth. Chronic inflammation, on the other hand,
              promotes neoplastic cell growth and may even be conducive to
              neovascularization. Thus, cancer-associated microbial pathogens must follow
              the "less is more" principle. According to this principle, only minor
              perturbations in cell proliferation and death are tolerated by the host, but in the
              long run, they are all that is necessary for tumorigenesis.

Key words:    oncogenes; cell proliferation; apoptosis; cytotoxic immunity; acute
              inflammation; tumor neovascularization

*Climb Mount Fuji,*
*O snail,*
*but slowly, slowly.*
ISSA KOBAYASHI

## 1.      INTRODUCTION

When George Klein introduced the winner of the 1966 Nobel Prize in Physiology or Medicine to the Swedish Royal Academy, he remarked that the trail-blazing discovery of Peyton Rous, the eponymous avian sarcoma virus (RSV), had not been met with universal acclaim. "The notion that virus diseases must be infectious and cancer not due to infectious processes was so deeply ingrained that there was a tendency to explain all virus tumours as strange exceptions. The Rous sarcomas were regarded as bird tumours, of no importance for mammals" (Klein, 1972). However, according to Professor Klein, "the situation changed radically in the 1950s," and the study of tumour viruses has become "a central area of modern cancer research." Several developments were responsible for this change.

## 1.1     The Golden Age of tumor virology

Intriguingly, several groups have demonstrated that RSV is also oncogenic in rodents (Zilber 1961b; Svoboda, 1986). In subsequent years, a number of other oncogenic retroviruses have been isolated (Weiss *et al.*, 1984) including several murine sarcoma viruses (Levy and Leclerc, 1977) which induce cancerous growth in experimental animals within weeks or months of infection. These findings led to the emergence of the genetic concept of cancer (Zilber, 1961a; Huebner and Todaro, 1969). Its essence is that tumors are caused by abnormal transfer and activation of genetic material. The transfer can occur vertically through the germ line or horizontally, by transducing viruses. The role of viruses in this process was experimentally confirmed by 1989 Nobelists Harold Varmus and Michael Bishop, who demonstrated (jointly with Dominique Stehelin and Peter Vogt) that RNA-containing retroviruses could capture, activate, and transmit cellular oncogenes (Stehelin *et al.*, 1976). Also identified in the 70's were DNA tumor viruses (papova-, adeno-, etc.) that cause malignant tumors in rodents after a very short latency (Tooze, 1979).

## 1.2 	Acutely transforming viruses and Koch's postulates

Not only did these viruses appear to be connected to cancer, they also clearly fulfilled Koch's postulates:

> ➤ The pathogen occurs in every case of the disease in question and under circumstances which can account for the pathological changes and clinical course of the disease.
> ➤ The pathogen occurs in no other disease as a fortuitous and non-pathogenic parasite.
> ➤ After being fully isolated from the body and repeatedly grown in pure culture, the pathogen can induce the disease anew. (quoted from Falkow, 2004).

Indeed, most spontaneous sarcomas and other tumors arising in laboratory animals have a viral etiology, and isolates of avian and murine sarcoma viruses are certainly not spurious pathogens. Finally, successes in studying these viruses have to do with the fact that they can be readily propagated in cell cultures, purified, and even molecularly cloned, without the loss of their transforming potential.

Subsequently, rapid advances in molecular biology and genetics allowed identification of discrete transforming genes which are responsible for autonomous, asocial proliferation of host cells. These genes are now known as oncogenes, and their bearers are acutely oncogenic in experimental animals, i.e. are capable of inducing rapid tumor formation. Undoubtedly, these discoveries were enormously influential and had a significant impact not only on cancer research but on all of cell and molecular biology. Yet, the contribution of the acutely transforming viruses to naturally occurring tumors is surprisingly modest.

## 2. 	WHY AREN'T ONCOGENE-BEARING VIRUSES TUMORIGENIC IN NATURAL HOSTS?

### 2.1 	Oncogenic viruses in search of diseases

In Table 1, we summarize the data on representative acutely transforming oncogenic viruses of avian and mammalian species, including primates. Their salient feature is that they encode dedicated oncoproteins (often dispensable for replication) [column 2] that trigger neoplastic transformation in various cell culture systems and transgenic contexts. Yet, hardly any of them are associated with neoplastic diseases in natural hosts [column 3]. Avian leukosis-sarcoma retroviruses exemplify this finding.

*Table 1.* Archetypal acutely transforming viruses

| VIRUS | PRINCIPAL ONCOPROTEIN | NEOPLASTIC PHENOTYPE IN EXPERIMENTAL SETTINGS & TIME BEFORE TUMOR ONSET | ROLE IN NATURALLY OCCURRING TUMORS |
|---|---|---|---|
| **RNA VIRUSES (retroviruses)** | | | |
| Rous sarcoma virus (RSV) | Src, a non-receptor tyrosine kinase, is essential for the oncogenic function of RSV (Martin, 1970), efficiently transforms chicken embryo fibroblasts (Radke and Martin, 1979), and is tumorigenic in a transgenic context (astrocytoma) (Weissenberger et al., 1997). | Transforms chicken fibroblasts *in vitro*, induces mesenchymal tumors *in vivo* (Weiss et al.,1984), is oncogenic in rodents (Svoboda, 1986; Zilber, 1961b), and induces experimental gliomas following intracerebral inoculation in dogs (Haguenau, 1981). | RSV re-isolation in the field has not been reported, although its helper virus (avian leukosis virus) is a common chicken pathogen (Aiello, 1998). |
| MC29 and related viruses | Myc, a nuclear phosphoprotein/ transcription factor, which possesses transforming activity in various cell types *in vitro* (Small et al., 1987; Thomas-Tikhonenko et al., 2004) and *in vivo* (Adams et al., 1985; Felsher and Bishop, 1999; D'Cruz et al., 2001; Yu and Thomas-Tikhonenko, 2002). | Original isolates induced myelo-cytomatosis (Ivanov et al., 1964). Late isolates and viruses like FH3 (Chen et al., 1989) induce a broad range of tumors of myeloid, non-myeloid and non-hematopoietic origin (see for instance Tikhonenko and Linial, 1992 and 1993). | Same as for RSV, although many strains have been isolated from birds deliberately infected with the helper virus in experimental settings. |

| | | | |
|---|---|---|---|
| Turkey reticulo-endothe-liosis virus, strain T | Rel (Wilhelmsen et al., 1984), which belongs to the NF-κB transcription factor family (Kieran et al., 1990; Ghosh et al., 1990). | REV-T induces an invariably fatal leukemia in chickens with a latency period of 7-10 days (Moore and Bose, Jr., 1988). v-Rel immortalizes lymphoid cells in vitro and REV-T-transformed cells are tumorigenic in histo-compatible birds (Hrdlickova et al., 1994) | The REV-T strain, which is responsible for an acute reticulum cell neoplasia in experimentally inoculated chicks, was isolated in 1958 from a diseased turkey (Bose, Jr. and Levine, 1967), but does not occur commonly in the field (Aiello, 1998). Field cases of chronic lymphoma do occur but are not caused by the REV-T strain. |
| Ableson murine leukemia (Ab-MuLV) | Abl, a non-receptor tyrosine kinase with many different substrates. v-Abl transform both hematopoietic and fibroblastic cells in vitro (reviewed by Shore et al., 2002). | The transduction of Abl by the helper murine leukemia virus reduces tumor latency from 3 months to 3 weeks (Cook, 1982). Mainly pre-B cell leukemias are formed in vivo with infiltration of the marrow, meninges, and lymph nodes. | None, although a related Bcr-Abl protein is crucial for the pathogenesis of chronic myelogenous leukemia, at least in part via activation of the NF-κB pathway (Hamdane et al.,1997; Reuther et al., 1998). |
| Spleen focus-forming virus (SFFV) | gp55, a viral glycoprotein capable of binding to the erythropoietin receptor (Li et al., 1990). | The primary consequence of SFFV infection is rapid-onset polyclonal erythroblastosis (Kabat, 1989). The gp55 gene is capable of inducing neoplastic proliferation of erythroid progenitor cells in vitro (Aizawa et al., 1990). | The two known strains of SFFV (SFFV-Friend and -Rauscher) are laboratory isolates. |

## DNA VIRUSES

| | | | |
|---|---|---|---|
| Non-primate polyoma-viruses | Large-T/middle-T antigens were among the first proteins with demonstrated ability to transform mammalian cells *in vitro* (Sachs and Medina, 1961). Insertion of the middle-T coding sequence into RSV in place of *src* results in oncogenesis in chicks (Kornbluth, *et al.*, 1986). | Injection of mouse polyomavirus into newborn rodents causes the insurgency of diverse tumors (quoted from Iacoangeli *et al.*, 1995), although strains vary in their ability to induce tumor formation in lab mice (Dawe *et al.*, 1987). Mice transgenic for HaPV develop epitheliomas as well (quoted from Scherneck *et al.*, 2001). Epithelioma-derived HaPV particles induce lymphomas and leukemia in animals from other colonies with short latency (4-8 weeks) (Graffi *et al.*, 1969). | Murine polyomavirus is common, but non-pathogenic in wild mice (quoted from Iacoangeli *et al.*, 1995). Although hamster polyomavirus was isolated from an epithelioma, the source of the virus is one research hamster colony in Berlin (Scherneck *et al.*, 2001). In general, in rodents, epitheliomas seldom arise from natural infection (Aiello, 1998). Avian polyomavirus is associated with delayed feathering, hemorrhages and non-neoplastic GI and skin pathologies (Aiello, 1998). |
| Primate polyoma-viruses (SV40, JCV, BKV) | Large-T antigen disables two key tumor suppressors (p53 and Rb) while small T-antigen perturbs protein phosphatase 2A, resulting in neoplastic transformation of human cells *in vitro* and *in vivo* (Hahn *et al.*, 2002; Chen *et al.*, 2004). | All polyomaviruses readily transform rodent (Todaro and Green, 1966) and human (Todaro *et al.*, 1966) fibroblasts *in vitro* and induce tumor formation in rodents (White and Khalili, 2004). Mice expressing SV40 large T transgenically develop tumors within the choroid plexus (Brinster *et al.*, 1984). Large T | Inadvertent exposure of humans to SV40 (as polio vaccine contaminant) has not resulted in wide-spread neoplastic diseases. Some connection with rare tumor mesothelioma is yet to be confirmed (zur Hausen, 2003; Gazdar *et al.*, 2002). JCV in natural hosts (humans) is associated with progressive multifocal leukoencelopathy (PML), a degenerative, non-neoplastic disease, while its connection to |

| | | | |
|---|---|---|---|
| | antigens of JCV and BKV are also tumorigenic in transgenic mice (Small et al., 1986). | | medulloblastoma remains tenuous (Safak and Khalili, 2003). Likewise, BKV is primarily linked to nephropathy (White and Khalili, 2004). |
| Bovine papilloma virus (BPV) | E5 (golgi transmembrane protein), capable of activating the PDGF receptor. Interestingly, E5 of human papillomaviruses fails to induce focus formation (Suprynowicz et al., 2005). | BPV induces tumors in inoculated hamsters (Robl and Olson, 1968) and BPV-transformed mouse C127 cells are tumorigenic in nude mice (Dvoretzky et al., 1980). BPV E5 transforms epithelial cells in culture (DiMaio et al., 1986). | In their natural hosts, BPV causes rapid formation of papilloma, i.e. mostly benign tumors that are thought to regress spontaneously (Campo, 2002). |
| Marek's disease herpes virus (MDV) | Meq, is a leucine zipper-containing transcription factor (Jones et al., 1992), which heterodimerizes with the Jun oncoprotein and is recruited to AP1 sites in gene promoters (Levy et al., 2003; Liu and Kung, 2000). This gene is not present in non-oncogenic serotypes 2 and 3 (Venugopal, 2000). | The whole virus transforms T-lymphocytes in vivo (Schat et al., 1991) and induces tumors after a short (3-4 weeks) latency. Mutants lacking Meq are replication-competent but do not cause lymphomas (Lupiani et al., 2004). | In the field, MDV causes Marek's disease, a common lymphoproliferative disease of poultry (Venugopal, 2000). Its tumorigenicity in natural hosts sets it apart from other acutely oncogenic viruses. This exception might stem from the ability of MDV to induce immunosuppression (see below). |

Most of them (except RSV) are replication-defective and require the presence of a helper virus, avian leukosis virus (ALV) (Weiss *et al.*, 1984). While ALV is a common poultry pathogen in the field, neither RSV nor MC29 have been re-isolated in natural settings. The same holds for DNA tumor viruses. For example, while murine polyomavirus readily induces tumors in newborn rodents and its T-antigens were among the first proteins with demonstrated ability to transform NIH3T3 cells, polyomavirus is common but non-pathogenic in wild mice. Its relative, SV40, is also a rather benign primate virus. Famously, millions of people in the U.S.A. were inadvertently exposed to it when polio vaccine was produced in monkey cells. However, its tenuous connection to some rare neoplasms notwithstanding, SV40 didn't turn out to be a major cancer-inducing pathogen. This, of course, raises the following question: why can oncogene-bearing viruses not cause tumors under natural, non-laboratory conditions?

## 2.2    How hard can it be to make a "real" tumor?

One possible explanation for the oncogenic viruses' "ineptness" under natural conditions is that one-hit neoplasms observed in experimental animals are not "real" cancers, but rather proliferative diseases. This theory is given credence by the observation that although oncoprotein-encoding transgenes do cause tumor formation, the latency of the neoplastic disease is generally long, consistent with the participation of additional genetic events. For example, Eμ-Myc mice expressing Myc in immature B-cells quickly develop benign enlargements of lymph nodes (Adams *et al.*, 1985), but it is subsequent mutations in the p53 pathway that yield full-fledged clonal B-lymphomas (Schmitt *et al.*, 1999).

Similar examples can be found in the realm of virally-induced tumors. Spleen focus-forming virus (SFFV) encodes a truncated env glycoprotein, gp55, capable of binding with high affinity to the erythropoietin receptor (Li *et al.*, 1990). This results in activation of erythroid signal transduction pathways and ensuing growth factor-independent proliferation of erythroid precursors. However, this transformed state depends on the continuous presence of gp55 and therefore is not truly malignant (Ruscetti, 1999). Complete neoplastic transformation requires additional activation of the protooncogene Sfpi-1. In murine erythroleukemias, this task is accomplished, with low frequency and long latency, via random insertional mutagenesis by non-acutely transforming Friend-MuLV, which serves as a helper virus for SFFV (Kabat, 1989).

Last but not least, the idea that "real" tumors require multiple genetic events gained support during attempts to generate neoplastic cells of human origin. The high-profile paper by Weinberg and co-workers estimates that at least four events are needed for neoplastic conversion of human cells (Hahn *et al.*, 1999). While two of these events (inactivation of the p53 and Rb tumor suppressors) presumably can be accomplished by a single protein (SV40 large T-antigen), activation of the Ras oncoprotein and telomerase, a frequent target of the Myc oncoprotein (Wang *et al.*, 1998), were also required. The multi-hit nature of spontaneous human neoplasms is also well-recognized (Knudson, 2001). One corollary of this genetic complexity is that full-fledged neoplasms cannot be caused (in Koch's sense) by any one virus, unless it carries multiple oncogenes. The best a microbial pathogen can hope for is to introduce some genetic aberrations and wait patiently for subsequent hits to occur by other means. It appears that cancer-associated viruses and other microbial pathogens do just that.

## 2.3 Re-writing Koch's postulates: causation versus predisposition

The association between viruses and certain human cancers have been known for a long time. As early as 1964, Epstein and Barr observed virus-like particles in lymphoblasts cultured from Burkitt's lymphoma (Epstein *et al.*, 1964); the eponymous virus (EBV) later proved to be a herpesvirus. In Table 2, we present data on other archetypal viruses associated with neoplastic disease in natural hosts. However, it is important to realize that these associations are not absolute. There are EBV-negative cases of Burkitt's lymphomas, especially in AIDS patients (Gaidano and Dalla-Favera, 1995). Conversely, in the majority of people, EBV infection, rather fortunately, leads to mononucleosis, a relatively benign lymphoproliferative disease (Beers and Berkow, 1999). In a recent review, it is estimated that only one percent of EBV-infected individuals develop Burkitt's lymphoma, less than one percent of HPV16-infected individuals develop cervical cancer, and no more than 10 percent of HBV-infected individuals develop hepatocellular carcinoma (Vakkila and Lotze, 2004). Moreover, in many cases neoplasms develop years and sometimes decades after the onset of viral infection. A good example is adult T-cell leukemia which can develop 20 years after infection with human T-lymphotropic virus I (Gallo and Reitz, 1985). Therefore, with respect to most agents in Table 2, the word "causation" should be used with utmost caution (Pagano *et al.*, 2004), and "predisposition" might be a better term, especially for pathogens like HBV whose genes are not even present in the full-fledged neoplasms.

Table 2. Microbial pathogens associated with neoplastic growth

| PATHOGEN | DISEASE | RESPONSIBLE GENES/ PROTEINS | TRANSFORMING ACTIVITY UNDER EXPERIMENTAL CONDITIONS | TUMOR INCIDENCE AND LATENCY |
|---|---|---|---|---|
| Assorted leukemia, mammary tumor, reticuloendo-theliosis, and lymphoprolife-rative disease viruses | Lymphoma, mammary adeno-carcinoma | Long terminal repeats (LTR) containing strong transcriptional enhancers | Not transforming *in vitro*. Tumorigenesis *in vivo* is based on the insertional activation of cellular proto-oncogenes (Myc, Wnt-1, etc.). | Common pathogens in the field (Aiello, 1998; Payne, 1998), but with tumor latency averaging many months (Weiss *et al.*, 1984). |
| Jaagsiekte sheep retrovirus | Ovine pulmonary carcinoma (adenoma-tosis) | Env | Morphological transformation of NIH3T3 cells, but no tumorigenic conversion (Maeda *et al.*, 2001). Mechanisms of tumorigenesis *in vivo* are largely unknown (reviewed in Fan *et al.*, 2003; Rosenberg, 2001). | Respiratory exudates from affected sheep are infectious. Cloned virus induced pulmonary adenomatosis in 50% of infected newborn lambs 4 months post-infection (Palmarini *et al.*, 1999). The incubation period after natural infection extends over months until sheep are 3-4 years old (Aiello, 1998). |

| Human papilloma-viruses 16 and 18 | Cervical cancer | E6 and E7, inhibitors of the p53 and Rb pathways, respectively | Poorly transforming *in vitro*, require cooperation with Ras (Storey *et al.*, 1988; Phelps *et al.*, 1988). Tumorigenesis *in vivo* is based on inactivation of p53 and Rb. | Latency period is probably measured in decades, so that the mean age for developing cervical cancer is ~50 years (Beers and Berkow, 1999). |
|---|---|---|---|---|
| Epstein-Barr virus | Burkitt's and Hodgkin lymphoma, nasopharyngeal carcinoma | EBNA-1, the only protein consistently expressed in B-lymphomas (Young and Rickinson, 2004). Another protein called LMP transforms MEFs (Wang *et al.*, 1985), but is often down-regulated in tumors. | Efficiently immortalizes B-cells *in vitro* (Humme *et al.*, 2003), but antagonizes the effects of the Myc oncoprotein (Pajic *et al.*, 2001) and shows no oncogenicity in cell culture assays (reviewed in Young and Rickinson, 2004). Tumorigenesis *in vivo* is most likely based on suppression of apoptosis (Kennedy *et al.*, 2003). EBV-positivity also correlates with expression of the Tcl-1 protooncogene (Bell and Rickinson, 2003). | In mice, transgenically expressed EBNA-1 leads to lymphomagenesis, but tumors are clonal (i.e. rely on secondary mutations) and arise after a long latency (Wilson *et al.*, 1996). In humans, EBV infection is common. 95% of the adult population in the U.S. has had an EBV infection (Beers and Berkow, 1999). |
| HHV6 | EBV-negative Hodgkin and non-Hodgkin lymphomas | DR7, putative inhibitor of p53 (Kashanchi *et al.*, 1997). | Although some HHV6 molecular clones appear to transform keratinocytes *in vitro* (Razzaque *et al.*, 1993), no transforming events have ever been detected after HHV-6 infection *in vitro* (De Bolle *et al.*, 2005). | Unknown |

| Virus | Disease | Oncogenic mechanism | Notes |
|---|---|---|---|
| HHV8 (KSHV) | Kaposi sarcoma (of endothelial cell origin), also lymphoproliferative disorders (PEL and MCD) | LANA-1 (binding to Rb and p53), v-cyclin (promotes cell cycle) and v-FLIP (inhibits apoptosis; activates NF-κB) (reviewed in Jenner and Boshoff, 2002). | All genes with oncogenic properties are only expressed during the lytic cycle (Hayward, 2003). This list includes vGPCR, which promotes endothelial cell malignization (Montaner et al., 2003). | In the USA and Europe, >90% of KS cases are found among homosexual and bisexual men with AIDS. The virus may be detected several years before the development of KS (Beers and Berkow, 1999). |
| HTLVI | Adult T-cell leukemia | Tax, multifunctional nuclear protein capable of suppressing apoptosis (reviewed in Kfoury, et al. 2005), in part via induction of NF-κB (Kawakami et al., 1999; Mori et al., 2001). | Tax is not transforming in vitro or oncogenic in transgenic mice (Nerenberg, M.I., 1990). Tumorigenesis in vivo is most likely based on suppression of apoptosis | Only a limited number of infected individuals will develop leukemia many years after infection (Nicot, 2005) |
| HBV | Hepatocellular carcinoma | HBx transactivator. This protein binds (Feitelson et al., 1993) and inactivates p53 (Wang et al., 1994), thus preventing apoptosis in vitro (Wang et al., 1995) and in a transgenic mouse model (Ueda et al., 1995). | Hbx is not transforming in vitro or oncogenic in transgenic mice (Lee et al., 1990). Tumorigenesis in vivo is most likely based on the suppression of apoptosis (Bouchard and Schneider, 2004). The liver disease has an immunologic component (cytotoxic T-cells) in transgenic mice (Chisari, 1996). | The risk of developing hepatocellular carcinoma is more than one hundredfold higher among HBV carriers. The exact duration of latency is unknown. No genetic traces of HBV exist in the resultant tumors. |

| Bacterium *Helicobacter pylori* | Gastric cancer (Peek and Blaser, 2002) | cagA (Hatakeyama, 2004), which is phosphorylated by Src and activates SHP2, a protein tyrosine phosphatase (Higashi *et al.*, 2002). | cagA induces "hummingbird phenotype" and scattering in gastric epithelium (Segal *et al.*, 1999), but its sustained activation leads to apoptosis not transformation (Tsutsumi *et al.*, 2003) | Gastric cancers develop in approximately 3% of the infected individuals (Uemura *et al.*, 2001). No genetic traces of *H.pylori* exist in the resultant tumors. |

## 2.4 Re-writing Koch's postulates: cell survival versus cell expansion

The "predisposing" nature of tumorigenic viruses comes as no surprise if one considers the following. The vast majority of pathogens associated with neoplastic disease do not possess transforming activity in cell culture. The proteins responsible for cancer predisposition usually improve cell survival, either via inactivation of p53 or activation of the NF-κB pathway. For example, the NF-κB-activating properties are shared by biochemically unrelated proteins such as v-FLIP of Kaposi sarcoma herpesvirus (HHV8/KSHV) and Tax of human T-cell leukemia virus I (column 3 in Table 2). Whichever acutely transforming oncoproteins might be encoded by these pathogens, they are usually not expressed in full-fledged neoplasms. The prime examples of this reticence are the LMP1 protein of EBV and the vGPCR of HHV8/KSHV. Rather curiously, the latter is essential for lytic infection, not immortalization.

## 3. PLAYING HIDE-AND-SEEK WITH THE IMMUNE SYSTEM

## 3.1 The importance of not being seen

The other notable feature of successful cancer-associated pathogens is their apparent desire not to be recognized by the immune system. For example, EBV employs several strategies to render host cells invisible: silencing of the majority of its proteins except EBNA-1 (see Table 2), downregulation of cell-adhesion molecules, and down-regulation of major histocompatibility complex (MHC) class I expression necessary for efficient antigen presentation (quoted from Tindle, 2002). Human papillomaviruses also employ a variety of tricks to render their E7 proteins tolerogenic, including altered codon usage (Tindle, 2002). We have already mentioned in Table 1 that the unique ability of Marek's disease virus to induce tumors in natural hosts correlates with its ability to induce profound immunosuppression (reviewed in Schat and Markowski-Grimsrud, 2001).

Clearly tumorigenic viruses go to extreme lengths to avoid recognition by the immune system in order to protect themselves from elimination. However, since viruses and many other microorganisms are obligatory intracellular parasites, they have a vested interest in protecting virus-harboring host cells, which also happen to be seeds of future neoplasms. In other words, the failure of the immune system is a triumph for both the virus and the nascent tumor cell. A corollary of this concept is that immunocompromised individuals would be at risk for virus-associated cancers. And they indeed are: in North America both Burkitt's lymphoma and Kaposi sarcoma strike mainly AIDS patients (Boshoff and Weiss, 2002). But is it simply because tumorigenic viruses can replicate uncontrollably or also because tumor cells expressing viral antigens are allowed to flourish? Two lines of evidence suggest that the second scenario plays as important a role as the first.

The first line of evidence comes from studies of experimental animal strains, in which tumorigenesis is driven by a single viral protein, not the infectious agent. In the most recent example, it has been shown that expression of the Jaagsiekte sheep retrovirus Env protein in lungs of mice, by using a replication-incompetent adeno-associated virus vector, results in pulmonary carcinomas in immunodeficient but not immunocompetent mice (Wootton *et al.*, 2005). The second line of evidence comes from various population studies suggesting that immunocompromised patients are at greater risk even for cancers of non-viral etiology. Examples include a two to four-fold increase in incidence of de novo malignant melanomas, a three-fold increase in non-Kaposi's sarcomas, and increased relative risks for colon, pancreatic, lung, endocrine, and urinary tract tumors in transplant patients as compared to the general population (Dunn *et al.*, 2002). Another study at the University of Pittsburgh demonstrated a twenty five-fold higher prevalence of lung cancer in a group of over 600 transplant patients (Pham *et al.*, 1995). These and similar studies are commonly construed to mean that many instances of neoplastic growth can be attributed to the breakdown of immune surveillance. Yet at the same time, the very existence of tumor surveillance, let alone its exact mechanisms, have been a subject of much debate over the past century.

## 3.2 The concept of immunosurveillance: a brief history

As early as 1909, Paul Ehrlich proposed that the immune system was responsible for identifying and destroying many nascent carcinomas, thus shielding the body against a high incidence of tumors. Yet, immunologists did not have the ability to confirm this proposition in the first decade of the 20th century. However, the field of immunology developed quickly over the next half century, providing useful animal models and a better understanding that could finally help substantiate this intriguing idea. Studies on allograft rejection and transplantation, and the discovery of tumor specific antigens, are good examples of major steps made in the field in the early 20th century.

In 1957, two scientists, Sir Macfarlane Burnet and Lewis Thomas, adopted Ehrlich's idea and coined the term "cancer immunosurveillance" (reviewed in Imai *et al.*, 2000; Ikeda *et al.*, 2002). The concept was defined by Burnet in the following words: "In large, long-lived animals, like most of the warm-blooded vertebrates, inheritable genetic changes must be common in somatic cells and a proportion of these changes will represent a step toward malignancy. It is an evolutionary necessity that there should be some mechanism for eliminating or inactivating such potentially dangerous mutant cells and it is postulated that this mechanism is of immunological character" (quoted from Dunn *et al.*, 2002).

## 3.3     Immunosurveillance: beyond virally-induced tumors

The immunosurveillance hypothesis was met with considerable resistance over the first few years as initial experiments aimed at corroborating it failed. Research groups using thymectomy on neonatal mice or various pharmacological methods to induce immunosuppression were not able to show consistent increases in the incidence of induced or spontaneous tumors in immunocompromised mice (reviewed in Dunn *et al.*, 2002). On the other hand, these mice were highly susceptible to virally-induced tumors and spontaneous lymphomas when compared to controls. However, this could be explained simply by the greater likelihood of infection with transforming viruses. Alternatively, it was postulated that the increased incidence of lymphomas was due to chronic antigenic stimulation from bacterial or viral infections leading to lymphocytic proliferation and the eventual transformation of these immune cells (reviewed in Dunn *et al.*, 2002). In the aggregate, these experiments neither confirmed nor invalidated the hypothesis of immunosurveillance, and new models of immuno-suppression were necessary.

Coincidentally, the late 1960s saw the development of athymic nude mice allowing for experiments in animals lacking all thymus-derived immune cells (Flanagan, 1966; Pantelouris, 1968). Using this model in a pathogen-free environment and the chemical carcinogen methylcholanthrene (MCA), Osias Stutman showed that nude mice did not form more chemically-induced tumors than control euthymic mice, nor did they form them any faster (Stutman, 1974 and 1979). These mice were also not more likely to develop spontaneous nonviral tumors (Rygaard and Povlsen, 1976). Unfortunately for its proponents, the immunosurveillance concept was at variance with these results and was therefore shelved for a number of years.

Later, however, it was recognized that nude mice actually possess functional αβ T-cell-receptor-bearing lymphocytes and though their repertoire is limited, the animals are not completely immunosuppressed

(Hunig and Bevan, 1980; Ikehara, *et al.*, 1984; Maleckar and Sherman, 1987). In addition, natural killer (NK) cells were discovered in the 1970s and were found to develop independently of the thymus such that athymic nude mice would also possess these important first-responder cells (Herberman and Holden, 1978). Though this discovery proved insufficient to fully revive the immunosurveillance hypothesis, it was followed by several key findings which helped bring the concept back into a more favorable light. First, perforin-deficient mice were found to be more susceptible to the formation of MCA-induced tumors than wild-type mice (van den Broek *et al.*, 1996; Street *et al.*, 2001). Because cytotoxic T and NK cells release perforin in order to kill their target cells, this finding suggested that these cells are involved in anti-tumor effects. Subsequently, both SCID mice and Rag-null mice were found to have increased tumor incidences as compared to their wild-type counterparts (Engel *et al.*, 1997; Shankaran, *et al.*, 2001). SCID mice lack the active subunit of DNA-dependent protein kinase such that they cannot generate rearranged lymphocyte receptors and therefore are unable to adapt their immune response to specific antigens. Rag-null mice lack the recombination activating genes 1 or 2 such that they cannot rearrange any of their lymphocyte antigen receptors and are deficient in all T, B, and NKT cells. In fact, all Rag2 null mice eventually develop spontaneous tumors as compared to only 30 percent of the age-matched wild-type control mice. Moreover, while half of the tumors affecting the Rag2 null mice are malignant, all tumors found in the wild-type mice are benign. The Rag2-null mice also develop more MCA-induced tumors and do so more quickly than controls.

## 3.4 Immunosurveillance: supporting data from the study of human tumors.

One important piece of evidence in support of the immunosurveillance concept is that infiltration of spontaneous tumors with cytotoxic cells is associated with better clinical outcomes. While such evidence was slow to emerge, several recent studies seem to provide evidence for such an association. In a study from the University of Pennsylvania, tumor-infiltrating lymphocytes (TIL) were detected in just 50 percent of ovarian cancers. However, patients with TIL-positive neoplasms had a five-year overall survival rate of 38 percent, compared to 4.5 percent among patients with TIL-negative tumors (Zhang *et al.*, 2003). Very similar results were obtained on patients with gastric cancer (Ishigami *et al.*, 2000), esophageal carcinomas (Schumacher *et al.*, 2001), and other neoplasms (reviewed in Vakkila and Lotze, 2004). Curiously, among colon cancer cohorts, TIL seem to only benefit patients whose tumors exhibit microsatellite instability

(Guidoboni *et al.*, 2001), but not patients with other types of colon cancers (Nanni *et al.*, 2002). Additional supportive evidence was offered by the Saitama cohort study which followed the general Japanese population for 11 years (Imai *et al.*, 2000). It showed that people with medium and high cytotoxic activity of their peripheral-blood lymphocytes were less likely to develop cancer, whereas those with low cytotoxic activity were significantly more likely to do so (Nakachi *et al.*, 2004). Thus, lymphocytes appear to be beneficial to the cancer patient, but their protective mechanism is poorly defined. It is still unclear whether they work mainly through direct cytotoxicity to cancer cells or through production of infection-induced cytokines. Could it be that the milieu created by infection is simply not conducive to tumor growth?

## 4. NON-IMMUNE FUNCTIONS OF THE IMMUNE SYSTEM VERSUS THE TUMOR

### 4.1 An infected animal is an inhospitable host for the tumor

In 1971, chronic infection with the intracellular protozoan pathogens *Toxoplasma* and *Besnoitia* was shown to be protective not only against the intracellular bacterium *Listeria*, but also against murine tumors, both transplanted and spontaneous (Hibbs *et al.*, 1971). In fact, macrophages isolated from the peritoneum of mice chronically infected with *Toxoplasma* and *Besnoitia* and from mice injected with *Mycobacterium butyricum* were found to be cytotoxic to syngeneic, allogeneic, and xenogeneic cancer cells *in vitro* (Hibbs *et al.*, 1972a and 1972b; Hibbs, 2002). Later, this was also shown using *Listeria monocytogenes* (North and Havell, 1988; Youdim and Sharman, 1976) and *Corynebacterium parvum* (Keller *et al.*, 1990). Most recently it was demonstrated that rejection of cells expressing papillomavirus protein E7 in syngeneic hosts could be substantially enhanced by infection with Listeria or injection with bacterial endotoxin (Frazer *et al.*, 2001). In summary, these experiments suggested a link between infection and anti-tumor immunity. It was, however, still unclear whether or not activated immune cells were actually responsible for defending the organism against naturally occurring tumors (Paglia and Guzman, 1998).

## 4.2    Suppression of tumorigenesis during acute infection: cytotoxicity is dispensable

This link between acute infection and anti-tumor defense prompted the Thomas-Tikhonenko laboratory, in collaboration with Dr. Christopher Hunter, to study the effect of *Toxoplasma gondii* infection on tumor formation. *T. gondii* is an obligate intracellular parasite that infects mice acutely, causing a strong Th1 immune response over the first two weeks of infection (Hunter and Reichmann, 2002). After infection with the pathogen, the mice were injected subcutaneously with non-immunogenic B16 melanoma cells (Fidler, 1975) which are not known to be immunogenic unless engineered to overexpress GM-CSF (Dranoff *et al.*, 1993). Nevertheless, mice infected with *Toxoplasma* did not develop melanomas while control uninfected mice did (Hunter *et al.*, 2001). This apparent inability of normally non-immunogenic cancer cells to form tumors during an acute *Toxoplasma* infection raised an important question: is tumor surveillance promoted in parasite-infected animals to such an extent as to inhibit tumor growth, or is a non-immune mechanism responsible for the observed tumor suppression?

Genetically modified mice were used to answer this intriguing question. It was known that macrophages from *T. gondii*-infected animals produce TNFα and nitric oxide (NO), two important molecules involved in macrophage cytotoxicity to tumor cells (Klostergaard, 1993; Xie and Fidler, 1998). B16 melanoma cells are not sensitive to TNFα, but they are readily killed by NO (Klostergaard *et al.*, 1991). Thus, mice lacking inducible NO-synthase (iNOS) could be used to study the role of macrophages in tumor suppression (Laubach *et al.*, 1995). Surprisingly, while iNOS-null mice are deficient in macrophage function, inhibition of tumor growth was still observed, challenging the hypothesis that cytotoxic macrophages might be essential for tumor immunity (Hibbs *et al.*, 1972a and 1972b). This, however, did not exclude a role for cytotoxic lymphocytes in tumor suppression. To test the involvement of TIL, two models were used: scid-beige and perforin knock-out mice. Scid-beige mice lack cytotoxic T- and NK cells (MacDougall *et al.*, 1990). Perforin knock-out mice have lymphocytes, but their cytolytic functions are impaired (Kagi *et al.*, 1994). Interestingly, when the above experiment was repeated in these two mouse models, tumor suppression was not alleviated despite the absence of the major immune effector mechanisms (Hunter *et al.*, 2001).

These results did not conform to the tacitly accepted model that cytotoxic immunity is a central player in tumor suppression during infection. Seeking an alternative explanation, we hypothesized that infection-induced pro-inflammatory cytokines such as interferons and interleukin-12, which are known to possess anti-angiogenic properties (Pepper *et al.*, 1996), could be blocking tumor neovascularization.

## 4.3     Suppression of tumorigenesis during acute infection: the importance of anti-angiogenesis

To verify this hypothesis, Matrigel pellets embedded with pro-angiogenic cells were implanted into infected or control mice to measure angiogenesis. After one week, the implants in control mice were high in hemoglobin content, indicating considerable stimulation of new vessel formation. Strikingly, hemoglobin levels measured in *T. gondii*-infected animals were 50-100 fold lower than the controls, and on histopathological examination no vascular channels were observed (Hunter *et al.*, 2001). To extend this observation to tumor neovascularization, tumor-bearing mice were injected either with fluorescently labeled lectin to identify endothelial cells lining blood vessels (Thurston *et al.*, 1996) or with EF5 which stains hypoxic areas of the tissue (Evans *et al.*, 1997). In addition, tumor sections were stained with an anti-CD31 monoclonal antibody which binds to endothelial cells lining blood capillaries. While tumors in control mice revealed robust vasculature without any apparent hypoxia, tumors that developed during the acute phase of *T. gondii* infection were not only lacking in functional vasculature, but were also completely devoid of solitary endothelial cells. In addition, extensive cores of hypoxia ringed with necrosis were found in these latter samples. The areas of deficient angiogenesis, hypoxia, and necrosis overlapped consistently, supporting a role for infection-mediated anti-angiogenesis in tumor growth inhibition.

It was also noteworthy that no protective effect was afforded by chronic infection, a sequel to acute infection with *T. gondii* (Hunter and Reichmann, 2002). Chronic infections are accompanied by chronic inflammation whose purpose is to repair the damage to tissue incurred during the acute response. Thus, it involves tissue regeneration or fibrosis (Fantone and Ward, 1999), two processes associated with new vessel growth (Martinez-Hernandez, 1999). Consequently, a variety of pro-angiogenic molecules is produced during chronic inflammation (Jackson *et al.*, 1997), ranging from prostaglandin E2 (Form and Auerbach, 1983) to vascular endothelial growth factor (VEGF) (Sunderkotter *et al.*, 1994). On the other hand, formation of new blood vessels during acute inflammation could have detrimental effects: exaggerated edema, increase in the number of inflammatory cells, more profound tissue damage from neutrophils, and increased likelihood of hematogenic spread of the infectious agent. Thus, it would make sense if most critical regulators of acute inflammation, under certain conditions, were to inhibit angiogenesis (Thomas-Tikhonenko and Hunter, 2003). Still, the question remained: which infection-induced molecules are crucial for both anti-angiogenesis and tumor-suppression? Since viral and non-viral infections alike entail the production of interferons, we focused our subsequent research on this particular family of Th1 cytokines.

## 4.4  Interferons and anti-angiogenesis

We studied the role of inflammatory cytokines released during infection to elucidate the mechanism underlying its anti-angiogenic effects. Tumor growth repression occurred consistently during acute infection with Th1 response-inducing pathogens such as *T. gondii* (Hunter and Reichmann, 2002), *Listeria monocytogenes* (Weiskirch and Paterson, 1997) and lymphocytic choriomeningitis virus (LCMV) (Zinkernagel *et al.*, 1999; Zajac *et al.*, 1998) but not during infection with Th2 response-inducing parasites like *Schistosoma mansoni* (Hoffmann *et al.*, 2002). Notably, chronic infection with LCMV also had no effect, and the lack of anti-tumor protection correlated with greatly diminished Th1 responses (Rankin *et al.*, 2004). This directed our focus to Th1 cytokines. To confirm their importance in the anti-tumor effects, mice lacking IL-10 (Kuhn *et al.*, 1993), a Th1 response repressor (Moore *et al.*, 2001), were infected with *T. gondii* and injected with the same B16 melanoma cells. Tumors in these infected IL-10 null mice were even smaller than those in the infected wild-type animals. The mutant mice also had increased levels of IFNγ. Conversely, mice lacking IFNγ no longer showed the anti-vascularization effects. Restoration of angiogenesis was also observed in animals deficient in STAT1 (Rankin *et al.*, 2004), a transcription factor activated by ligation of type I (α and β) and type II (γ) interferon receptors (Stark *et al.*, 1998).

Consistent with our results, there are compelling data to suggest that both type I and type II interferons possess anti-angiogenic properties (Pepper *et al.*, 1996; Ellis and Fidler, 1996; Sidky and Borden, 1987), and IFNα has been used for the treatment of pediatric hemangioma, an endothelium-derived benign neoplasm (Ezekowitz *et al.*, 1992). The anti-angiogenic effects of type I interferons stem from their ability to inhibit expression of two potent angiogenic inducers: basic fibroblast growth factor (bFGF) (Singh *et al.*, 1995; Vermeulen *et al.*, 1997) and interleukin-8 (Oliveira *et al.*, 1992; Singh *et al.*, 1996). Type II interferon directly inhibits endothelial cell proliferation (Friesel *et al.*, 1987; Norioka *et al.*, 1992) and is responsible for the production of anti-angiogenic chemokines IP-10 (Strieter *et al.*, 1995; Angiolillo *et al.*, 1995) and MIG (Sgadari *et al.*, 1997; Vicari and Caux, 2002).

## 4.5    Anti-tumoral effects of interferons: indirect & direct

In addition to their angiogenic properties, both type I and type II interferons are regarded as components of tumor surveillance (Gresser and Belardelli, 2002; Ikeda *et al.*, 2002) and govern, to a large extent, all the above-described anti-tumoral effects of cytotoxic immunity. For example, IFNγ-insensitive (STAT1-null) mice lacking the p53 tumor suppressor gene were found to develop spontaneous tumors more quickly than IFNγ-sensitive p53-null mice (13.7 weeks versus 18.5 weeks) (Kaplan *et al.*, 1998). Interestingly, the types of tumors were also different. While the vast majority of IFNγ-sensitive mice succumbed only to lymphoid tumors, over a third of the IFNγ-insensitive mice bore non-lymphoid neoplasms.

Yet some of the most potent anti-tumoral effects of interferon have to do with its ability to kill tumor cells directly. The exact molecular mechanisms of cell killing by interferons are incompletely understood but are thought to include induction of death ligands (e.g., TRAIL) and receptors thereof (reviewed in Barber, 2000; Clemens, 2003). Thus, viruses (including tumorigenic ones) go to great lengths to inhibit IFN signaling in infected cells. The prime example of this survival strategy is inhibition by the KSHV/HHV8 viral interferon regulatory factor (vIRF) protein of host interferon responses (Gao *et al.*, 1997). As an added bonus, vIRF also inhibits p53 function and thus blocks the intrinsic apoptotic pathway (Nakamura *et al.*, 2001).

## 5.    TAKE HOME MESSAGES FOR PATHOGENS WITH ONCOGENIC ASPIRATIONS

➢ Don't focus solely on promoting the cell cycle. Host cell expansion can be achieved more subtly by improving cell survival. Simply having NF-κB on your side goes a long way.

➢ Stay invisible to the immune system. To this end, express the bare minimum of your own genes since acutely transforming proteins (even of cellular origin) can elicit immune responses. If you have to express a multitude of proteins to support your life cycle, assign some of them to the suppression of immune responses.

➢ Attempt to establish chronic infection. Accompanying chronic inflammation is conducive to cell expansion and neovascularization. In contrast, acute infection results in the inhibition of angiogenesis.

➢ Interferons are not only the pathogen's worst enemies; they also have potent anti-tumoral effects. Direct or indirect inhibition of interferon responses will greatly aid tumorigenesis.

# 6.    REFERENCES

Adams, J.M. *et al.* (1985). The c-myc oncogene driven by immunoglobulin enhancers induces lymphoid malignancy in transgenic mice. *Nature* **318**: 533-538.

Aiello, S.E. (editor) (1998). The Merck Veterinary Manual. Merck & Co. Inc., Whitehouse Station, NJ.

Aizawa, S. *et al.* (1990). Env-derived gp55 gene of Friend spleen focus-forming virus specifically induces neoplastic proliferation of erythroid progenitor cells. *EMBO J.* **9**: 2107-2116.

Angiolillo, A.L. *et al.* (1995). Human interferon-inducible protein-10 is a potent inhibitor of angiogenesis *in vivo. J. Exp. Med.* **182**: 155-162.

Barber, G.N. (2000). The interferons and cell death: guardians of the cell or accomplices of apoptosis? *Sem. Cancer Biol.* **10**: 103-111.

Beers, M.H. and Berkow, R. (1999). The Merck Manual of Diagnosis and Therapy. Merck & Co. Inc., Whitehouse Station, NJ.

Bell, A. and Rickinson, A.B. (2003). Epstein-Barr virus, the TCL-1 oncogene and Burkitt's lymphoma. *Trends Microbiol.* **11**: 495-497.

Bose, H.R., Jr. and Levine, A.S. (1967). Replication of the reticuloendotheliosis virus (strain T) in chicken embryo cell culture. *J. Virol.* **1**: 1117-1121.

Boshoff, C. and Weiss, R. (2002). AIDS-related malignancies. *Nat. Rev. Cancer* **2**: 373-382.

Bouchard, M.J. and Schneider, R.J. (2004). The enigmatic X gene of hepatitis B virus. *J. Virol.* **78**: 12725-12734.

Brinster, R.L. *et al.* (1984). Transgenic mice harboring SV40 T-antigen genes develop characteristic brain tumors. *Cell* **37**: 367-379.

Campo, M.S. (2002). Animal models of papillomavirus pathogenesis. *Virus Res.* **89**: 249-261.

Charlton, B.R. (editor) (2000). Whiteman and Bickford's Avian disease manual. American Association of Avian Pathologists, Kenneth Square, PA.

Chen, C. *et al.* (1989). FH3, a v-myc avian retrovirus with limited transforming ability. *J.Virol.* **63**: 5092-5100.

Chen, W. *et al.* (2004). Identification of specific PP2A complexes involved in human cell transformation. *Cancer Cell* **5**: 127-136.

Chisari, F.V. (1996). Hepatitis B virus transgenic mice: models of viral immunobiology and pathogenesis. *Curr. Top. Microbiol. Immunol.* **206**: 149-173.

Clemens, M.J. (2003). Interferons and apoptosis. *J. Interferon Cytokine Res.* **23**: 277-292.

Cook, W.D. (1982). Rapid thymomas induced by Abelson murine leukemia virus. *Proc. Natl Acad. Sci. U.S.A* **.79**: 2917-2921.

D'Cruz, C.M. *et al.* (2001). c-MYC induces mammary tumorigenesis by means of a preferred pathway involving spontaneous Kras2 mutations. *Nature Med.* **7**: 235-239.

Dawe, C.J. *et al.* (1987). Variations in polyoma virus genotype in relation to tumor induction in mice. Characterization of wild-type strains with widely differing tumor profiles. *Am. J. Pathol.* **127**: 243-261.

De Bolle *et al.* (2005). Update on human herpesvirus 6 biology, clinical features, and therapy. *Clin. Microbiol. Rev.* **18**: 217-245.

DiMaio, D. *et al.* (1986). Translation of open reading frame E5 of bovine papillomavirus is required for its transforming activity. *Proc. Natl Acad. Sci. U.S.A.* **83**: 1797-1801.

Dranoff, G. *et al.* (1993). Vaccination with irradiated tumor cells engineered to secrete murine granulocyte-macrophage colony-stimulating factor stimulates potent, specific, and long-lasting anti-tumor immunity. *Proc.Natl Acad.Sci.U.S.A.* **90**: 3539-3543.

Dunn, G.P. *et al.* (2002). Cancer immunoediting: from immunosurveillance to tumor escape. *Nat. Immunol.* **3**: 991-998.

Dvoretzky, I. *et al.* (1980). A quantitative *in vitro* focus assay for bovine papillomavirus. *Virology* **103**: 369-375.

Ellis, L.M. and Fidler, I.J. (1996). Angiogenesis and metastasis. *Eur. J. Cancer* **32A**: 2451-2460.

Engel, A.M. *et al.* (1997). MCA sarcomas induced in scid mice are more immunogenic than MCA sarcomas induced in congenic, immunocompetent mice. *Scand. J. Immunol.* **45**: 463-470.

Epstein, M.A. *et al.* (1964). Virus particles in cultured lymphoblasts from Burkitt's lymphoma. *Lancet* **1**: 702.

Evans, S.M. *et al.* (1997). Imaging hypoxia in diseased tissues. *Adv.Exp.Med.Biol.* **428**: 595-603.

Ezekowitz, R.A.B. *et al* .(1992). Interferon α2A therapy for life-threatening hemangiomas of infancy. *N. Engl. J. Med.* **326**: 1456-1463.

Falkow, S. (2004). Molecular Koch's postulates applied to bacterial pathogenicity--a personal recollection 15 years later. *Nat. Rev. Microbiol.* **2**: 67-72.

Fan, H. *et al.* (2003). Transformation and oncogenesis by jaagsiekte sheep retrovirus. *Curr. Top. Microbiol. Immunol.* **275**:139-177.

Fantone, J.C. and Ward, P.A. (1999) in Pathology, edited by Rubin, E. and Farber, J.L., Lippincott-Raven, Philadelphia and New York, 37-75.

Feitelson, M.A. *et al.* (1993). Hepatitis B X antigen and p53 are associated *in vitro* and in liver tissues from patients with primary hepatocellular carcinoma. *Oncogene* **8**: 1109-1117.

Felsher, D.W. and Bishop, J.M. (1999). Reversible tumorigenesis by MYC in hematopoietic lineages. *Mol. Cell* **4**: 199-207.

Fidler, I.J. (1975). Biological behavior of malignant melanoma cells correlated to their survival *in vivo*. *Cancer Res.* **35**: 218-224.

Flanagan, S.P. (1966). 'Nude', a new hairless gene with pleiotropic effects in the mouse. *Genet. Res.* **8**: 295-309.

Form, D.M. and Auerbach, R. (1983). $PGE_2$ and angiogenesis. *Proc. Soc. Exp. Biol. Med.* **172**: 214-218.

Frazer, I.H. *et al.* (2001). Tolerance or immunity to a tumor antigen expressed in somatic cells can be determined by systemic proinflammatory signals at the time of first antigen exposure. *J. Immunol.* **167**: 6180-6187.

Friesel *et al.* (1987). Inhibition of endothelial cell proliferation by gamma-interferon. *J.Cell Biol.* **104**: 689-696.

Gaidano G. and Dalla-Favera, R. (1995). Molecular pathogenesis of AIDS-related lymphomas. *Adv. Cancer Res.* **67**: 113-153.

Gallo, R.C. and Reitz, M.S., Jr. (1985). The first human retroviruses: are there others? *Microbiol. Sci.* **2**: 97-98 and 101-104.

Gao, S.J. *et al.* (1997). KSHV ORF K9 (vIRF) is an oncogene which inhibits the interferon signaling pathway. *Oncogene* **15**: 1979-1985.

Gazdar *et al.* (2002). SV40 and human tumours: myth, association or causality? *Nat. Rev. Cancer* **2**: 957-964.

Ghosh, S. *et al.* (1990). Cloning of the p50 DNA binding subunit of NF-kappa B: homology to rel and dorsal. *Cell* **62**: 1019-1029.

Graffi, A. *et al.* (1969). Induction of transmissible lymphomas in Syrian hamsters by application of DNA from viral hamster papovavirus-induced tumors and by cell-free filtrates from human tumors. *Proc. Natl Acad. Sci. U.S.A.* **64**: 1172-1175.

Gresser, I. and Belardelli, F. (2002). Endogenous type I interferons as a defense against tumors. *Cytokine Growth Factor Rev.* **13**: 111-118.

Guidoboni, M. *et al.* (2001). Microsatellite instability and high content of activated cytotoxic lymphocytes identify colon cancer patients with a favorable prognosis. *Am. J. Pathol.* **159**: 297-304.

Haguenau, F. (1981). Comparative ultrastructure of human gliomas and experimental gliomas induced by Rous sarcoma virus (RSV). *Neurochirurgie* **27**: 251-253.

Hahn, W.C. *et al.* (1999). Creation of human tumour cells with defined genetic elements. *Nature* **400**: 464-468.

Hahn, W.C. *et al.* (2002). Enumeration of the simian virus 40 early region elements necessary for human cell transformation. *Mol. Cell. Biol.* **22**: 2111-2123.

Hamdane, M. *et al.* (1997). Activation of p65 NF-κB protein by p210BCR-ABL in a myeloid cell line (P210BCR-ABL activates p65 NF-κB). *Oncogene* **15**: 2267-2275.

Hatakeyama, M. (2004). Oncogenic mechanisms of the Helicobacter pylori CagA protein. *Nat. Rev. Cancer* **4**: 688-694.

Hayward, G.S. (2003). Initiation of angiogenic Kaposi's sarcoma lesions. *Cancer Cell* **3**: 1-3.

Herberman, R.B. and Holden, H.T. (1978). Natural cell-mediated immunity. *Adv. Cancer Res.* **27**: 305-377.

Hibbs, J.B., Jr. (2002). Infection and nitric oxide. *J.Infect.Dis.* **185**: S9-S17.

Hibbs *et al.* (1971). Resistance to murine tumors conferred by chronic infection with intracellular protozoa, Toxoplasma gondii and Besnoitia jellisoni. *J. Infect. Dis.* **124**: 587-592.

Hibbs *et al.* (1972a). Control of carcinogenesis: a possible role for the activated macrophage. *Science* **177**: 998-1000.

Hibbs *et al.* (1972b). Possible role of macrophage mediated nonspecific cytotoxicity in tumour resistance. *Nature New Biol.* **235**: 48-50.

Higashi, H. *et al.* (2002). SHP-2 tyrosine phosphatase as an intracellular target of Helicobacter pylori CagA protein. *Science* **295**: 683-686.

Hoffmann, K.F. *et al.* (2002). Cytokine-mediated host responses during schistosome infections: walking the fine line between immunological control and immunopathology. *Adv. Parasitol.* **52**: 265-307.

Hrdlickova, R. *et al.* (1994). *In vivo* evolution of c-rel oncogenic potential. *J. Virol.* **68**: 2371-2382.

Huebner, R.J. and Todaro, G.J. (1969). Oncogenes of RNA tumor viruses as determinants of cancer. *Proc. Natl Acad. Sci. U.S.A.* **64**: 1087-1094.

Humme, S. *et al.* (2003). The EBV nuclear antigen 1 (EBNA1) enhances B cell immortalization several thousandfold. *Proc. Natl Acad. Sci. U.S.A.* **100**: 10989-10994.

Hunig, T. and Bevan, M.J. (1980). Specificity of cytotoxic T cells from athymic mice. *J. Exp. Med.* **152**: 688-702.

Hunter, C.A. and Reichmann, G. (2002) 'Immunology of toxoplasma infection' in Toxoplasmosis. A comprehensive clinical guide. Joynson, D.H.M. and Wreghitt, T.G. (eds). Cambridge University Press, Cambridge, 43-57.

Hunter, C.A. *et al.* (2001). Cutting edge: Systemic inhibition of angiogenesis underlies resistance to tumors during acute toxoplasmosis. *J.Immunol.* **166**: 5878-5881.

Iacoangeli, A. *et al.* (1995). Role of mouse polyomavirus late region in the control of viral DNA replication: a review. *Biochimie* **77**: 780-786.

Ikeda, H. *et al.* (2002). The roles of IFNγ in protection against tumor development and cancer immunoediting. *Cytokine Growth Factor Rev.* **13**: 95-109.

Ikehara, S. *et al.* (1984). Functional T cells in athymic nude mice. *Proc. Natl Acad. Sci. U.S.A.* **81**: 886-888.

Imai, K. *et al.* (2000). Natural cytotoxic activity of peripheral-blood lymphocytes and cancer incidence: an 11-year follow-up study of a general population. *Lancet* **356**: 1795-1799.

Ishigami, S. *et al.* (2000). Clinical impact of intratumoral natural killer cell and dendritic cell infiltration in gastric cancer. *Cancer Lett.* **159**: 103-108.

Ivanov, X. *et al.* (1964). Experimental investigations into avian leucoses. V. Transmission, haematology and morphology of avian myelocytomatosis. *Bull. Inst. Pathol. Comp. Anim. Acad. Bulg. Sci.* **10**: 5-38.

Jackson, J.R. *et al.* (1997). The codependence of angiogenesis and chronic inflammation. *FASEB J.* **11**: 457-465.

Jenner, R.G. and Boshoff, C. (2002). The molecular pathology of Kaposi's sarcoma-associated herpesvirus. *Biochim. Biophys. Acta* **1602**: 1-22.

Jones, D. *et al.* (1992). Marek disease virus encodes a basic-leucine zipper gene resembling the fos/jun oncogenes that is highly expressed in lymphoblastoid tumors. *Proc. Natl Acad. Sci. U.S.A.* **89**: 4042-4046.

Kabat, D. (1989). Molecular biology of Friend viral erythroleukemia. *Curr. Top. Microbiol. Immunol.* **148**: 1-42.

Kagi, D. *et al.* (1994). Cytotoxicity mediated by T cells and natural killer cells is greatly impaired in perforin-deficient mice. *Nature* **369**: 31-37.

Kaplan, D.H. *et al.* (1998). Demonstration of an interferon gamma-dependent tumor surveillance system in immunocompetent mice. *Proc. Natl. Acad. Sci. U.S.A.* **95**: 7556-7561.

Kashanchi, F. *et al.* (1997). Human herpesvirus 6 (HHV-6) ORF-1 transactivating gene exhibits malignant transforming activity and its protein binds to p53. *Oncogene* **14**: 359-367.

Kawakami, A. *et al.* (1999). Inhibition of caspase cascade by HTLV-I tax through induction of NF-κB nuclear translocation. *Blood* **94**: 3847-3854.

Keller, R. *et al.* (1990). Resistance to a non-immunogenic tumor, induced by Corynebacterium parvum or Listeria monocytogenes, is abrogated by anti-interferon gamma. *Int. J.Cancer* **46**: 687-690.

Kennedy, G. *et al.* (2003). Epstein-Barr virus provides a survival factor to Burkitt's lymphomas. *Proc. Natl Acad. Sci. U.S.A.* **100**: 14269-14274.

Kfoury, Y. *et al.* (2005). Proapoptotic regimes for HTLV-I-transformed cells: targeting Tax and the NF-κB pathway. *Cell Death Differ* **12**: 871–877.

Kieran, M. *et al.* (1990). The DNA binding subunit of NF-kappa B is identical to factor KBF1 and homologous to the rel oncogene product. *Cell* **62**: 1007-1018.

Klein, G. (1972) in Nobel Lectures, Physiology or Medicine 1963-1970. Elsevier Publishing Company, Amsterdam.

Klostergaard, J. (1993). Macrophage tumoricidal mechanisms. *Res. Immunol.* **144**: 274-276.

Klostergaard, J. *et al.* (1991). Cellular models of macrophage tumoricidal effector mechanisms *in vitro*. Characterization of cytolytic responses to tumor necrosis factor and nitric oxide pathways *in vitro*. *J.Immunol.* **147**: 2802-2808.

Knudson, A.G. (2001). Two genetic hits (more or less) to cancer. *Nat. Rev. Cancer* **1**: 157-162.

Kornbluth, S. *et al.* (1986). Transformation of chicken embryo fibroblasts and tumor induction by the middle T antigen of polyomavirus carried in an avian retroviral vector. *Mol. Cell Biol.* **6**: 1545-1551.

Kuhn, R. *et al.* (1993). Interleukin-10-deficient mice develop chronic enterocolitis. *Cell* **75**: 263-274.

Laubach, V.E. *et al.* (1995). Mice lacking inducible nitric oxide synthase are not resistant to lipopolysaccharide-induced death. *Proc. Natl Acad. Sci. U.S.A.* **92**: 10688-10692.

Lee, T.H. *et al.* (1990). Hepatitis B virus transactivator X protein is not tumorigenic in transgenic mice. *J. Virol.* **64**: 5939-5947.

Levy, A.M. *et al.* (2003). Characterization of the chromosomal binding sites and dimerization partners of the viral oncoprotein Meq in Marek's disease virus-transformed T cells. *J. Virol.* **77**: 12841-12851.

Levy, J.P. and Leclerc, J.C. (1977). The murine sarcoma virus-induced tumor: exception or general model in tumor immunology? *Adv. Cancer Res.* **24**: 1-66.

Li, J.P. *et al.* (1990). Activation of cell growth by binding of Friend spleen focus-forming virus gp55 glycoprotein to the erythropoietin receptor. *Nature* **343**: 762-764.

Liu, J.L. and Kung, H.J. (2000). Marek's disease herpesvirus transforming protein MEQ: a c-Jun analogue with an alternative life style. *Virus Genes* **21**: 51-64.

Lupiani, B. *et al.* (2004). Marek's disease virus-encoded Meq gene is involved in transformation of lymphocytes but is dispensable for replication. *Proc. Natl Acad. Sci. U.S.A.* **101**: 11815-11820.

MacDougall, J.R. *et al.* (1990). Demonstration of a splenic cytotoxic effector cell in mice of genotype SCID/SCID.BG/BG. *Cell. Immunol.* **130**: 106-117.

Maeda, N. *et al.* (2001). Direct transformation of rodent fibroblasts by jaagsiekte sheep retrovirus DNA. *Proc. Natl Acad. Sci. U.S.A.* **98**: 4449-4454.

Maleckar, J.R. and Sherman, L.A. (1987). The composition of the T cell receptor repertoire in nude mice. *J. Immunol.* **138**: 3873-3876.

Martin, G.S. (1970). Rous sarcoma virus - a function required for maintenance of transformed state. *Nature* **227**: 1021.

Martinez-Hernandez, A. (1999) in Pathology. Rubin, E. and Farber, J.L. (eds). Lippincott-Raven, Philadelphia and New York: 76-103.

Montaner, S. *et al.* (2003). Endothelial infection with KSHV genes *in vivo* reveals that vGPCR initiates Kaposi's sarcomagenesis and can promote the tumorigenic potential of viral latent genes. *Cancer Cell* **3**: 23-36.

Moore, B.E. and Bose, H.R., Jr. (1988). Transformation of avian lymphoid cells by reticuloendotheliosis virus. *Mutat. Res.* **195**: 79-90.

Moore, K.W. *et al.* (2001). Interleukin-10 and the interleukin-10 receptor. *Annu. Rev. Immunol.* **19**: 683-765.

Mori, N. *et al.* (2001). Human T-cell leukemia virus type I tax protein induces the expression of anti-apoptotic gene Bcl-xL in human T-cells through nuclear factor-κB and c-AMP responsive element binding protein pathways. *Virus Genes* **22**: 279-287.

Nakachi, K. *et al.* (2004). Perspectives on cancer immuno-epidemiology. *Cancer Sci.* **95**: 921-929.

Nakamura, H. *et al.* (2001). Inhibition of p53 tumor suppressor by viral interferon regulatory factor. *J. Virol.* **75**: 7572-7582.

Nanni, O. *et al.* (2002). Role of biological markers in the clinical outcome of colon cancer. *Br. J. Cancer* **87**: 868-875.

Nerenberg, M.I. (1990). An HTLV-I transgenic mouse model: role of the tax gene in pathogenesis in multiple organ systems. *Curr. Top. Microbiol. Immunol.* **160**: 121-128.

Nicot, C. (2005). Current views in HTLV-I-associated adult T-cell leukemia/lymphoma. *Am. J. Hematol.* **78**: 232-239.

Norioka, K. *et al.* (1992). Inhibitory effects of cytokines on vascular endothelial cells: synergistic interactions among interferon-gamma, tumor necrosis factor-alpha, and interleukin-1. *J.Immunotherapy* **12**: 13-18.

North, R.J. and Havell, E.A. (1988). The Antitumor Function of Tumor Necrosis Factor (TNF). II. Analysis of the Role of Endogenous Tnf in Endotoxin-Induced Hemorrhagic Necrosis and Regression of An Established Sarcoma. *J. Exp. Med.* **167**: 1086-1099.

Oliveira, I.C. *et al.* (1992). Down-regulation of interleukin-8 gene expression in human fibroblasts - unique mechanism of transcriptional inhibition by interferon. *Proc. Natl Acad. Sci. U.S.A.* **89**: 9049-9053.

Pagano, J.S. *et al.* (2004). Infectious agents and cancer: criteria for a causal relation. *Sem. Cancer Biol.* **14**: 453-471.

Paglia, P. and Guzman, C.A. (1998). Keeping the immune system alerted against cancer. *Cancer Immunol. Immunother.* **46**: 88-92.

Pajic, A. *et al.* (2001). Antagonistic effects of c-myc and Epstein-Barr virus latent genes on the phenotype of human B cells. *Int. J. Cancer* **93**: 810-816.

Palmarini, M. *et al.* (1999). Jaagsiekte sheep retrovirus is necessary and sufficient to induce a contagious lung cancer in sheep. *J. Virol.* **73**: 6964-6972.

Pantelouris, E.M. (1968). Absence of thymus in a mouse mutant. *Nature* **217**: 370-371.

Payne, L.N. (1998). Retrovirus-induced disease in poultry. *Poult. Sci.* **77**: 1204-1212.

Peek, R.M., Jr. and Blaser, M.J. (2002). *Helicobacter pylori* and gastrointestinal tract adenocarcinomas. *Nat. Rev. Cancer* **2**: 28-37.

Pepper, M.S. *et al.* (1996). Angiogenesis-regulating cytokines: activities and interactions. *Curr. Top. Microbiol. Immunol.* **213**: 31-67.

Pham, S.M. *et al.* (1995). Solid tumors after heart transplantation: lethality of lung cancer. *Ann. Thorac. Surg.* **60**, 1623-1626.

Phelps, W.C. *et al.* (1988). The human papillomavirus type 16 E7 gene encodes transactivation and transformation functions similar to those of adenovirus E1A. *Cell* **53**: 539-547.

Radke, K. and Martin, G.S. (1979). Transformation by Rous sarcoma virus: effects of src gene expression on the synthesis and phosphorylation of cellular polypeptides. *Proc. Natl Acad. Sci. U.S.A.* **76**: 5212-5216.

Rankin, E.B. *et al.* (2004). An essential role of Th1 responses and interferon gamma in infection-mediated suppression of neoplastic growth. *Cancer Biol. Ther.* **2**: 687-693.

Razzaque, A. *et al.* (1993). Neoplastic transformation of immortalized. human epidermal keratinocytes by two HHV-6 DNA clones. *Virology* **195**: 113-120.

Reuther, J.Y. *et al.* (1998). A requirement for NF-κB activation in Bcr-Abl-mediated transformation. *Genes Dev.* **12**: 968-981.

Robl, M.G. and Olson, C. (1968). Oncogenic action of bovine papilloma virus in hamsters. *Cancer Res.* **28**: 1596-1604.

Rosenberg, N. (2001). New transformation tricks from a barnyard retrovirus: implications for human lung cancer. *Proc. Natl Acad. Sci. U.S.A.* **98**: 4285-4287.

Ruscetti, S.K. (1999). Deregulation of erythropoiesis by the Friend spleen focus-forming virus. *Int. J. Biochem. Cell Biol.* **31**: 1089-1109.

Rygaard, J. and Povlsen, C.O. (1976). The nude mouse vs the hypothesis of immunological surveillance. *Transplant. Rev.* **28**: 43-61.

Sachs, L. and Medina, D. (1961). *In vitro* transformation of normal cells by polyoma virus. *Nature* **189**: 457-458.

Safak, M. and Khalili, K. (2003). An overview: Human polyomavirus JC virus and its associated disorders. *J. Neurovirol.* **9**: 3-9.

Schat, K.A. *et al.* (1991). Transformation of T-lymphocyte subsets by Marek's disease herpesvirus. *J. Virol.* **65**: 1408-1413.

Schat, K.A. and Markowski-Grimsrud, C.J. (2001). Immune responses to Marek's disease virus infection. *Curr. Top. Microbiol. Immunol.* **255**: 91-120.

Scherneck, S. *et al.* (2001). The hamster polyomavirus - a brief review of recent knowledge. *Virus Genes* **22**: 93-101.

Schmitt, C.A. *et al.* (1999). INK4a/ARF mutations accelerate lymphomagenesis and promote chemoresistance by disabling p53. *Genes Dev.* **13**: 2670-2677.

Schumacher, K. *et al.* (2001). Prognostic significance of activated CD8(+) T cell infiltrations within esophageal carcinomas. *Cancer Res.* **61**: 3932-3936.

Segal, E.D. *et al.* (1999). Altered states: involvement of phosphorylated CagA in the induction of host cellular growth changes by *Helicobacter pylori*. *Proc. Natl Acad. Sci. U.S.A.* **96**: 14559-14564.

Sgadari, C. *et al.* (1997). Mig, the monokine induced by interferon-gamma, promotes tumor necrosis *in vivo*. *Blood* **89**: 2635-2643.

Shankaran, V. *et al.* (2001). IFN gamma and lymphocytes prevent primary tumour development and shape tumour immunogenicity. *Nature* **410**: 1107-1111.

Shore, S.K. *et al.* (2002). Transforming pathways activated by the v-Abl tyrosine kinase. *Oncogene* **21**: 8568-8576.

Sidky, Y.A. and Borden, E.C. (1987). Inhibition of angiogenesis by interferons: effects on tumor- and lymphocyte-induced vascular responses. *Cancer Res.* **47**: 5155-5161.

Singh, R.K. *et al.* (1995). Interferons α and β down-regulate the expression of basic fibroblast growth factor in human carcinomas. *Proc. Natl Acad. Sci. U.S.A.* **92**: 4562-4566.

Singh, R.K. *et al.* (1996). Interferon-β prevents the upregulation of interleukin-8 expression in human melanoma cells. *J. Interferon Cytokine Res.* **16**: 577-584.

Small, J.A. *et al.* (1986). Early regions of JC virus and BK virus induce distinct and tissue-specific tumors in transgenic mice. *Proc. Natl Acad. Sci. U.S.A.* **83**: 8288-8292.

Small, M.B. *et al.* (1987). Neoplastic transformation by the human gene N-myc. *Mol. Cell. Biol.* **7**: 1638-1645.

Stark, G.R. *et al.* (1998). How cells respond to interferons. *Ann. Rev. Biochem.* **67**: 227-264.

Stehelin, D. *et al.* (1976). DNA related to the transforming gene(s) of avian sarcoma viruses is present in normal avian DNA. *Nature* **260**: 170-173.

Storey, A. *et al.* (1988). Comparison of the *in vitro* transforming activities of human papillomavirus types. *EMBO J.* **7**: 1815-1820.

Street, S.E. *et al.* (2001). Perforin and interferon-gamma activities independently control tumor initiation, growth, and metastasis. *Blood* **97**: 192-197.

Strieter, R.M. *et al.* (1995). Interferon gamma-inducible protein 10 (IP-10), a member of the C-X-C chemokine family, is an inhibitor of angiogenesis. *Biochem. Biophys. Res. Comm.* **210**: 51-57.

Stutman, O. (1974). Tumor development after 3-methylcholanthrene in immunologically deficient athymic-nude mice. *Science* **183**: 534-536.

Stutman, O. (1979). Chemical carcinogenesis in nude mice: comparison between nude mice from homozygous matings and heterozygous matings and effect of age and carcinogen dose. *J. Natl Cancer Inst.* **62**: 353-358.

Sunderkotter, C. *et al.* (1994). Macrophages and angiogenesis. *J. Leukoc. Biol.* **55**: 410-422.

Suprynowicz, F.A. *et al.* (2005). Are transforming properties of the bovine papillomavirus E5 protein shared by E5 from high-risk human papillomavirus type 16? *Virology* **332**: 102-113.

Svoboda, J. (1986). Rous sarcoma virus. *Intervirology* **26**: 1-60.

Thomas-Tikhonenko, A. and Hunter, C.A. (2003). Infection and cancer: the common vein. *Cytokine Growth Factor Rev.* **14**: 67-77.

Thomas-Tikhonenko, A. *et al.* (2004). Myc-transformed epithelial cells down-regulate clusterin which inhibits their growth *in vitro* and carcinogenesis *in vivo*. *Cancer Res* **64**: 3126-3136.

Thurston, G. *et al.* (1996). Permeability-related changes revealed at endothelial cell borders in inflamed venules by lectin binding. *Amer. J. Physiol.* **271**: H2547-H2562.

Tikhonenko, A.T. and Linial, M. (1993). Transforming variants of the avian myc-containing retrovirus FH3 arise prior to phenotypic selection. *J. Virol.* **67**: 3635-3638.

Tikhonenko, A.T. and Linial, M. (1992). gag as well as myc sequences contribute to the transforming phenotype of the avian retrovirus FH3. *J. Virol.* **66**: 946-955.

Tindle, R.W. (2002). Immune evasion in human papillomavirus-associated cervical cancer. *Nat. Rev. Cancer* **2**: 59-65.

Todaro, G.J. and Green, H. (1966). High frequency of SV40 transformation of mouse cell line 3T3. *Virology* **28**: 756-759.

Todaro, G.J. *et al.* (1966). Susceptibility of human diploid fibroblast strains to transformation by SV40 virus. *Science* **153**: 1252-1254.

Tooze, J. (editor), (1979). DNA tumor viruses. Cold Spring Harbor Laboratory Press, Cold Spring Harbor, NY.

Tsutsumi, R. *et al.* (2003). Attenuation of Helicobacter pylori CagA x SHP-2 signaling by interaction between CagA and C-terminal Src kinase. *J. Biol. Chem.* **278**: 3664-3670.

Ueda, H. *et al.* (1995). Functional inactivation but not structural mutation of p53 causes liver cancer. *Nat. Genet.* **9**: 41-47.

Uemura, N. *et al.* (2001). *Helicobacter pylori* infection and the development of gastric cancer. *N. Engl. J. Med.* **345**: 784-789.

Vakkila, J. and Lotze, M.T. (2004). Inflammation and necrosis promote tumour growth. *Nat. Rev. Immunol.* **4**: 641-648.

van den Broek, M.E. *et al.* (1996). Decreased tumor surveillance in perforin-deficient mice. *J. Exp. Med.* **184**: 1781-1790.

Venugopal, K. (2000). Marek's disease: an update on oncogenic mechanisms and control. *Res. Vet. Sci.* **69**: 17-23.

Vermeulen, P.B. *et al.* (1997). Serum basic fibroblast growth factor and vascular endothelial growth factor in metastatic renal cell carcinoma treated with interferon alfa-2b. *J. Natl. Cancer Inst.* **89**: 1316-1317.

Vicari, A.P. and Caux, C. (2002). Chemokines in cancer. *Cytokine & Growth Factor Rev* **13**: 143-154.

Wang, D. *et al.* (1985). An EBV membrane protein expressed in immortalized lymphocytes transforms established rodent cells. *Cell* **43**: 831-840.

Wang, J. *et al.* (1998). Myc activates telomerase. *Genes Dev.* **12**: 1769-1774.

Wang, X.W. *et al.* (1994). Hepatitis B virus X protein inhibits p53 sequence-specific DNA binding, transcriptional activity, and association with transcription factor ERCC3. *Proc. Natl Acad. Sci. U.S.A.* **91**: 2230-2234.

Wang, X.W. *et al.* (1995). Abrogation of p53-induced apoptosis by the hepatitis B virus X gene. *Cancer Res.* **55**: 6012-6016.

Weiskirch, L.M. and Paterson, Y. (1997). *Listeria monocytogenes*: a potent vaccine vector for neoplastic and infectious disease. *Immunol. Rev.* **158**: 159-169.

Weiss R. *et al.* (editors) (1984). RNA tumor viruses. Cold Spring Harbor Laboratory Press, Cold Spring Harbor, NY

Weissenberger, J. *et al.* (1997). Development and malignant progression of astrocytomas in GFAP-v-src transgenic mice. *Oncogene* **14**: 2005-2013.

White, M.K. and Khalili, K. (2004). Polyomaviruses and human cancer: molecular mechanisms underlying patterns of tumorigenesis. *Virology* **324**: 1-16.

Wilhelmsen, K.C. *et al.* (1984). Nucleic acid sequences of the oncogene v-rel in reticuloendotheliosis virus strain T and its cellular homolog, the proto-oncogene c-rel. *J. Virol.* **52**: 172-182.

Wilson, J.B. *et al.* (1996). Expression of Epstein-Barr virus nuclear antigen-1 induces B cell neoplasia in transgenic mice. *EMBO J.* **15**: 3117-3126.

Wootton, S.K. *et al.* (2005). Sheep retrovirus structural protein induces lung tumours. *Nature* **434**: 904-907.

Xie, K. and Fidler, I.J. (1998). Therapy of cancer metastasis by activation of the inducible nitric oxide synthase. *Cancer Metast. Rev.* **17**: 55-75.

Youdim, S. and Sharman, M. (1976). Resistance to tumor growth mediated by Listeria monocytogenes: collaborative and suppressive macrophage-lymphocyte interactions *in vitro*. *J.Immunol.* **117**: 1860-1865.

Young, L.S. and Rickinson, A.B. (2004). Epstein-Barr virus: 40 years on. *Nat. Rev. Cancer* **4**: 757-768.

Yu, D. and Thomas-Tikhonenko, A. (2002). A non-transgenic mouse model for B-cell lymphoma: *in vivo* infection of p53-null bone marrow progenitors by a Myc retrovirus is sufficient for tumorigenesis. *Oncogene* **21**: 1922-1927.

Zajac, A.J. *et al.* (1998). Viral immune evasion due to persistence of activated T cells without effector function. *J. Exp. Med.* **188**: 2205-2213.

Zhang, L. *et al.* (2003). Intratumoral T cells, recurrence, and survival in epithelial ovarian cancer. *N. Engl. J. Med.* **348**: 203-213.

Zilber, L.A. (1961a). On interaction between tumor viruses and cells - a virogenetic concept of tumorigenesis. *J. Natl Cancer Inst.* **26**: 1311-&.

Zilber, L.A. (1961b). Pathogenicity of Rous sarcoma virus for rats and rabbits. *J. Natl Cancer Inst.* **26**: 1295-1309.

Zinkernagel, R.M. *et al.* (1999). General and specific immunosuppression caused by antiviral T-cell responses. *Immunol. Rev.* **168**: 305-315.

zur Hausen, H. (2003). SV40 in human cancers - an endless tale? *Int. J. Cancer* **107**: 687.

# Chapter 9

# CYTOKINES AS MEDIATORS AND TARGETS FOR CANCER CACHEXIA

Josep M. Argilés, Sílvia Busquets and Francisco J. López-Soriano
*Departament de Bioquímica i Biologia Molecular, Facultat de Biologia, Universitat de Barcelona, Barcelona, Spain.*

Abstract:      The cachexia syndrome, characterized by a marked weight loss, anorexia, asthenia and anaemia, is invariably associated with the growth of a tumour and leads to a malnutrition status caused by the induction of anorexia or decreased food intake. In addition, the competition for nutrients between the tumour and the host results in a state of accelerated catabolism, which promotes severe metabolic disturbances in the patient. The search for the cachectic factor(s) started a long time ago, and many scientific and economic efforts have been devoted to its discovery, but we are still a long way from a complete answer. The present review aims to evaluate the different molecular mechanisms and catabolic mediators (both humoural and tumoural) that are involved in cancer cachexia and to discuss their potential as targets for future clinical investigations.

Keywords:      cytokines; tumour-derived factors; transcriptional factors; therapeutic strategies.

# 1.     INTRODUCTION

The cachectic syndrome, characterized by a marked weight loss, anorexia, asthenia and anaemia, is often associated with the presence and growth of a tumour and leads to a status of malnutrition due to the induction of anorexia or decreased food intake. In addition, the competition for nutrients between the tumour and the host leads to accelerated starvation which promotes severe metabolic disturbances in the host, including hypermetabolism, which leads to decreased energetic efficiency. Although the search for the cachectic factor(s) started a long time ago, and although many scientific and economic efforts have been devoted to its discovery, we are still a long way from knowing the whole truth.

Perhaps the most common manifestation of advanced malignant disease is the development of cancer cachexia. Indeed, cachexia occurs in the majority of cancer patients before death, and it is responsible for the deaths of 22% of cancer sufferers. Abnormalities associated with cancer cachexia include anorexia, weight loss, muscle loss and atrophy, anaemia and alterations in carbohydrate, lipid and protein metabolism (see Fearon and Moses, 2002 and Costelli and Baccino, 2000 for reviews). The degree of cachexia is inversely correlated with the survival time of the patient and the condition always implies a poor prognosis.

The aim of the present chapter is to summarize and update the role of catabolic mediators (cytokines and tumour-derived factors) in cancer cachexia since research based on these compounds may be of great relevance to future clinical investigations.

# 2.     CYTOKINES AS MEDIATORS

Cytokines have a key role as the main humoural factors involved in cancer cachexia. Thus a large number of them may be responsible for the metabolic changes associated with the cancer wasting syndrome (Figure 1). Anorexia may play an important role by accounting for malnutrition, invariably associated with cancer cachexia. But are cytokines involved in the induction of anorexia? Cytokines such as interleukin-1 (IL-1) and tumour necrosis factor-$\alpha$ (TNF) have been suggested as involved in cancer-related anorexia, possibly by increasing the levels of corticotropin-releasing hormone (CRH), a central nervous system neurotransmitter that suppresses food intake and the firing of glucose-sensitive neurons, which would also decrease food intake. However, many other mediators have been suggested as involved in cancer-induced anorexia. Leptin (an adiposity signal to the hypothalamus that is a member of the cytokine family) does not seem to play a role, at least in experimental models (López-Soriano *et al.*, 1999; Sato *et al.*, 2002). In human subjects, cancer anorexia does not seem to be due to dysregulation of leptin production (Kowalczuk *et al.*, 2001). Indeed, leptin concentrations are not elevated in cancer patients losing weight (Tessitore *et*

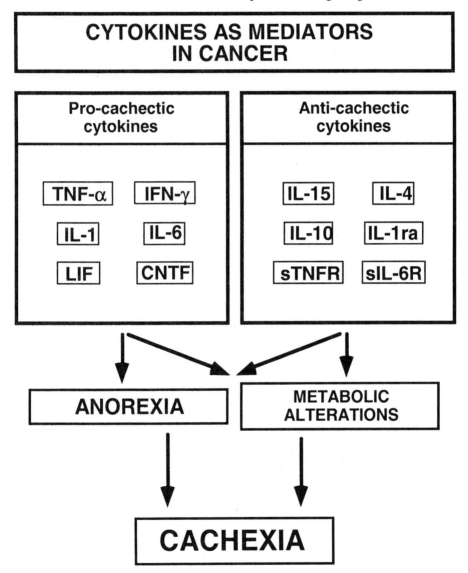

*Figure 1.* Cytokines as catabolic mediators in cancer. Both pro-cachectic and anti-cachectic cytokines are involved in mediating anorexia and metabolic changes characteristic of the cachectic state.

*al.*, 2000; Brown *et al.*, 2001) and are inversely related to the intensity of the inflammatory response (Aleman *et al.*, 2002) as well as the levels of pro-inflammatory cytokines (Mantovani *et al.*, 2000 and 2001). The concentrations of the peptide seem to be dependent only on the total amount of adipose tissue present in the patient. Cytokines can have a role in cancer-induced anorexia since they modulate gastric motility and emptying, either directly in the gastrointestinal system or via the brain, by altering efferent signals that regulate satiety. IL-1, in particular, has been clearly associated with the induction of anorexia (Plata-Salaman, 2000), by blocking neuropeptide Y (NPY)-induced feeding. The levels of this molecule (a feeding-stimulating peptide) are reduced in anorectic tumour-bearing rats (Chance *et al.*, 1994) and a correlation between food intake and brain-IL-1 has been found in anorectic rats with cancer. The mechanism involved in the attenuation of NPY activity by cytokines may be related to an inhibition of cell firing rates, to an inhibition of NPY synthesis or an attenuation of its postsynaptic effects (King *et al.*, 2000). Other mediators have been proposed (Laviano *et al.*, 2002) including changes in the circulating levels of free tryptophan. These may induce changes in serotonin brain concentrations and, consequently, cause changes in food intake. Bing *et al.* (2001) have also suggested that some tumour-derived compounds may induce the anorexia associated with tumour burden.

Different experimental approaches have demonstrated that cytokines are able to stimulate weight loss. Nevertheless, the results obtained have to be carefully interpreted. Thus, episodic TNF administration has proved unsuccessful at inducing cachexia in experimental animals. Indeed, repetitive TNF administrations initially induce a cachectic effect, although tolerance to the cytokine soon develops and food intake and body weight return to normal. Other studies have shown that escalating doses of TNF are necessary to maintain the cachectic effects. In an elegant experiment, Oliff *et al.* (1987), after transfecting the human TNF gene in CHO cells that were later implanted in *nude* mice, clearly showed that the expression and release of the cytokine leads to a massive body weight loss that is characterized by profound anorexia.

Strassman *et al.* (1993) have shown that treatment with an anti-mouse interleukin-6 (IL-6) antibody can reverse the key parameters of cachexia in murine colon adenocarcinoma tumour-bearing mice. These results seem to indicate that, at least in certain types of tumours, IL-6 could have a more direct involvement than TNF in the cachectic state. Similar results were obtained in a mouse model that reproduces the cachexia associated with multiple myeloma (Barton *et al.*, 2000; Barton and Murphy, 2001) and in a murine model of intracerebral injection of human tumours (Negri *et al.*, 2001). Conversely, studies using incubated rat skeletal muscle have clearly shown that IL-6 has no direct effect on muscle proteolysis (García-Martínez *et al.*, 1994).

Another interesting candidate for a cachexia inducer is interferon-γ (IFN-γ), which is produced by activated T and NK cells and possesses biological activities that overlap with those of TNF. Matthys *et al.* (1991), using a monoclonal antibody against IFN-γ, were able to reverse the wasting syndrome associated with the growth of the Lewis lung carcinoma in mice, thus indicating that endogenous production of IFN-γ occurs in the tumour-bearing mice and is instrumental in bringing about some of the metabolic changes characteristic of cancer cachexia. The same group has also demonstrated that severe cachexia develops rapidly in nude mice inoculated with CHO cells constitutively producing IFN-γ, as a result of the transfection of the corresponding gene.

Other cytokines, such as the leukemia inhibitory factor (LIF), transforming growth factor-β (TGF-β) or IL-1 have also been suggested as mediators of cachexia. Thus, mice engrafted with tumours secreting LIF develop severe cachexia. Concerning IL-1, although its anorectic and pyrogenic effects are well-known, administration of IL-1 receptor antagonist (IL-1ra) to tumour-bearing rats did not result in any improvement in the degree of cachexia, thus suggesting that its role in cancer cachexia may be secondary to the actions of other mediators. Interestingly the levels of both IL-6 and LIF have been shown to be increased in patients with different types of malignancies.

Cyliary neurotrophic factor (CNTF) is a member of the family of cytokines which include IL-6 and LIF and which is produced predominantly by glial cells of the peripheral nervous system; however, this cytokine also seems to be expressed in skeletal muscle. Henderson *et al.* (1996) have demonstrated that CNTF induces potent cachectic effects and acute-phase proteins (independent of the induction of other cytokine family members) in mice implanted with C6 glioma cells, genetically modified to secrete this cytokine. The cytokine, however, exerted divergent direct effects dependent on the dose and the time of exposure on *in vitro* muscle preparations (Wang and Forsberg, 2000).

If anorexia is not the only factor involved in cancer cachexia, it becomes clear that metabolic abnormalities leading to a hypermetabolic state must have a very important role. Interestingly, injection of low doses of TNF either peripherally or into the brain of laboratory animals elicits rapid increases in metabolic rate which are not associated with increased metabolic activity but rather with an increase in blood flow and thermogenic activity associated with uncoupling protein (UCP1) of brown adipose tissue (BAT). Interestingly, during cachectic states, there is an increase in BAT thermogenesis both in humans and experimental animals. Until recently, the

UCP1 protein (present only in BAT) was considered to be the only mitochondrial protein carrier that stimulates heat production by dissipating the proton gradient generated during respiration across the inner mitochondrial membrane and therefore uncoupling respiration from ATP synthesis. Interestingly, two additional proteins sharing the same function, UCP2 and UCP3, have been described. While UCP2 is expressed ubiquitously, UCP3 is expressed abundantly and specifically in skeletal muscle in humans and also in BAT of rodents. Our research group has demonstrated that both UCP2 and UCP3 mRNAs are elevated in skeletal muscle during tumour growth and that TNF is able to mimic the increase in gene expression (Busquets *et al.*, 1998). In addition, TNF is able to induce uncoupling of mitochondrial respiration as recently shown in isolated mitochondria (Busquets *et al.*, 2003).

Several cytokines have been shown to mimic many of the metabolic abnormalities found in cancer patients during cachexia. Among these metabolic disturbances, changes in lipid metabolism, skeletal muscle proteolysis and apoptosis as well as acute-phase protein synthesis have been described (see Argilés and López-Soriano, 1998 for a review). Concerning muscle wasting, it seems that administration of TNF to rats results in increased skeletal muscle proteolysis associated with an increase in both gene expression and higher levels of free and conjugated ubiquitin, both in experimental animals and humans (Baracos, 2000). In addition, the *in vivo* action of TNF during cancer cachexia does not seem to be mediated by IL-1 or glucocorticoids. Other cytokines such as IL-1 or IFN-γ are also able to activate ubiquitin gene expression. Therefore, TNF, alone or in combination with other cytokines (Alvarez *et al.*, 2002), seems to mediate most of the changes concerning nitrogen metabolism associated with cachectic states. In addition to the massive muscle protein loss during cancer cachexia, similar to that observed in skeletal muscle of chronic heart failure patients suffering from cardiac cachexia (Sharma and Anker, 2002), muscle DNA is also decreased, leading to DNA fragmentation and consequently apoptosis (Van Royen *et al.*, 2000; Belizario *et al.*, 2001). Interestingly, TNF can mimic the apoptotic response in muscle of healthy animals (Carbó *et al.*, 2002).

## 3. OTHER MEDIATORS: TUMOUR-DERIVED FACTORS

In addition to humoural factors, tumour-derived molecules have also been suggested as mediators of cancer cachexia. Firstly, cancer cells are capable of producing cytokines constitutively. These cytokines may act on the cancer cells in an autocrine manner or on the supporting tissues such as fibroblasts and blood vessels to produce an environment conducive to cancer growth (Dunlop and Campbell, 2000). In addition to tumour-produced cytokines, which may have a more important role in the anorexia-cachexia syndrome than those produced by the host (Cahlin *et al.*, 2000), several compounds have been reported to have an important role in mimicking the metabolic changes associated with the cachectic state.

The first evidence of tumour-derived catabolic factors came from studies with Krebs-2 carcinoma cells in mice. Inactive extracts of these cells were able to induce cachexia once injected in normal non-tumour-bearing mice (Costa and Holland, 1966). Similarly, Kitada *et al.* (1981) purified a low molecular weight proteinaceous material from extracts of thymic lymphoma in AKR mice that showed lipolytic activity in rat adipocyte suspensions. Thus, extracts of thymic lymphoma, conditioned medium from thymic lymphoma cell lines, and serum from lymphoma-bearing mice, caused lipid mobilization in experimental animals. Toxohormone L, a polypeptide of approximately 75 kD, was isolated from the ascites fluid of patients with hepatoma as well as sarcoma-bearing mice (Masuno *et al.*, 1981). It induces lipid mobilization, immunosuppression and involution of the thymus.

Tisdale's group at Aston University have described and characterized a lipid-metabolizing factor (LMF) which is able to induce lipolysis in adipose tissue, this being associated with stimulation of adenylate cyclase activity (Khan and Tisdale, 1999). This factor was originally purified from a cachexia-inducing mouse colon adenocarcinoma (MAC16), but it has also been found in the urine of cancer patients, suggesting that it is able to induce lipid mobilization and catabolism in cachectic cancer patients (Hirai *et al.*, 1998). In fact, LMF is homologous to the plasma protease Zn-alpha2-glycoprotein (ZAG) in amino acid sequence, electrophoretic mobility and immunoreactivity. The 2.8 Å cristal structure of ZAG resembles a class I major histocompatibility complex (MHC) heavy chain although it does not bind class I light chain beta2-microglobulin. The ZAG structure includes a large groove analogous to class I MHC peptide binding grooves. Instead of a peptide, the ZAG groove contains a nonpeptidic compound that may be implicated in lipid metabolism under pathological conditions. Hirai *et al.* (1997) also suggest that LMF can have a role in initiating hepatic glycogenolysis during experimental cancer cachexia through an increase in cyclic AMP in liver.

Anemia-inducing factor (AIS) is a protein of approximately 50 kD, secreted by malignant tumour tissues, that depresses erythrocyte and immunocompetent cell functions. AIS is able to reduce food intake as well as an increase in body weight and body fat in rabbits. In addition, it shows an important lipolytic activity (Ishiko *et al.*, 1999).

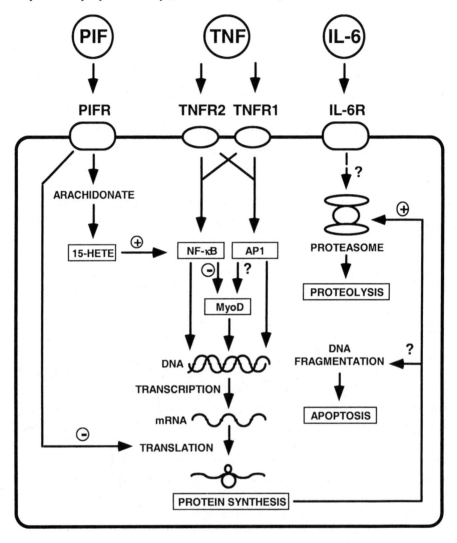

*Figure 2.* Interactions between pro-inflamatory cytokines and PIF. Both humoral (TNF and IL-6) and tumoural (PIF) factors have been shown to be able to activate intracellular muscle proteolysis by different mechanisms, possibly sharing common pathways.

Todorov *et al.* (1996) have purified and characterized a 24 kD proteoglycan, present both in experimental animals (Lorite *et al.*, 1997) and in the urine of cachectic patients (Wigmore *et al.*, 2000), which seems to account for increased muscle protein degradation and decreased protein synthesis (Lorite *et al.*, 1997). This compound, known as PIF (proteolysis-inducing factor), is able to activate protein degradation specifically through stimulation of the ATP/proteasome-dependent pathway (Lorite *et al.*, 1998). The compound, when injected into healthy animals, is able to mimic the muscle wasting associated with experimental cancer cachexia. *In vitro* studies on C2C12 myoblasts have shown that eicosapentaenoic acid (EPA) is able to block PIF action on proteolysis in addition to suggesting that PIF acts intracellularly via the arachidonate metabolite 15-hydroxyeicosatetraenoic acid (15-HETE) (Smith *et al.*, 1999). In addition, PIF is able to increase NF-κB expression in cultured cells (M. Tisdale, personal communication) (Fig. 2). In conclusion, PIF may have a constitutive role in normal states and become altered or overproduced during cancer cachexia. Therefore, it may induce important effects in both muscle protein catabolism and acute phase proteins (APP) synthesis in this pathological state.

# 4.    INTRACELLULAR SIGNALING

At the moment, there are few studies describing the involvement of different transcription factors in muscle wasting. Penner *et al.* (2001) reported an increase in both NF-κB and AP-1 during sepsis in experimental animals. Recent data from our laboratory do not support an involvement of NF-κB in skeletal muscle during cancer cachexia (unpublished data). However, tumour burden results in a significant increase in the binding activity of AP-1. Interestingly, inhibition of NF-κB (Busquets *et al.*, 2001) is not able to revert muscle wasting in cachectic tumour-bearing animals. However, inhibition of AP-1 results in a partial reversal of protein degradation in skeletal muscle associated with tumour growth (Moore-Carrasco *et al.*, unpublished data). The increase in NF-κB observed in skeletal muscle during sepsis can be mimicked by TNF. Indeed TNF addition to C2C12 muscle cultures results in a short-term increase in NF-κB (Fernández-Celemin *et al.*, 2002; Li *et al.*, 1998). Whether or not this increase in NF-κB promoted by TNF is associated with increased proteolysis and/or increased apoptosis in skeletal muscle remains to be established. In relation with AP-1 activation, TNF has been shown to increase *c-jun* expression in C2C12 cells (Brenner *et al.*, 1989). Interestingly, overexpression of *c-jun* mimics the observed effect of TNF upon differentiation. Indeed, it results in decreased myoblast differentiation

(Thinakaran *et al.*, 1993). Tumour mediators, PIF in particular, also seem to be able to increase NF-κB expression in cultured muscle cells, this possibly being linked with increased proteolysis (M. Tisdale, personal communication) (Figure 2). Other transcription factors that have been reported to be involved in muscle changes associated with catabolic conditions include c/EBPβ and δ, which are increased in skeletal muscle during sepsis (Penner *et al.*, 2002), PW-1 and PGC-1. TNF decreases MyoD content in cultured myoblasts (Guttridge *et al.*, 2000) and blocks differentiation by a mechanism which seems to be independent of NF-κB and which involves PW-1, a transcriptional factor related to p53-induced apoptosis (Coletti *et al.*, 2002). The action of the cytokines on muscle cells, therefore, seems to rely most likely on satellite cells blocking muscle differentiation or, in other words, regeneration.

Finally the transcription factor PGC-1 has been associated with the activation of UCP-2 and UCP-3 as well as increased oxygen consumption by cytokines in cultured myotubes (Puigserver *et al.*, 2001). This transcription factor is involved as an activator of PPAR-γ in the expression of uncoupling proteins.

## 5. CYTOKINES AS TARGETS

Bearing in mind the fact that both anorexia and metabolic disturbances are involved in cancer cachexia, the development of different therapeutic strategies has focused on these two factors. Unfortunately, counteracting anorexia either pharmacologically or nutritionally has led to rather disappointing results in the treatment of cancer cachexia. It is basically for this reason that the strategies mentioned below rely on neutralizing the metabolic changes induced by the tumour, which are ultimately responsible for the weight loss. Therefore, taking into account the involvement of cytokines in cachexia, different therapeutic strategies have been based on either blocking their synthesis or action.

As previously mentioned, the cytokines that have been implicated in this cachectic response are TNF, IL-1, IL-6 and IFN-γ. Interestingly, these cytokines share the same metabolic effects and their activities are closely interrelated. In many cases, these cytokines exhibit synergic effects when administered together (Evans *et al.*, 1989). Therefore, therapeutic strategies have been based on either blocking their synthesis or their action (Yamamoto *et al.*, 1998).

# 5.1 Blocking synthesis

### 5.1.1 Pentoxifylline

Pentoxifylline (Figure 3), a methylxantine derivative, is a phosphodiesterase inhibitor that inhibits TNF synthesis by decreasing gene transcription. This drug was originally used for the treatment of various types of vascular insufficiency because of its haemorheological activity, thought to be based on its ability to reduce blood viscosity and increase the filterability of blood cells. While several studies using animal models suggest that pentoxifylline is able to decrease the cytokine-induced toxicity of antineoplasic agents while preserving antitumour treatment efficacy (Balazs and Kiss, 1994), clinical studies have shown that the drug failed to improve appetite or to increase the weight of cachectic patients (Goldberg *et al.*, 1995). In addition, pentoxifylline has also been used in the treatment of cachectic AIDS patients with very poor results since it did not influence the weight of the subjects (Dezube *et al.*, 1993). In fact, the patients frequently reported gastrointestinal side effects. However, the reported clinical trials have been relatively small and, therefore, larger randomized studies are necessary to assess the efficacy of pentoxifylline in the treatment of cancer cachexia.

### 5.1.2 Rolipram

Rolipram (Figure 3) is a type IV phosphodiesterase inhibitor that has been shown to decrease TNF production by LPS-stimulated human monocytes (Semmler *et al.*, 1993). This compound has previously been used in the treatment of endogenous depression in both animals and man, and it may have therapeutic activity in disease states where TNF seems to play a role in the pathogenesis, such as in endotoxic shock (Badger *et al.*, 1994).

### 5.1.3 Thalidomide

Thalidomide ($\alpha$-N-phthalimidoglutaramide) (Figure 3) is a drug unfortunately associated with tragedy. Indeed, its use as a sedative in pregnant women caused over 10,000 cases of severe malformations in newborn children. However, a certain revival has affected the drug since it has been demonstrated to suppress TNF production in monocytes *in vitro* (Sampaio *et al.*, 1991) and to normalize elevated TNF levels *in vivo* (Sampaio *et al.*, 1993). Apparently thalidomide activity is due to a selective destabilization of TNF mRNA (Moreira *et al.*, 1993). The drug has successfully been used to counteract high cytokine levels in tuberculosis patients (Klausner *et al.*, 1996). A significant improvement in quality of life and weight gain occurs in AIDS patients given relatively low doses of

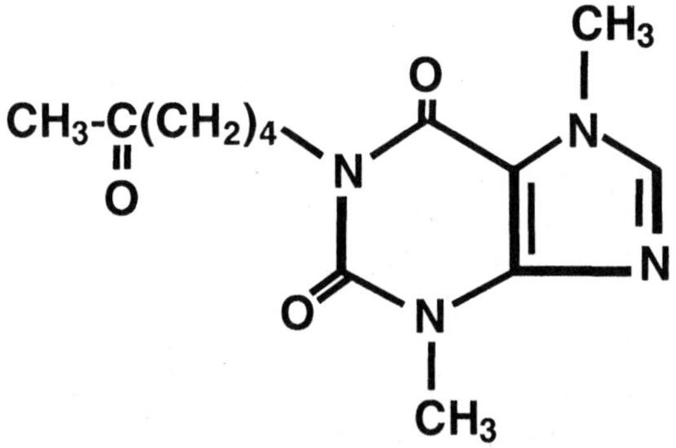

**PENTOXIFYLLINE**

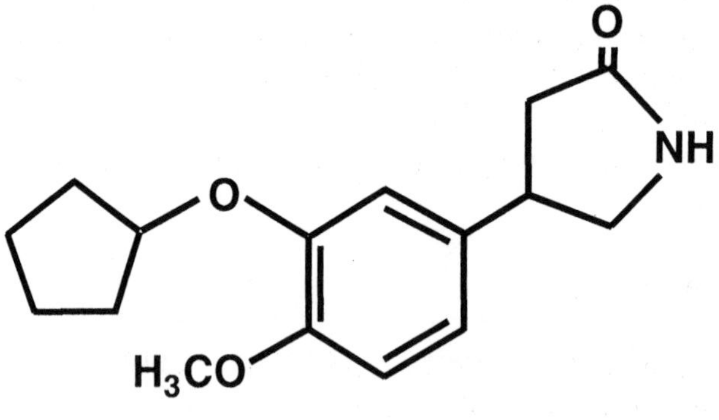

**ROLIPRAM**

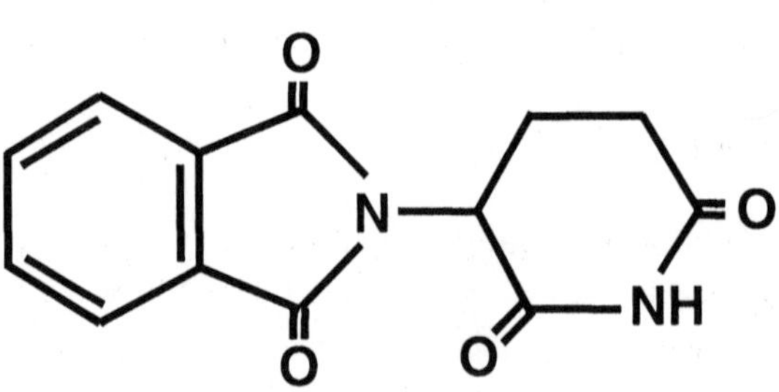

**THALIDOMIDE**

*Figure 3.* Chemical structures of some of the compounds used to treat cachexia based on cytokines.

thalidomide (Klausner *et al.*, 1996). Its usefulness in the treatment of cancer cachexia remains to be established, but it could potentially have a certain role in counteracting TNF-mediated metabolic changes. In addition, thalidomide therapy has been shown to improve insomnia and restlessness as well as nausea in advanced cancer patients, and it has improved appetite as well, resulting in an enhanced feeling of well-being in one-half to two-thirds of patients studied (Bruera *et al.*, 1999). Indeed, a recent pilot study carried out in 10 patients affected by oesophageal cancer revealed that thalidomide was able to reverse the loss of weight and lean body mass over a 2-week trial period (Khan *et al.*, 2003). In chronic heart failure, a recent study shows that thalidomide is able, in addition to decreasing TNF levels, to increase cardiac performance (Gullestad *et al.*, 2002).

### 5.1.4 Blocking action

#### 5.1.4.1 Antibodies and soluble receptors

The use of anti-cytokine antibodies (either mono or polyclonal) and cytokine receptor antagonists or soluble receptors has led to very interesting results. Thus, in rats bearing the Yoshida AH-130 ascites hepatoma (a highly cachectic tumour) anti-TNF therapy resulted in a partial reversal of the abnormalities associated with both lipid (Carbó *et al.*, 1994) and protein metabolism (Costelli *et al.*, 1993). In humans, however, clinical trials using anti-TNF treatment have led to poor results in reverting the protein waste associated with sepsis (Reinhart *et al.*, 1996). Concerning chronic heart failure, several clinical trials involving anti-TNF strategies, such as etanercept (soluble TNF receptor) or infliximab (monoclonal antibody against TNF) have led to poor results in the clinical output of the patients (Anker and Coats, 2002). Concerning IL-6, experimental models have proven that the use of antibodies is highly effective in preventing tumour-induced waste (Yasumoto *et al.*, 1995). Strassman *et al.* (1993) have demonstrated that the experimental drug suramine (which prevents the binding of IL-6 to its cell surface receptor, as demonstrated by radioreceptor-binding assays and affinity binding experiments) partially blocks (up to 60%) the catabolic effects associated with the growth of colon-26 adenocarcinoma in mice. In humans, administration of an anti-IL-6 monoclonal antibody to patients with AIDS, and suffering from an immunoblastic or a polymorphic large-cell lymphoma, resulted in a very positive effect on fever and cachexia (Emilie *et al.*, 1994). Concerning other cytokines, anti-IFN-γ therapy has also been effective in reverting cachexia in mice bearing Lewis lung carcinoma (Matthys *et al.*, 1991) but there is a lack of clinical data. On the other hand, blocking IL-1 actions by means of the IL-

1 receptor antagonist (IL-1ra) in tumour-bearing rats had no effect on either body weight or reversal of metabolic changes (Costelli *et al.*, 1995).

It has to be pointed out here that routine use of anti-cytokine antibodies is, at present, too expensive due to the fact that this type of therapy requires a very large number of antibody molecules in order to block cytokine action completely.

### 5.1.4.2    Anti-inflammatory cytokines

The degree of the cachectic syndrome is dependent not only on the production of the above-mentioned cytokines, known as catabolic pro-inflammatory cytokines, but also on anti-inflammatory cytokines, such as IL-4, IL-10 and IL-12.

Mori *et al.* (1996) have demonstrated that the administration of IL-12 to mice bearing colon-26 carcinoma alleviates the body weight loss and other abnormalities associated with cachexia, such as adipose tissue wasting and hypoglycaemia. These anticachectic properties are seen at low doses of IL-12, insufficient to inhibit tumour growth. The effects of IL-12 seem to be dependent on a significant decrease of IL-6 (Mori *et al.*, 1996), a cytokine which is responsible for the cachexia associated with this tumour model (Tanaka *et al.*, 1990; Fujimoto-Ouchi *et al.*, 1995). A similar action has been described for INF-γ. Administration of this cytokine promoted a decrease in both IL-6 mRNA levels in the tumour and serum IL-6 levels, resulting in an amelioration of cachexia in murine model of malignant mesothelioma (Bielefeldt-Ohmann *et al.*, 1995).

Interleukin-15 (IL-15) has been reported to be an anabolic factor for skeletal muscle (Quinn *et al.*, 1995) and experiments carried out in our laboratory clearly demonstrate that the cytokine is able to reverse most of the abnormalities associated with cancer cachexia in a rat tumour model (Carbó *et al.*, 2000).

## 6.    INTERFERING WITH TRANSCRIPTION FACTORS

Concerning therapeutic strategies based on events related to transcription factors in muscle wasting, several points can be raised. First, Kawamura *et al.* (1999 and 2001) reported that the use of an oligonucleotide that competes with an NF-κB-binding site can revert cachexia in a mouse experimental model without affecting the growth of the primary tumour. This treatment, however, reduces metastasic capacity in the colon-26 adenocarcinoma model. In spite of this, administration of curcumin to tumour-bearing rats was unable to block muscle wasting. This suggests that

NF-κB is not involved in the cachectic response in this tumour model (Busquets *et al.*, 2001).

As we have previously said, AP-1 is clearly involved in muscle wasting during sepsis (Penner *et al.*, 2001) and also in cancer. Interestingly, administration of SP-100030 (Signal Pharmaceuticals, San Diego), an inhibitor of both NF-κB and AP-1, results in a partial blockade of muscle wasting in rats bearing the AH-130 Yoshida ascites hepatoma, a highly cachectic rat tumour (unpublished data).

## 7. CONCLUDING REMARKS

Because metabolic alterations often appear soon after the onset of tumour growth, appropriate treatment, although not aimed at achieving immediate eradication of the tumour mass, could influence the course of the patient's clinical state or, at least, prevent the steady erosion of dignity that the patient may feel in association with the syndrome. This would no doubt contribute to improving the patient's quality of life and, possibly, prolong survival. Although exploration of the role that cytokines play in the host response to invasive stimuli is an endeavour that has been underway for many years, considerable controversy still exists over the mechanisms of lean tissue and body fat dissolution that occur in patients with either cancer or inflammation and whether humoural factors regulate this process. A better understanding of the role of cytokines, both host and tumour-derived (Cahlin *et al.*, 2000), interfering with the molecular mechanisms accounting for protein wasting in skeletal muscle is essential for the design of future effective therapeutic strategies. In any case, understanding the humoural response to cancer and modifying cytokine actions pharmacologically may prove very suitable and no doubt future research will concentrate on this interesting field. Finally, understanding the intracellular signalling mechanisms, particulary transcription factors, may also be very important for the design of effective therapeutic approaches.

## 8. REFERENCES

Aleman, M.R. *et al.* (2002). Leptin role in advanced lung cancer. A mediator of the acute phase response or a marker of the status of nutrition? *Cytokine.* **19**: 21-26.

Alvarez, B. *et al.* (2002). Tumor necrosis factor-alpha exerts interleukin-6-dependent and - independent effects on cultured skeletal muscle cells. *Biochim. Biophys. Acta.* **1542**: 66-72.

Anker, S.D. and Coats, A.J. (2002). How to RECOVER from RENAISSANCE? The significance of the results of RECOVER, RENAISSANCE, RENEWAL and ATTACH. *Int. J. Cardiol.* **86**: 123-130.

Argilés, J.M. and López-Soriano, F.J. (1998). Catabolic proinflammatory cytokines. *Curr. Opin. Clin. Nutr. Metab. Care.* **1**: 245-251.

Badger, A.M. *et al.* (1994). Beneficial effects of the phosphodiesterase inhibitors BRL 61063, pentoxifylline, and rolipram in a murine model of endotoxin shock. *Circ. Shock* **44**: 188-195.

Balazs, C. and Kiss, E. (1994). Immunological aspects of the effect of pentoxifylline. *Acta Microbiol. Immunol. Hung.* **41**: 121-126.

Baracos, V.E. (2000). Regulation of skeletal-muscle-protein turnover in cancer-associated cachexia. *Nutrition.* **16**: 1015-1018.

Barton, B.E. *et al.* (2000). A model that reproduces syndromes associated with human multiple myeloma in nonirradiated SCID mice. *Proc. Soc. Exp. Biol. Med.* **223**: 190-197.

Barton, B.E. and Murphy, T.F. (2001). Cancer cachexia is mediated in part by the induction of IL-6-like cytokines from the spleen. *Cytokine.* **16**: 251-257.

Belizario, J.E. *et al.* (2001). Cleavage of caspases-1, -3, -6, -8 and -9 substrates by proteases in skeletal muscles from mice undergoing cancer cachexia. *Br. J. Cancer.* **84**: 1135-1140.

Bielefeldt-Ohmann, H. *et al.* (1995). Interleukin-6 involvement in mesothelioma pathobiology: inhibition by interferon alpha immunotherapy. *Cancer Immunol. Immunother.* **40**: 241-250.

Bing, C. *et al.* (2001). Cachexia in MAC16 adenocarcinoma: suppression of hunger despite normal regulation of leptin, insulin and hypothalamic neuropeptide Y. *J. Neurochem.* **79**: 1004-1012.

Brenner, D.A. *et al.* (1989). Prolonged activation of jun and collagenase genes by tumor necrosis factor-alpha. *Nature.* **337**: 661-663.

Brown, D.R. *et al.* (2001). Weight loss is not associated with hyperleptinemia in humans with pancreatic cancer. *J. Clin. Endocrinol. Metab.* **86**: 162-166.

Bruera, E. *et al.* (1999) Thalidomide in patients with cachexia due to terminal cancer: preliminary report. *Ann. Oncol.* **10**: 857-859.

Busquets, S. *et al.* (1998). In the rat, TNF-$\alpha$ administration results in an increase in both UCP2 and UCP3 mRNAs in skeletal muscle: a possible mechanism for cytokine-induced thermogenesis? *FEBS Lett.* **440**: 348-350.

Busquets, S. *et al.* (2001). Curcumin, a natural product present in turmeric, decreases tumor growth but does not behave as an anticachectic compound in a rat model. *Cancer Lett.* **167**: 33-38.

Busquets, S. *et al.* (2003). Tumour necrosis factor-alpha uncouples respiration in isolated rat mitochondria. *Cytokine.* **22**: 1-4.

Cahlin, C. *et al.* (2000). Experimental cancer cachexia: the role of host-derived cytokines interleukin (IL)-6, IL-12, interferon-gamma, and tumor necrosis factor alpha evaluated in gene knockout, tumor-bearing mice on C57 Bl background and eicosanoid-dependent cachexia. *Cancer Res.* **60**: 5488-5493.

Carbó, N. *et al.* (1994). Anti-tumour necrosis factor-alpha treatment interferes with changes in lipid metabolism in a tumour cachexia model. *Clin. Sci.* **87**: 349-355.

Carbó, N. *et al.* (2000). Interleukin-15 antagonizes muscle protein waste in tumour-bearing rats. *Br. J. Cancer.* **83**: 526-531.

Carbó, N. *et al.* (2002). TNF-$\alpha$ is involved in activating DNA fragmentation in murine skeletal muscle. *Br. J. Cancer.* **86**: 1012-1016.

Chance, W.T. *et al.* (1994). Hypothalamic concentration and release of neuropeptide Y into microdialysates is reduced in anorectic tumor-bearing rats. *Life Sci.* **54**: 1869-1874.

Coletti, D. *et al.* (2002). TNFalpha inhibits skeletal myogenesis through a PW1-dependent pathway by recruitment of caspase pathways. *EMBO J.* **21**: 631-642.

Costa, G. and Holland, J.F. (1966). Effects of Krebs-2 carcinoma on the lipid metabolism of male Swiss mice. *Cancer Res.* **22**: 1081-1083.

Costelli, P. *et al.* (1993). Tumor necrosis factor-alpha mediates changes in tissue protein turnover in a rat cancer cachexia model. *J. Clin. Invest.* **92**: 2783-2789.

Costelli, P. *et al.* (1995). Interleukin-1 receptor antagonist (IL-1ra) is unable to reverse cachexia in rats bearing an ascites hepatoma (Yoshida AH-130). *Cancer Lett.* **95**: 33-38.

Costelli, P. and Baccino, F.M. (2000). Cancer cachexia: from experimental models to patient management. *Curr. Opin. Clin. Nutr. Metab. Care.* **3**: 177-181.

Dezube, B.J. *et al.* (1993). Pentoxifylline decreases tumor necrosis factor expression and serum triglycerides in people with AIDS. NIAID AIDS Clinical Trials Group. *J. Acquir. Immune. Defic. Syndr.* **6**: 787-794.

Dunlop, R.J. and Campbell, C.W. (2000). Cytokines and advanced cancer. *J. Pain Symptom Manage.* **20**: 214-232.

Emilie, D. *et al.* (1994). Administration of an anti-interleukin-6 monoclonal antibody to patients with acquired immunodeficiency syndrome and lymphoma: effect on lymphoma growth and on B clinical symptoms. *Blood.* **84**: 2472-2479.

Evans, R.D. *et al.* (1989). Metabolic effects of tumour necrosis factor-alpha (cachectin) and interleukin-1. *Clin. Sci.* **77**: 357-364.

Fearon, K. and Moses, A. (2002). Cancer cachexia. *Int. J. Cardiol.* **85**: 73-81.

Fernandez-Celemin, L. *et al.* (2002). Inhibition of muscle insulin-like growth factor I expression by tumor necrosis factor-alpha. *Am. J. Physiol.* **283**: E1279-E1290.

Fujimoto-Ouchi, K. *et al.*. (1995). Establishment and characterization of cachexia inducing and non-inducing clones of murine colon 26 carcinoma. *Int. J. Cancer.* **61**: 522-528.

García-Martínez, C. *et al.* (1994). Interleukin-6 does not activate protein breakdown in rat skeletal muscle. *Cancer Lett.* **76**:1-4.

Goldberg, R.M. *et al.* (1995). Pentoxifylline for treatment of cancer anorexia and cachexia? A randomized, double-blind, placebo-controlled trial. *J. Clin. Oncol.* **13**: 2856-2859.

Gullestad, L. *et al.* (2002). Effect of thalidomide in patients with chronic heart failure. *Am. Heart J.* **144**: 847-850.

Guttridge, D.C. *et al.* (2000). NF-kappaB-induced loss of MyoD messenger RNA: possible role in muscle decay and cachexia. *Science.* **289**: 2363-2366.

Henderson, J.T. *et al.* (1996). Physiological effects of CNTF-induced wasting. *Cytokine.* **8**: 784-793.

Hirai, K. *et al.* (1997). Mechanism of depletion of liver glycogen in cancer cachexia. *Biochem. Biophys. Res. Commun.* **241**: 49-52.

Hirai, K. *et al.* (1998). Biological evaluation of a lipid-mobilising factor isolated from the urine of cancer patients. *Cancer Res.* **58**: 2359-2365.

Ishiko, O. *et al.* (1999). Lipolytic activity of anemia-inducing susbtance from tumor-bearing rabbits. *Nutr. Cancer.* **33**: 201-205.

Kawamura, I. *et al.* (1999). Intratumoral injection of oligonucleotides to the NF-kappaB binding site inhibits cachexia in a mouse tumor model. *Gene Ther.* **6**: 91-97.

Kawamura, I. *et al.* (2001). Intravenous injection of oligodeoxynucleotides to the NF-kappaB binding site inhibits hepatic metastasis of M5076 reticulosarcoma in mice. *Gene Ther.* **8**: 905-912.

Khan, S. and Tisdale, M.J. (1999). Catabolism of adipose tissue by a tumour-produced lipid metabolising factor. *Int. J. Cancer.* **80**: 444-447.

Khan, Z.H. *et al.* (2003). Oesophageal cancer and cachexia: the effect of short-term treatment with thalidomide on weight loss and lean body mass. *Aliment. Pharmacol. Ther.* **17**: 677-682.

King, P.J. *et al.* (2000). Effect of cytokines on hypothalamic neuropeptide Y release *in vitro*. *Peptides.* **21**: 143-146.

Kitada, S. *et al.* (1981). Characterization of a lipid mobilizing factor from tumors. *Prog. Lipid Res.* **20**: 823-826.

Klausner, J.D. *et al.* (1996). The effect of thalidomide on the pathogenesis of human immunodeficiency virus type 1 and M. tuberculosis infection. *J. Acquir. Immune. Defic. Syndr. Hum. Retrovirol.* **11**: 247-257.

Kowalczuk, A. *et al.* (2001). Plasma concentration of leptin, neuropeptide Y and tumour necrosis factor alpha in patients with cancers, before and after radio- and chemotherapy. *Pol. Arch. Med. Wewn.* **106**: 657-668.

Laviano, A. *et al.* (2002). Neurochemical mechanisms for cancer anorexia. *Nutrition.* **18**: 100-105.

Li, Y.P. *et al.* (1998). Skeletal muscle myocytes undergo protein loss and reactive oxygen-mediated NF-kappaB activation in response to tumor necrosis factor alpha. *FASEB J.* **12**: 871-880.

López-Soriano, J. *et al.* (1999). Leptin and tumour growth in the rat. *Int. J. Cancer.* **81**: 726-729.

Lorite, M.J. *et al.* (1997). Induction of muscle protein degradation by a tumour factor. *Br. J. Cancer.* **76**: 1035-1040.

Lorite, M.J. *et al.* (1998). Mechanism of muscle protein degradation induced by a cancer cachectic factor. *Br. J. Cancer.* **78**: 850-856.

Mantovani, G. *et al.* (2000). Serum levels of leptin and proinflammatory cytokines in patients with advanced-stage cancer at different sites. *J. Mol. Med.* **78**: 554-561.

Mantovani, G. *et al.* (2001). Serum values of proinflammatory cytokines are inversely correlated with serum leptin levels in patients with advanced stage cancer at different sites. *J. Mol. Med.* **79**: 406-414.

Masuno, H. *et al.* (1981). Purification and characterization of a lipolytic factor (toxohormone L) from cell free fluid of ascites sarcoma 180. *Cancer Res.* **41**: 284-288.

Matthys, P. *et al.* (1991). Anti-interferon-γ antibody treatment, growth of Lewis lung tumours in mice and tumour-associated cachexia. *Eur. J. Cancer.* **27**: 182-187.

Moreira, A.L. *et al.* (1993). Thalidomide exerts its inhibitory action on tumor necrosis factor alpha by enhancing mRNA degradation. *Exp. Med.* **177**: 1675-1680.

Mori, K. *et al.* (1996). Murine interleukin-12 prevents the development of cancer cachexia in a murine model. *Int. J. Cancer.* **67**: 849-855.

Negri, D.R. *et al.* (2001). Role of cytokines in cancer cachexia in a murine model of intracerebral injection of human tumours. *Cytokine.* **15**: 27-38.

Oliff, A. *et al.* (1987). Tumors secreting human TNF/cachectin induce cachexia in mice. *Cell.* **50**: 555-563.

Penner, C.G. *et al.* (2001) The transcription factors NF-kappaB and AP-1 are differentially regulated in skeletal muscle during sepsis. *Biochem. Biophys. Res. Commun.* **281**: 1331-1336.

Penner, G. *et al.* (2002). C/EBP DNA-binding activity is upregulated by a glucocorticoid-dependent mechanism in septic muscle. *Am. J. Physiol.* **282**: R439-R444.

Plata-Salaman, C.R. (2000). Central nervous system mechanisms contributing to the cachexia-anorexia syndrome. *Nutrition.* **16**: 1009-1012.

Puigserver, P. *et al.* (2001). Cytokine stimulation of energy expenditure through p38 MAP kinase activation of PPARgamma coactivator-1. *Mol. Cell.* **8**: 971-982.

Quinn, L.S. *et al.* (1995). Interleukin-15: a novel anabolic cytokine for skeletal muscle. *Endocrinology.* **136**: 3669-3672.

Reinhart, K. *et al.* (1996). Assessment of the safety and efficacy of the monoclonal anti-tumor necrosis factor antibody fragment, MAK 195F, in patients with sepsis and septic shock: a multicenter, randomized, placebo-controlled, dose-ranging study. *Crit. Care Med.* **24**: 733-742.

Sampaio, E.P. *et al.* (1993). The influence of thalidomide on the clinical and immunologic manifestation of erythema nodosum leprosum. *J. Infect. Dis.* **168**: 408-414.

Sampaio, E.P. *et al.* (1991). Thalidomide selectively inhibits tumor necrosis factor alpha production by stimulated human monocytes. *J. Exp. Med.* **173**: 699-703.

Sato, T. *et al.* (2002). Does leptin really influence cancer anorexia? *Nutrition.* **18**: 82-83.

Semmler, J. *et al.* (1993). The specific type IV phosphodiesterase inhibitor rolipram suppresses tumor necrosis factor-alpha production by human mononuclear cells. *Int. J. Immunopharmacol.* **15**: 409-413.

Sharma, R. and Anker, S.D. (2002). Cytokines, apoptosis and cachexia: the potential for TNF antagonism. *Int. J. Cardiol.* **85**: 161-171.

Smith, H.J. *et al.* (1999). Effects of a cancer cachectic factor on protein synthesis/degradation in murine C2C12 myoblasts: modulation by eicosapentaenoic acid. *Cancer Res.* **59**: 5507-5513.

Strassmann, G. *et al.* (1993). Suramin interferes with interleukin-6 receptor binding *in vitro* and inhibits colon-26-mediated experimental cancer cachexia *in vivo. J. Clin. Invest.* **92**: 2152-2159.

Tanaka, Y. *et al.* (1990). Experimental cancer cachexia induced by transplantable colon 26 adenocarcinoma in mice. *Cancer Res.* **50**: 2290-2295.

Tessitore, L. *et al.* (2000). Leptin expression in colorectal and breast cancer patients. *Int. J. Mol. Med.* **5**: 421-426.

Thinakaran, G. *et al.* (1993). Expression of c-jun/AP-1 during myogenic differentiation in mouse C2C12 myoblasts. *FEBS Lett.* **319**: 271-276.

Todorov, P. *et al.* (1996). Characterization of a cancer cachectic factor. *Nature.* **22**: 739-742.

Van Royen, M. *et al.* (2000). DNA fragmentation occurs in skeletal muscle during tumour growth: a link with cancer cachexia? *Biochem. Biophys. Res. Commun.* **270**: 533-537.

Wang, M.C. and Forsberg, N.E. (2000). Effects of ciliary neurotrophic factor (CNTF) on protein turnover in cultured muscle cells. *Cytokine.* **12**: 41-48.

Wigmore, S.J. *et al.* (2000). Characteristics of patients with pancreatic cancer expressing a novel cancer cachexia factor. *Br. J. Surgery.* **87**: 53-58.

Yamamoto, N. *et al.* (1998). Effect of FR143430, a novel cytokine suppressive agent, on adenocarcinoma colon26-induced cachexia in mice. *Anticancer Res.* **18**: 139-144.

Yasumoto, K. *et al.* (1995). Molecular analysis of the cytokine network involved in cachexia in colon26 adenocarcinoma-bearing mice. *Cancer Res.* **55**: 921-927.

Chapter 10

# TARGETING NF-κB IN ANTICANCER ADJUNCTIVE CHEMOTHERAPY

*Dedicated to the memory of Valerie Fincham.*
*Everything in the laboratory she touched turned into gold.*

Burkhard Haefner
*Department of Oncology, Johnson&Johnson Pharmaceutical Research and Development, Beerse, Belgium*

Abstract: After more than three decades of its declaration, the war against cancer still appears far from being won. Although there have been decisive victories in a few battles, such as the one against testicular cancer, the overall result is sobering. Hopes for an imminent cure had been raised among the public by the promises of molecular biology, combinatorial chemistry and high-throughput screening. These promises have manifested themselves in the widely proclaimed strategy of rationally targeted anticancer drug discovery, which may be summarized as the 'one-gene-one target-one drug' approach. Over the years, however, it has gradually become clear that, in most cases, treatment of cancer with a single drug may at best delay progression of the disease but is unlikely to lead to a cure. Thus, it appears that rationally targeted monotherapy will have to be replaced by rationally targeted combination therapy. Inhibitors of NF-κB look likely to become an important weapon in the anticancer combination therapy arsenal.

Key words: NF-κB; combination therapy; kinase inhibitor; proteasome inhibitor; Gleevec; Velcade

# 1.    INTRODUCTION

A commentary in the July 2003 issue of the Cleveland Clinic Journal of Medicine by Maurie Markman, chairman of the Department of Hematology/Medical Oncology and The Cleveland Clinic Taussig Cancer Center, raised the question if we are winning or losing the war against cancer (Markman, 2003). An answer to this question was given eight months later by Clifton Leaf, Executive Editor of Fortune Magazine and cancer survivor, who, in a provocative article (Leaf, 2004), spelled out why we may be far from winning this war. While there may not be the cancer epidemic proclaimed by some (Fisher *et al.*, 1995; Regenstein, 2002; Eaton 2002; Chambon and Beuzard, 2004), it is a sad and undeniable fact that, despite the billions spent on cancer research around the world since president Nixon declared war on this dreadful disease in 1971, long-term survival of advanced forms of cancer has hardly increased and the percentage of people dying of cancer in the developed world has hardly changed, even when adjusted for age, in the 33 years which have since elapsed (Leaf, 2004; Stewart and Kleihues, 2003; Cancer Facts and Figures 2004).

Clearly, a new strategy for the treatment of cancer is urgently needed, as Michael Baum, professor emeritus of surgery at University College London, already pointed out in a 2002 article in Prospect (Baum, 2002). But what could this new strategy be? Most likely, a single strategy will not be enough to win the war against cancer. As the great British immunologist Sir Peter Medawar once correctly remarked: 'Cancer is not one disease and there will not be one cure for it!'. Indeed, although it has been possible to identify common features shared by practically all types of cancer, such as genetic instability and unchecked proliferation, different sets of genetic lesions may give rise to individual tumours outwardly appearing as belonging to the same type of cancer. This tremendous complexity inherent to cancer is amplified by the characteristic genetic instability of cancer cells, a hallmark of the disease (Hanahan and Weinberg, 2000). The consequent evolution in multiple directions towards ever increasing malignancy manifests itself in markedly different responses to standard anticancer therapy shown by different patients suffering from a particular type of cancer (Watters and McLeod, 2003). This complicating fact indicates that what is required are therapeutic regimens tailored to the individual tumour and the specific set of molecular defects which gave rise to it (Carr *et al.*, 2004). However, personalized therapy is unlikely to be sufficient to win this war because of the considerable robustness and ability to develop resistance, which is another characteristic feature of tumours. This results from their composition of heterogenous and continuously evolving populations of cells. Because the only way to cure a cancer is to destroy every last one of these cells, a single drug will not be able to achieve this unless an Achilles heel, a drug target on which all cancer cells depend for survival, can be found. (Angiogenesis and telomerase were put forward as having this property, but, so far at least, Medawar's insight is still valid.) Obviously, the millions of cancer patients around the world fighting for their lives have no time to wait for this to happen.

## 2.      NF-κB: FRIEND OR FOE OF CANCER CELLS?

Until a few years ago, it had been widely believed that NF-κB activation was a critical step in an antiapoptotic cellular response to insult or injury, i.e. that the transcription factor protects cells from damage or death induced by noxious or toxic stimuli such as cytotoxic drugs. It has since become clear that this notion is too simplistic (Kucharczak *et al.*, 2003). In 2000, Kevin Ryan and colleagues published data suggesting that NF-κB activation is critical to p53-induced apoptosis (Ryan *et al.*, 2000). It became immediately clear that, if correct, these results would have important implications for the targeting of this transcription factor in anticancer drug discovery. Initially, however, they were met with some resistance including suggestions that this study may have been flawed. Inder Verma and co-workers countered the proposal of a proapoptotic function for NF-κB with the observation that apoptosis induced by p53 in response to treatment with the chemotherapeutic drug doxorubicin is increased in fibroblasts from IKKα/β double knockout mice which lack NF-κB activity (Tergaonkar *et al.*, 2002). Reintroduction of IKKβ into these cells was found to decrease p53 stabilization and cell death induced by the drug. This effect was abrogated by co-expression of a transdominant negative mutant of IκB. These findings are in stark contrast to those of Ryan and co-workers and point to a role for NF-κB in the suppression of chemotherapy-induced p53-dependent apoptosis and consequently in the acquisition of resistance to cytotoxic drugs by cancer cells. The prevailing view of the function of NF-κB in the regulation of cell survival and apoptosis seemed vindicated - but not for long. Shortly after the article by Verma's group had been published, a novel protein, overexpressed in the majority of human hepatocellular carcinomas, was identified, which stimulates export of NF-κB from the nucleus and inhibits p53-dependent apoptosis (Higashitsuji *et al.*, 2002). Since then, more publications supporting a proapoptotic role for NF-κB in p53-induced cell death have appeared, including one which claims that stabilization of p53 is a mechanism by which NF-κB can induce apoptosis (Fujioka *et al.*, 2004a), and one which shows that IKK is not required by p53 for the activation of the transcription factor (Bohuslav *et al.*, 2004), thus drawing into doubt the results of Verma and colleagues. In fact, the idea of IKK being indispensable for NF-κB activation has recently been refuted by a number of researcher including Verma himself (Tergaonkar *et al.*, 2003). This has considerable consequences for the discovery of inhibitors of NF-κB activation which is currently almost exclusively focusing on compounds inhibiting IKK. "So, who is right, then?", the confused drug discovery scientists, looking to acadaemia for some guidance in his attempt to find novel, validated targets for the treatment of cancer, may ask. The answer is that both schools, the one arguing that NF-κB's function is to suppress apoptosis and the other proposing that the transcription factor actually promotes apoptosis, may be right. As so often in cellular regulation, it all appears to depend on the circumstances.

## 2.1     A model for NF-κB in apoptosis regulation

A revised model for the role of NF-κB in the regulation of apoptosis, and consequently in cancer, has been put forward by Neil Perkins in a recent review article (Perkins, 2004) in answer to the question if NF-κB is a tumour promoter or suppressor, or, to put it differently, a friend or foe of cancer cells (Shishodia and Aggarwal, 2004). The proposed tumour suppressor function of NF-κB is linked to the ability of the transcription factor to behave differently in normal cells as opposed to cancer cells. In the early stages of tumourigenesis, aberrant and potentially tumour-promoting activation of NF-κB caused by DNA damage or dysregulation of the networks which control its activity or expression is thought to be counteracted by simultaneous activation of tumour suppressors, such as p53, ARF, p16INK4a and PTEN, which inhibit its transactivation function. This turns the transcription factor into a repressor rather than an activator of antiapoptotic and proliferation-promoting gene expression. As cells progress down the road to cell transformation and tumour formation, they loose tumour suppressor functions which, in this model, allows NF-κB to exert its antiapoptotic, tumour-promoting effects. As a consequence, drug discovery scientists may have to rethink the idea that inhibition of NF-κB is a suitable strategy *per se* for fighting cancer. However, if the only requirement for a tumour suppressor function of NF-κB to manifest itself was inhibition of the transactivation activity of the transcription factor by tumour suppressor proteins, achieving the same by administration of a drug preventing nuclear translocation, DNA binding or stimulation of gene expression by NF-κB, could not be expected to have any unwanted effects such as stimulating precancerous cells to become fully malignant. Unfortunately for drug discovery, there does not appear to be such a simple way out of the dilemma.

## 2.2      Complicating complexities

Tumour suppressor proteins p53 and ARF have been found to turn NF-κB into a repressor of antiapoptotic genes by inducing it to change binding partners and associate with histone deacetylase 1 (HDAC1), a transcriptional repressor, rather than with co-activators such as p300/CBP, two highly homologous acetyltransferases (Rocha *et al.*, 2003; Campbell *et al.*, 2004). Consequently, only a drug inhibiting NF-κB without interfering with its ability to such complexes at promoters would be free from the danger of inducing tumour progression rather than cancer cell death. Clearly, inhibitors of IKK or the proteasome preventing degradation of IκB and consequently accumulation of NF-κB in the nucleus do not fall into this category. Interfering with covalent modification, i.e. phosphorylation and acetylation, of p65, required for the protein to achieve its full transactivation potential at promoters in the nucleus, may be a more promising strategy. The phosphorylation of p65 by Msk1, for example, has been shown to stimulate association of NF-κB with p300/CBP (Vermeulen *et al.*, 2003). Inhibition of this protein serine/threonine kinase may therefore be expected to reduce binding of this transcriptional co-activator and consequently NF-κB-dependent gene expression. Moreover, unbound p65 molecules may become free to bind to HDAC1 further reducing NF-κB-mediated transactivation. Alas, the binding of HDAC1 and consequent antiapoptotic gene repression is unlikely to be the whole story of apoptosis stimulation by NF-κB. The transcription factor has been found not only to drive antiapoptotic gene expression but also to be able to induce expression of proapoptotic genes such as Fas, Fas ligand, caspase 11 and p53 (Loop and Pahl, 2003). This truly proapoptotic function of NF-κB appears to be dependent on the cellular context, i.e. the activating stimulus, the kinetics of its activation, the activity state of other signaling pathways, and the cell type.

## 2.3      Could NF-κB inhibitors cause more problems than they might solve?

The observation that NF-κB inhibition in combination with expression of a Ras oncogene induces human epidermal neoplasia in a mouse model has given support to the concern that inhibition of the transcription factor may, under certain circumstances, be tumourigenic in humans (Dajee *et al.*, 2003).

However, several points have to be made with respect to this finding. First, human skin does not consist of keratinocytes alone, but also contains immune cells, unlike in the model used. Second, human beings are not normally immune-deficient, as were the mice employed in this model. Third, small molecule inhibitors are rarely as potent in inhibiting NF-κB as is the degradation resistant IκB used in these experiments. Fourth, NF-κB inhibitors would not be given long-term when used in cancer therapy. Generally speaking, the danger that inhibition of NF-κB may result in the progression of cells carrying precancerous lesions to full-blown cancer because of the abrogation of the proposed tumour suppressor function of the transcription factor is of little concern to those who are planning to develop NF-κB inhibitors as anticancer drugs. This is because the first worry of cancer patients and their doctors is how to fight the cancer at hand and not the possibility that additional cancers may arise in the future as a side effect of chemotherapy as long as the drugs administered are effective. After all, the currently used DNA-damaging anticancer drugs and radiotherapy are far from being free from this concern, either. The proteasome inhibitor Velcade (bortezomib, PS-341) (Fig. 1) is a case in point. Although its efficacy cannot exclusively be attributed to inhibition of NF-κB activation, it is clear that the therapeutic benefit it confers to patients suffering from multiple myeloma, a cancer fatal in the overwhelming majority of cases, far outweighs the risk of inducing novel tumours by interfering with activation of the transcription factor. Moreover, targeting the proteasome, itself, had been predicted by many scientists as likely to have catastrophic consequences for normal cells. Fortunately for multiple myeloma patients, there were drug discovery researchers and managers at Millennium Pharmaceuticals bold enough to throw caution to the wind and embark on a program for the discovery of proteasome inhibitors which has been extraordinarily successful (National Institutes of Health Office of Technology Transfer, 2003). For those drug companies planning to develop NF-κB inhibitors for long-term use in the treatment of chronic inflammatory disease, however, it is a different story. They would be well-advised not to ignore the potential long-term risks inhibition of NF-κB may entail.

## 3.    HISTORY AND FUTURE PROSPECTS OF COMBINATION ANTICANCER THERAPY

Attempts to treat cancer are almost as old as medicine itself (Porter, 1997; Nutton, 2004; The History of Cancer). The first documentary evidence for a treatment of cancer comes from an Egyptian papyrus dating back to 1600 B.C., which describes the cauterization of breast tumours. The text states that despite this treatment, the illness proved incurable. Ancient physicians, such as Hippocrates (460-370 B.C.), who gave the disease its name, observed that cancer was incurable by surgery once it had spread. If the tumour could be removed at an earlier stage, however, surgical cures of breast cancer could apparently be achieved already at the time of Galen (A.D. 129-216). The first real progress in cancer treatment was made only after anesthesia and antisepsis had been invented which allowed more elaborate and radical surgical procedures to be developed in the nineteenth century. A high degree of local control and palliation could thus be achieved but mortality remained high. Surgery still remains the mainstay of treatment for many types of cancer, today, but has since been supplemented with chemo-and radiotherapy. Radiotherapy became widely used as cancer treatment after the discovery of X-rays by Roentgen in 1896. In the United States, it was championed by Ewing who opposed the use of Coley's toxin, a bacterial preparation successfully employed to induce necrosis in certain types of tumour. Anticancer chemotherapy was first systematically investigated by Goodman and Gilman, working for the U.S. Army, who, during World War II, studied agents related to mustard gas. A compound named nitrogen mustard was found to have activity against lymphoma and became the model for a series of alkylating agents which kill rapidly proliferating cells by inducing DNA damage. Such cytotoxic drugs quickly replaced earlier potions used to treat cancer such as Fowler's solution, a solution of potassium arsenite which had been used for the treatment of leukemia (Waxman and Anderson, 2001). Shortly afterwards, Sidney Farber, a Boston surgeon, discovered the antileukemic effect of aminopterin, predecessor of methotrexate, an antimetabolite inhibiting nucleotide biosynthesis and still commonly used anticancer drug.

## 3.1    The emergence of combination therapy

In the early 1970s, surgical oncologist Bernard Fisher pioneered the use of chemotherapy after surgery which can, at best, achieve local control. Such adjuvant chemotherapy, the post-surgical administration of anticancer drugs to destroy residual cancer cells, was first tested in breast cancer where it proved effective (Wolmark and Fisher, 1985). Adjunctive chemotherapy, i.e. the use of a multiple drugs simultaneously was first used successfully in the treatment of leukemias and lymphomas some of which showed a complete response. Administration and dosing of such anticancer drug combinations has since been optimized and novel combinations have been tested in clinical trials. Currently, combinations of novel and established anticancer drugs are usually tested in such studies. Cocktails consisting entirely of experimental drugs have been successfully used to control the replication and spread of HIV, which like cancer cells, has a high mutation rate. A similar approach may be a strategy for the treatment of cancer with a high chance of achieving a cure even of advanced forms of the disease. However, legal and regulatory issues need to be addressed before such combinations can be brought to the market. For example, concerns have been raised that in cases when different drugs found to be working well in combination belong to different companies, an agreement on who owns the right to the combination may often not be reachable (Leaf, 2004). It would be possible to avoid such problems if anticancer drugs with multiple molecular targets can be identified. Such 'combination therapies in one pill' are nothing new. Aspirin is a well-known example of a drug for which multiple targets have over the years been described. Among them are, most prominently, cyclooxygenase (Levesque and Lafont, 2000) and also IKKβ (Yin *et al.*, 1998). Although these enzymes are inhibited only at micromolar concentrations, their combined, moderate, inhibition is apparently sufficient to produce the potent antiinflammatory effects of the drug.

## 4.    MULTI-TARGETED PROTEIN KINASE INHIBITORS

Owing to the apparent impossibility to find completely specific protein kinase inhibitors, a new strategy in the field of kinase inhibitor drug discovery is to look for so-called mixed (Celgene) or multi-kinase (Methylgene) inhibitors which act on a set of kinases relevant to the disease to be treated (Investigational Drugs database). In order to be able to do this in a rational fashion, prior knowledge of the 'right' combination of kinases would be required. However, such sets of kinases are currently only identifiable by profiling after the fact, i.e. after the compound has shown activity in disease models. This may change in the near future. Generation of protein-protein interaction maps and computer simulations of the dynamics of cellular regulatory networks is a hotly pursued area of Systems Biology promising to revolutionize drug target identification and validation (Davidov *et al.*, 2003; Butcher *et al.*, 2004). This integrative and quantitative approach to the study of cellular signal transduction and regulation may also convert traditional combination anticancer chemotherapy from a mostly 'trial-and-error' to a more rational strategy by enabling the *a priori* identification of combinations of anticancer drugs whose mechanisms of action are most likely to beneficially complement each other.

Even cancer drugs which have proven highly effective as monotherapy, such as Gleevec (imatinib mesylate) (Fig.1), may show enhanced efficacy when administered in combination with another drug having the same or a different relevant target. This is because the chronic myelogenous leukemia (CML) cells this compound is supposed to kill develop resistance to the drug, most often by mutations in the gene for the target kinase, Bcr-Abl, or by its overexpression (Nimmanapalli and Bhalla, 2002; Azam *et al.*, 2003; Cools *et al.*, 2005). BMS-354825 (Fig. 1) is a novel Bcr-Abl inhibitor which eliminated the vast majority of Gleevec-resistant CML strains against which it was tested (Shah *et al.*, 2004; Lombardo *et al.*, 2004; Doggrell, 2005). The compound was originally aimed at Src, prototype of a family of protein tyrosine kinase implicated in the pathogenesis of a variety of cancers. The highly homologous Src-family kinase Lyn has been found to be activated in some cases of Gleevec-resistant CML thus causing a form of resistance to the drug which does not depend on mutation or overexpression of Bcr-Abl (Donato *et al.*, 2003). Inhibition of Lyn by BMS-354825 may, as a consequence, also help overcome this form of resistance to Gleevec. Moreover Src-family kinases Lyn, Hck and Fgr have been found to be required for Bcr-Abl-induced B-cell acute lymphoblastic leukemia which may thus be another indication for this compound (Hu *et al.*, 2004). BMS-354825 may therefore be an example of a multi-targeted kinase inhibitor acting on a set of protein kinases causally involved in the pathogenesis of two forms of leukemia. Administration of Gleevec and BMS-354825 in combination may prevent CML cells from becoming resistant to either of them because they may be targeting Bcr-Abl in sufficiently different ways for resistance against both drugs to require different mutations to occur. The occurrence of such mutations simultaneously would be much more unlikely than that of a single mutation conferring resistance to Gleevec. In this context, it is important to note that treatment of CML patients with just BMS-354825 is unlikely to result in a cure, either, because the compound has been found to be inactive against a common mutant (T351I) form of Bcr-Abl causing Gleevec resistance (O'Hare *et al.*, 2005; Burgess *et al.*, 2005). However, this form of the kinase is inhibited by a series of other, multi-targeted protein kinase inhibitors including ONO12380 (Fig. 1), which does not target the ATP binding pocket of Bcr-Abl, as do Gleevec and BMS-354825, but the substrate binding site (Gumireddy *et al.*, 2005), and like BMS-354825, is reported to also be active against Lyn. (Undoubtedly, CML cells are likely to find a way to develop resistance against each single one of these novel compounds, as well.)

A logic similar to that of combining different Bcr-Abl inhibitors in newly diagnosed patients applies to combinations of Gleevec with the proteasome inhibitor Velcade, which has been found to be active against Gleevec-sensitive as well as resistant CML. It may in future be possible to discover multi-target anticancer drugs which, similar to aspirin, do not only act on kinases but also on other types of enzymes. As a matter of fact, one such compound has already been reported. Researchers at McGill University and M.D. Anderson Cancer Center have identified ZR-2002 (Fig. 1) as an irreversible inhibitor of the epidermal growth factor receptor protein tyrosine kinase and as a DNA damage-inducing agent (Brahimi *et al.*, 2004; Rachid *et al.*, 2005). This compound may thus fall between the two categories of novel, targeted anticancer drugs and classical cytotoxics. Anticancer drugs are also used in combination with radiotherapy. Some of these compounds act as radiosensitizers when administered concurrently with irradiation (Caffo, 2001). Others are employed as adjuvants to eradicate any cancer cells which survived exposure to the X-rays. Combinations of drugs, such as the mitotic spindle poison paclitaxel plus a platinum-derived drug, have shown improved efficacy in clinical trials when used to sensitize cancer cells to irradiation in a kind of 'double combination therapy' (Constantinou *et al.*, 2003).

## 4.1    Synthetic lethality

It has been argued that certain targeted anticancer drugs exert their cytotoxic effect by way of synthetic lethality, i.e. by exploiting genetic lesions of cancer cells, which, on their own, are not lethal but which, in combination with the drug, will drive the cells over the edge between proliferation and programmed cell death, on which they are thought to exist in delicate balance, and induce them to undergo apoptosis (Garber, 2002 and 2004). Indeed, it has been observed that cancer cells lacking functional tumour suppressor PTEN are exquisitely sensitive to the rapamycin derivative CCI-779 (Neshat *et al.*, 2001; Shi *et al.*, 2002) and that antibodies activating the TRAIL receptor can trigger apoptosis in myc-overexpressing tumours but not in others, supporting this concept (Wang *et al.*, 2004). Could drugs selected on the basis of their ability to kill cancer cells carrying specific genetic aberrations not present in normal cells be the solution to the cancer problem? May be, but, in all likelihood, a single one of these drugs will not be sufficient to kill all, genetically heterogenous, populations of cells present in a single tumour, because not all of them will carry the critical lesion. In fact, the critical component may not be a genetic defect but the abnormal dependence on such proteins or protein complexes as Hsp90 and the proteasome, respectively, whose activities appear to prevent cancer cells from being overwhelmed by abnormally folded proteins produced by the expression of defective genes. Furthermore, there may be cancer cells which carry the lesion on which the drug depends for its cytotoxic activity but which at the same time are resistant to the drug because they pump it out as quickly as it enters the cell or because they have undergone a rewiring of their protein-protein interaction network which allows them to survive the effect of the drug. The realization that there are cancer cells carrying genetic lesions which are not lethal by themselves but which, in combination with a second disturbance, such as a drug, will kill these cells, points to the following possibility: there may be compounds which when tested on their own will not be cytotoxic but when administered together with another molecule showing similar behaviour on its own, will have dramatic therapeutic effects. Are we missing all these synergistically active combinations of compounds because we will never be able to pick them up in our *in vitro* screens for the inhibition of a single molecular activity where each individual compound may well have shown activity but then failed to do so in subsequent cellular assays? Clifton Leaf would probably argue that this is most likely the case. If so, is there anything we can do about it?

## 4.2 Screening for combinations

Say our compound library has 100,000 molecules. Testing them in all possible combinations of 2 would mean, we would have to run $5 \times 10^9$ assays. Even if we were able to use 3456 well assay plates, we would have to screen over 1,4 million plates. Clearly the costs of such an enterprise would be forbidding even if the necessary capacity in terms of available screening robots and manpower existed. If we wanted to test the library in combinations of 3 or more, the project would become astronomically difficult to put into practice and would require the budget of the NASA space program. In the future, however, we may find ways round these problems using compound library profiling technology provided by the novel field of chemical genomics which has made it its goal to test large compound collections in an almost as large a number of assays, molecular and cellular (Strausberg and Schreiber, 2003). Such efforts will provide every compound with a long 'CV' listing every activity or absence of it in all these assays similar to, but much more comprehensive than, the databases already existing within the pharmaceutical industry. This alone, however, would not bring us much further. What would be needed in addition to this data is a detailed understanding of which combinations of activities (an activity being the modulation of a target molecule or cellular process) will synergistically interact to produce enhanced therapeutic effects in a given disease situation. This would enable us to bring down the number of combinations of molecules to be tested to feasible levels. Molecular interaction maps and computer modeling of cellular regulatory processes may in the future help us obtain such knowledge (Uetz and Finley, 2005; Bhalla, 2004). In the case of cancer, additional data from extensive molecular profiling of tumours would be required as a further precondition because of the heterogeneity of individual tumours at the molecular level (Sorlie, 2004). This may appear as science fiction, today, but given that it took mankind less than seven decades to go from becoming airborne in a motorized airplane for the first time to setting foot on the moon, who can say what productive combinations of talent and expertise in biology, chemistry, computer science and engineering will make possible in the 21st century in the field of biomedical research?

A first step into the direction of rational and systematic combination screening has been made by researchers at CombinatoRx. They tested roughly 120,000 two-compound combinations of reference-listed drugs. For this purpose, they used a custom-designed robotic screening and informatics system in combination high-throughput screening (cHTS). As a result, they identified drug combinations with novel and unexpected activities including glucocorticoid and antiplatelet agents suppressing TNFα production in human peripheral blood mononuclear cells (PBMC) as well as antipsychotic and antiprotozoal agents inhibiting tumour growth in mice (Borisy *et al.*, 2003). This combination screening approach may therefore be expected to enable the rapid discovery of novel multicomponent therapeutics consisting of established and/or experimental drugs. Moreover, integration of cHTS into chemical genomics programs may become useful for the exploration of biological networks.

## 5. CLASSES OF NF-κB INHIBITORS IN DEVELOPMENT

Compounds aimed at NF-κB activation currently in development within the pharmaceutical and biotech industry fall into three major classes depending on the target against which they have been screened: protein kinase inhibitors, inhibitors of NF-κB-mediated reporter gene expression, also called transactivation inhibitors, and proteasome inhibitors (Haefner 2005). Among all of these compounds, only one of the latter class, Millennium Pharmaceutical's Velcade, has so far reached the market.

## 5.1 Kinase inhibitors

Despite there now being multiple protein kinases which have been identified as regulators of NF-κB activation, including IKK, GSK-3β, MSK-1, and Src, and which therefore constitute potential drug targets, drug discovery research has so far been focusing on IKK. In this section, I will present two exemplary IKK inhibitors because they are central to my argument that targeting single proteins or processes is likely to be less efficacious than aiming drugs at multiple targets.

Scientists at Signal Pharmaceuticals, now a subsidiary of Celgene, were among the first researchers to purify the IKK complex and to identify its two principal components IKKα and β (Mercurio *et al.*, 1997). Soon after this, they began to look for IKK inhibitors in collaboration with Serono. One compound they identified, SPC-839 (Fig. 1), a quinazoline analogue, is 200 times more active against IKKβ ($IC_{50} = 62$ nM) than α, inhibits NF-κB transactivation and cytokine production in Jurkat cells as well as TNFα production and paw oedema formation in rats (Investigational Drugs database). The compound also has significant activity against Jun N-terminal kinase 2 (JNK2) ($IC_{50} = 600$ nM).

Derivatives of the alkaloid β-carboline are another series of early IKK inhibitors (Investigational Drugs database; Castro *et al.*, 2003). Starting from the lead compound 5-bromo-6-methoxy-β-carboline, which had been found to be a nonspecific inhibitor of IKK, Millennium Pharmaceuticals, in collaboration with Aventis, investigated the structure-activity relationship (SAR) of β-carbolines with the aim of optimizing potency and selectivity. One of the analogues, named PS-1145 (Fig. 1), was selected for further investigation. In immune complex kinases assays performed on lysates of TNFα-stimulated HeLa cells, PS-1145 showed inhibition of endogenous IKK ($IC_{50} = 150$ nM). Moreover, IκB phosphorylation and NF-κB DNA binding in these cells were found to be inhibited in a dose-dependent manner. *In vivo*, the compound reduced LPS-induced TNFα production in mice by 60% at 5 hours post-challenge when given orally at 50 mg/kg 1 hour prior to LPS administration. In multiple myeloma cells (MMCs), PS-1145 blocked TNFα-induced phosphorylation of IκB, NF-κB activation, and ICAM-1 expression. The compound also inhibited proliferation and promoted TNFα-induced apoptosis in these cells. Furthermore, it reduced secretion of IL-6, a growth factor for MMCs, by bone marrow stromal cells (BMSCs) in co-cultures of the two cell types (Hideshima *et al.*, 2002).

The only other protein kinase involved in NF-κB activation currently pursued as target for NF-κB inhibitors is NIK, a mitogen-activated protein kinase kinase kinase (MAP3K) necessary for IKKα activation by stimuli such as BAFF which regulates B-cell survival and maturation (Claudio *et al.*, 2002). It has been suggested that selective inhibition of this IKK isoform may therefore be beneficial in lupus erythematodes, in which BAFF levels have been found to be elevated (Kalled *et al.*, 2003), and related B-cell mediated autoimmune diseases. Inhibition of NIK can be expected to have a significant and fairly specific effect on IKKα activity, B cell maturation, and progression of lupus-like autoimmune diseases because, although this

MAP3K has been reported to also activate IKKβ, gene disruption analysis has shown that it is not required in the canonical pathway of NF-κB activation (Smith *et al.*, 2001). Until the recent disclosure by Aventis of a series of pyrazolo[4,3-*c*]isoquinoline NIK inhibitors, only Signal Pharmaceuticals, in collaboration with Serono, had announced their interest in this kinase as a drug target (Investigational Drugs database).

## 5.2    Transactivation inhibitors

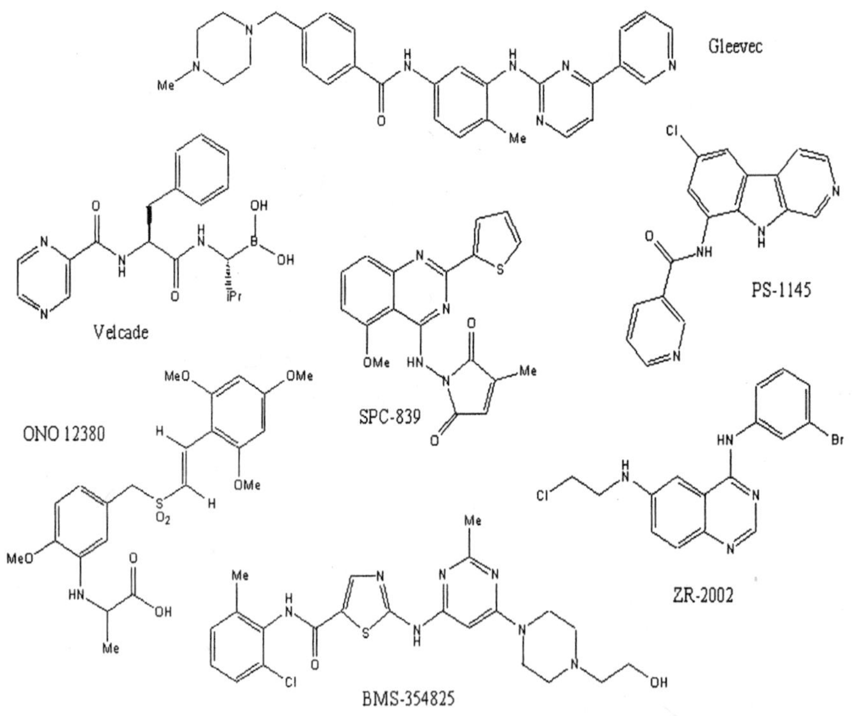

*Figure 1.* Structures of selected compounds mentioned in the text.

Since NF-κB is a transcription factor, an obvious way of screening for inhibitors of its activity are assays for NF-κB-dependent reporter gene expression. With the recent introduction of high-throughput screening platforms for eukaryotic cells, chemical libraries containing several hundred thousand small molecules can be screened in such cellular assays almost as rapidly as in activity assays for individual, isolated target proteins (Clemons,

2004). One of the advantages of such NF-кB transactivation assays is the potential for yielding inhibitors of all of the different drugable targets within the NF-кB signal transduction network. The major disadvantage is that it is not known *a priori* against which one of these targets a given hit is active, and that identification of the molecular target(s) of such a compound often requires considerable additional effort. However, hits which came out of HTS campaigns against isolated targets frequently show cellular and/or in *vivo* activities which cannot be explained by the predicted mechanism of action, and therefore also require further investigation. Moreover, as pointed out above, it is becoming increasingly clear that for pathological processes which are governed by complex intracellular events, targeting of a single cell component with a small molecule may not be sufficient for achieving maxiumum therapeutic efficacy. Cellular screening assays provide an opportunity for the discovery of compounds which act on multiple disease-relevant proteins.

Both NF-кB and AP-1 are transcription factors, which, either alone or in combination, regulate the expression of a large number of pro-inflammatory genes, and, therefore, AP-1 is also a potential target for anti-inflammatory drugs. Efforts at Signal Pharmaceuticals to identify inhibitors of both NF-кB- and AP1-driven gene expression in Jurkat cells have recently yielded quinazoline analogues (Palanki *et al.*, 2003). Interestingly, these compounds include SPC-839, which has previously been described as an inhibitor of IKK (see above). Until the recent publication of a mechanism for NF-kB-dependent AP-1 activation (Fujioka *et al.*, 2004b), it was difficult to envisage how the activity of this compound on AP-1-stimulated transcription could be due to IKK inhibition. However, inhibition of AP-1-dependent reporter gene expression is not a common feature of potent and supposedly selective IKKβ inhibitors suggesting that inhibition of this kinase alone cannot explain this activity of the compound. Moreover, the fact that inhibition of the activity of both transcription factors apparently occurs with identical potency (IC50 = 8 nM) suggests that there is another cellular target of this molecule. It is true that JNK-2, which SPC-839 has been reported to inhibit *in vitro*, albeit ten times less potently than IKKβ, is a protein kinase involved in AP-1 activation, but it is difficult to envisage how this activity of the compound could produce the much more potent inhibition of AP-1-dependent reporter gene expression observed. Likely cellular targets whose inhibition could be responsible for this effect are kinases of the MAP3K family (Hagemann and Blank, 2001), which can activate both MAP kinase pathways leading to AP-1 activation as well as IKK, and thus NF-кB (Schmidt *et al.*, 2003).

## 5.3 Proteasome inhibitors

Despite evidence for proteasome-independent NF-κB activation (Han *et al.*, 1999), IκB degradation by proteasomes still appears to be a critical event in response to most stimuli activating this transcription factor. Moreover, generation of the NF-κB subunits p50 and p52 is proteasome-dependent (Beinke and Ley, 2004). Proteasome inhibition has been shown to suppress NF-κB activity and to enhance chemo- and radiotherapy induced apoptosis in cancer cell lines and tumour models (Voorhees *et al.*, 2003; Russo *et al.*, 2001; Munshi *et al.*, 2004). Thus, inhibition of these proteolytic multiprotein complexes remains a valid strategy for targeting NF-κB in cancer and other diseases. This is borne out by the success of the Millennium proteasome inhibitor Velcade in the treatment of multiple myeloma, a B cell cancer in which chronic NF-κB activation has a major causative role. Velcade is a dipeptidyl boronic acid. Peptidyl boronates are potent and selective inhibitors of the 20S proteasome chymotrypsin-like activity. In cell culture and xenograft models of human cancers, the drug increases sensitivity to conventional chemotherapeutics and, as a consequence, overcomes chemoresistance (Adams, 2003; Investigational Drugs database). This observation has led to phase I and II combination trials (see below). Velcade not only inhibits growth in isolated human MMCs but, like PS-1145, also interferes with their survival-promoting interaction with BMSCs in co-cultures by blocking adhesion molecule expression, suppresses BMSC production of IL-6, and inhibits angiogenesis in xenografts (Hideshima *et al.*, 2002).

## 6. INHIBITORS OF NF-κB ACTIVATION AS EXAMPLES FOR MULTI-TARGETED DRUGS

Clearly, proteasome inhibition does not only affect NF-κB. The more specific inhibitor of NF-κB activation PS-1145 inhibits MMC proliferation much less potently than Velcade (Hideshima *et al.*, 2002). Thus, although inhibition of the transcription factor is thought to be critical for the efficacy of the drug in multiple myeloma, additional effects such as accumulation of cyclin-dependent kinase inhibitors (Cayrol and Ducommun, 1998) are likely to contribute and to be responsible for its greater potency as compared to PS-1145. Thus, Velcade, although not inhibiting multiple targets, still acts like a multi-targeted drug owing to the multiple functions of its target whose inhibition produces pleiotropic effects as a consequence. With some transactivation inhibitors, at least, it may be a similar story. We have found a series of compounds which inhibit NF-κB-dependent reporter gene expression and cytokine production in PBMC with nanomolar potency as well as *in vivo* apparently by targeting a set of protein kinases involved in NF-κB activation, each of these kinases being inhibited merely with micromolar potency. One conceivable explanation for this phenomenon may be a synergistic effect produced by the inhibition of NF-κB at multiple points along the activation pathway occupied by protein kinases, by the inhibition of kinases acting in parallel to phosphorylate and activate the transcription factor, or by a combination of both modes of inhibition (Fig. 2). Admittedly, until our compound has been tested against all known protein kinases, once this becomes possible, the verdict is still out if this is the actual mechanism of action or if a single protein kinase whose inhibition is responsible for the observed cellular effects of our molecule can be identified. Finally, molecules reported to be selective IKK inhibitors *in vitro* may show cellular and in *vivo* efficacy, which, on closer inspection, is likely to be produced by the modulation of additional targets, SPC-839 being one example for such compounds.

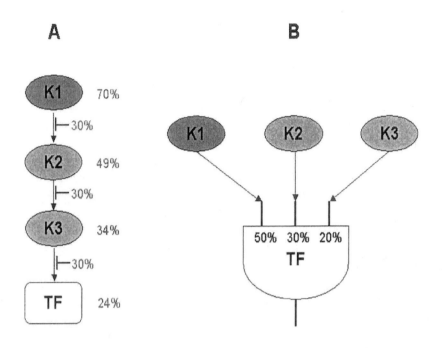

*Figure 2.* Predicted enhanced inhibitory effect on transcription factor activity due to inhibition of multiple upstream kinases forming (A) a regulatory chain (percentages activity to the right of the protein symbol) or (B) a multi-input motif. In the case of the multi-input motif, phosphorylation of the target transcription factor by each one of the upstream kinases may contribute to transcription factor activation to a different extent (50, 30 and 20 percent, respectively, in this example).

## 7.     NF-κB INHIBITION AS ADJUNCTIVE ANTICANCER CHEMOTHERAPY

Tumours are highly robust in that they are able to survive and proliferate in the face of repeated onslaughts with a diverse arsenal of cytotoxic drugs (Kitano, 2004). This robustness is a consequence of cellular heterogeneity, caused by genetic instability resulting in tremendous adaptability through selection of resistant populations of tumour cells, and of the activation by many cytotoxic drugs of stress response pathways leading to NF-κB activation as well as angiogenic and/or multidrug-resistance gene expression, in which the transcription factor is involved. Tumour robustness is a systems property since individual cancer cells often show fragility rather than robustness when compared to normal cells in that they are more sensitive to chemotherapeutic drugs. This is exemplified by the sensitivity of certain cancer cells to proteasome inhibitors, thought to be the result, at least to a certain extent, of their increased dependence on the removal of misfolded, nonfunctional proteins which they produce in increased amounts because of multiple genetic defects they have sustained. If all tumour cells were alike, finding an Achilles' heel whose targeting will kill them all would be much less of a challenge for drug discovery researchers. Therefore, effective treatment of cancer with radio- or chemotherapy, will become much more likely if the heterogeneity of tumours (Losi *et al.*, 2005) can be reduced. Treatment with single genotoxic agents, which may aggravate the situation by inducing further mutations in surviving tumour cells, or with other cytotoxic drugs, is unlikely to achieve this objective, even if a series of them is applied successively, because at best, each of these drugs may kill a different subpopulation of sensitive tumour cells but may not be able to prevent resistant clones to expand and take the place of the destroyed cells. Tumour heterogeneity will quickly be restored because of the genetic instability of the surviving tumour cells.

An alternative strategy, suggested by the success of a similar approach taken to the treatment of AIDS, is the application of a combination of anticancer drugs simultaneously. The rationale behind this strategy is that there may be many subpopulations of tumour cells resistant to one or the other drug, but far fewer which will be resistant, at the same time, to two or three of them. It is conceivable that some drug combinations may thus reduce tumour heterogeneity so much that only one, homogenuous, cell population is able to survive, which can then be delivered the final blow by administration of one further agent to which it is highly sensitive. Taking this strategy to its logical extremes, one might argue that all that is needed to kill every last tumour cell is the combination of a large enough number of different chemotherapeutic agents to reach a point where no tumour cell population able to withstand them all will be left. Apart from the likelihood of potentiation by this strategy not only of therapeutic efficacy but also of toxicity and consequent adverse effects, which may thus become intolerable, there is no guarantee that a single cancer cell cannot be resistant to a large number of available anticancer drugs. For example, it may be able to rid itself of these molecules before they can do any damage through the activation of efflux pumps, such as the P-glycoprotein, responsible for multidrug resistance (Borst *et al.*, 1999). While it is true that, conceptionally, this strategy has advantages over successive treatment with different chemotherapeutics, to make it a success will require targeting of the right proteins, especially those which make cancer cells resistant to multiple drugs. One such protein appears to be NF-κB (Thevenod *et al.*, 2000; Kuo *et al.*, 2002).

## 7.1     NF-κB and HDAC inhibitors

Activation of NF-κB is an important step in the response of cells to a large variety of toxic chemicals which include common cancer chemotherapeutics, as well as many novel, more specific cancer drugs currently in development such as HDAC inhibitors (Arts *et al.*, 2003). NF-κB activation induced by these drugs, or by radiotherapy, appears to protect cells from the damaging effects of these therapies (Orlowski and Baldwin, 2002) and is therefore likely to put a limit on their efficacy against cancer cells (Denlinger *et al.*, 2004), especially since many tumours show increased NF-κB activity already prior to treatment (Rayet and Gelinas, 1999). Consequently, induced or constitutive NF-κB activation is bound to confer cross-resistance, the ability of cancer cells to resist multiple cytotoxic drugs. HDAC inhibitors, for example, have recently been demonstrated to be limited in their ability to induce apoptosis in cancer cells by activating NF-κB via the PI 3-kinase/Akt pathway (Mayo *et al.*, 2003). Cells in which this pathway, or NF-κB itself, is inhibited before exposure to HDAC inhibitors show sensitization to apoptosis induction by these compounds suggesting that a combination of HDAC and NF-κB inhibitors may result in increased cancer cell killing in patients (Rundall *et al.*, 2004).

## 7.2     Lessons from Velcade

As described above, the proteasome inhibitor Velcade, whose cell killing effect on MMCs is thought to be largely due to inhibition of IκB degradation, and consequently of NF-κB activation, has been shown to synergize with other cancer drugs. One example is its potentiation of HDAC inhibitor-induced killing of chronic myelogenous leukaemia (CML) cells resistant to Gleevec and positive for Bcr-Abl (Yu *et al.*, 2003), a protein kinase which has been shown to depend on NF-κB activation for its ability to transform haematopoietic progenitor cells (Reuther *et al.*, 1998). Given that IκB degradation in response to anticancer drug treatment can occur independently of IKK (Tergaonkar *et al.*, 2003), inhibitors of the proteases catalyzing this proteolytic reaction appear much more suitable for use as adjuncts in anticancer chemotherapy than compounds inhibiting IKK. Indeed, Velcade has proved effective in both Gleevec-sensitive and resistant

Bcr-Abl-positive CML cells pointing to a potential benefit of the use of the two drugs in combination for the treatment of this form of leukaemia (Gatto *et al.*, 2003). Moreover, the proteasome inhibitor has been shown to increase sensitivity of MMCs, and to reverse resistance to a combination of the conventional DNA-damaging chemotherapeutic drugs doxorubicin and melphalan (Mitsiades *et al.*, 2003). This effect is thought to be due to inhibition, by Velcade, of the expression of NF-κB-dependent genes promoting cell survival, such as Bcl-2 and cIAP-2, and of genes involved in DNA repair including DNA-dependent protein kinase. Not only does Velcade overcome resistance to genotoxic agents but the drug also synergizes with the experimental, plant natural product-derived compound CDDO-imidazolide in the killing of Velcade-resistant MMCs (Chauhan *et al.*, 2004). These results lend further weight to the strategy of using Velcade in combination with conventional and experimental anticancer drugs to increase treatment efficacy in certain types of leukaemia. However, these leukaemias are not the only types of cancer in which Velcade enhances the efficacy of other drugs. Velcade has also been found to increase solid tumour cell killing induced by tumour necrosis factor-related apoptosis-inducing ligand (TRAIL), a member of the tumour necrosis factor family (Nencioni *et al.*, 2005; Lashinger *et al.*, 2005; Sayers and Murphy, 2005). TRAIL as well as agonistic anti-TRAIL receptor monoclonal antibodies are currently in development for the treatment of cancer (Bhojani *et al.*, 2003; French and Tschopp, 2003; Pukac *et al.*, 2005; Investigational drugs database), indicating that Velcade may also enhance treatment efficacy in combination with such biopharmaceuticals.

## 8.    CONCLUSION

A number of cancers have been shown to have an inflammatory component and a promising strategy for their prevention and treatment thus appears to be the inhibition of key regulators of the inflammatory response, most prominent among them the transcription factor NF-κB, frequently found to be dysregulated in premalignant inflammatory conditions, which have been poignantly described as 'wounds that do not heal' (Dvorak, 1986). Moreover, inhibition of NF-κB may also be therapeutically beneficial in the treatment of other types of cancer, i.e. malignancies in which tumour suppressor functions have been lost and NF-κB has become constitutively activated resulting in the suppression of cancer cell apoptosis. Owing to the complexity and mutability of tumours, however, in both cases, inhibition of this transcription factor alone is unlikely to have a decisive therapeutic effect. These key characteristics of tumours appear to be responsible for the limited efficacy of most conventional anticancer chemotherapeutic drugs and thus to form a barrier to effective drug treatment of cancer that may only be possible to be overcome by a combination of drugs each targeting a specific cellular macromolecule involved in tumourigenesis or by a single drug with a broader spectrum of relevant molecular targets. Ideally, such combination chemotherapy would be tailored to the profile of molecular lesions of the tumour to be eradicated. Available evidence suggests that within the pathways leading to the activation of NF-κB, promising targets for combination anticancer chemotherapy of a variety of malignancies can be found.

## 9. REFERENCES

Adams, J. (2003). Potential for proteasome inhibition in the treatment of cancer. *Drug. Discov. Today* **8**: 307-315.

Aggarwal, B.B. (2004). Nuclear factor-κB: the enemy within. *Cancer Cell* **6**: 203-208.

Amit, S. and Ben-Neriah, Y. (2003). NF-κB activation in cancer: a challenge for ubiquitination- and proteasome-based therapeutic approaches. *Semin. Cancer Biol.* **13**: 15-28.

Arts, J. *et al.* (2003). Histone deacetylase inhibitors: from chromatin remodeling to experimental cancer therapeutics. *Curr. Med. Chem.* **10**: 2343-2350.

Azam, M. *et al.* (2003). Mechanisms of autoinhibition and STI-571/imatinib resistance revealed by mutagenesis of Bcr-Abl. *Cell* **112**: 831-843.

Baum, M. (2002). A new strategy for cancer. *Prospect* February: 44-48.

Beinke, S. and Ley, S.C. (2004). Functions of NF-κB and NF-κB2 in immune cell biology. *Biochem. J.* **382**: 393-409.

Bhalla, U.S. (2004). Models of cell signaling pathways. *Curr. Opin. Genet. Dev.* **14**: 375-381.

Bhojani, M.S. *et al.* (2003). TRAIL and anti-tumor responses. *Cancer Biol. Ther.* **2** (4 Suppl. 1): S71-S78.

Bohuslav, J. *et al.* (2004). p53 induces NF-κB activation by an IκB kinase-independent mechanism involving phosphorylation of p65 by ribosomal S6 kinase 1. *J. Biol. Chem.* **279**: 26115-26125.

Borisy, A.A. *et al.* (2003). Systematic discovery of multicomponent therapeutics. *Proc. Natl Acad. Sci. USA* **100**: 7977-7982.

Borst, P. *et al.* (1999). The multidrug resistance protein family. *Biochem. Biophys. Acta* **1461**: 347-357.

Brahimi, F. *et al.* (2004). Multiple mechanisms of action of ZR2002 in human breast cancer cells: a novel combi-molecule designed to block signaling mediated by the Erb family of oncogenes and to damage genomic DNA. *Int. J. Cancer* **112**: 484-491.

Burgess, M.R. *et al.* (2005). Comparative analysis of two clinically active Bcr-Abl kinase inhibitors reveals the role of conformation-specific binding in resistance. *Proc. Natl Acad. Sci. USA* **102**: 3395-3400.

Butcher, E.C. *et al.* (2004). Systems biology in drug discovery. *Nat. Biotechnol.* **22**:1253-1259.

Caffo, O. (2001). Radiosensitization with chemotherapeutic agents. *Lung Cancer* **34**: S81-S90.

Campbell, K.J. *et al.* (2004). Active repression of antiapoptotic gene expression by RelA(p65) NF-κB. *Mol. Cell* **13**: 853-865.

Cancer Facts and Figures 2004. American Cancer Society.

Carr, K.M. *et al.* (2004). Genomic and proteomic approaches for studying human cancer: prospects for true patient-tailored therapy. *Hum. Genomics* **1**: 134-140.

Castro, A.C. *et al.* (2003). Novel IKK inhibitors: β-carbolines. *Bioorg. Med. Chem. Lett.* **13**: 2419-2422.

Cayrol, C. and Ducommun, B. (1998). Interaction with cyclin-dependent kinases and PCNA modulates proteasome-dependent degradation of p21. *Oncogene* **17**: 2437-2444.

Chambon, P. and Beuzard, M. (2004). Cancer. Les varies raisons d'une epidemie. *Science & Vie* June: 46-69.

Chauhan, D. *et al.* (2004). The bortezomib/proteasome inhibitor PS-341 and triterpenoid CDDO-Im induce synergistic anti-multiple myeloma (MM) activity and overcome bortezomibn resistance. *Blood* **103**: 3158-3166.

Claudio, E. *et al.* (2002). BAFF-induced NEMO-independent processing of NF-κB2 in maturing B cells. *Nat. Immunol.* **3**: 958-965.

Clemons, P.A. (2004). Complex phenotypic assays in high-throughput screening. *Curr. Opin. Chem. Biol.* **8**: 334-338.

Constantinou, M. *et al.* (2003). Paclitaxel and concurrent radiation in upper gastrointestinal cancers. *Cancer Invest.* **21**: 887-896.

Cools, J. *et al.* (2005). Resistance to tyrosine kinase inhibitors: calling on extra forces. *Drug Resist. Updat.* in press.

Dajee, M. *et al.* (2003). NF-κB blockade and oncogenic Ras trigger invasive human epidermal neoplasia. *Nature* **421**: 639-643.

Davidov, E. *et al.* (2003). Advancing drug discovery through systems biology. *Drug Discov. Today* **8**: 175-183.

Denlinger, C.E. *et al.* (2004). Modulation of antiapoptotic cell signaling pathways in non-small cell lung cancer: the role of NF-κB. *Semin. Thorac. Cardiovasc. Surg.* **16**: 28-39.

Doggrell, S.A. (2005). BMS-354825: a novel drug with potential for the treatment of imatinib-resistant chronic myeloid leukaemia. *Expert. Opin. Investig. Drugs* **14**: 89-91.

Donato, N.J. *et al.* (2003). Bcr-Abl independence and Lyn kinase overexpression in chronic myelogenous leukemia cells selected for resistance to STI571. *Blood* **101**: 690-698.

Dvorak, H.F. (1986). Tumors: wounds that do not heal. Similarities between tumor stroma generation and wound healing. *N. Engl. J. Med.* **315**: 1650-1659.

Eaton, D.L. (2002). 'Americas epidemic of chemicals and cancer – myth or fact?' in Chiras, D. Human Biology. Fourth Edition. Jones and Bartlett, Sudbury MA.

Fisher, A.C. *et al.* (1995). Update: is there a cancer epidemic in the United States? American Council of Science and Health.

French, L.E. and Tschopp, J. (2003). Protein-based therapeutic approaches targeting death receptors. *Cell Death Differ.* **10**: 117-123.

Fujioka, S. *et al.* (2004a). Stabilization of p53 is a novel mechanism for proapoptotic function of NF-κB. *J. Biol. Chem.* **279**: 27549-27559.

Fujioka, S. *et al.* (2004b). NF-κB and AP-1 connection: mechanism of NF-κB-dependent regulation of AP-1 activity. *Mol. Cell. Biol.* **24**: 7806-7819.

Garber, K. (2002). Synthetic lethality: killing cancer with cancer. *J. Natl Cancer Inst.* **94**: 1666-1668.

Garber, K. (2004). Running interference: pace picks up on synthetic lethality research. *J. Natl Cancer Inst.* **96**: 982-983.

Gatto, S. *et al.* (2003). The proteasome inhibitor PS-341 inhibits growth and induces apoptosis in Bcr/Abl-positive cell lines sensitive and resistant to imatinib mesylate. *Haematologica* **88**: 853-863.

Gumireddy, K. *et al.* (2005). A non-ATP-competitive inhibitor of Bcr-Abl overrides imatinib resistance. *Proc. Natl Acad. Sci. USA* **102**: 1992-1997.

Haefner, B. (2005). The transcription factor NF-κB as drug target. *Progress in Medicinal Chemistry* **43**: 137-188.

Hagemann, C. and Blank J.L. (2001). The ups and downs of MEK kinase interactions. *Cell. Signal.* **13**, 863-875.

Han, Y. *et al.* (1999). Tumor necrosis factor-α-inducible IκBα proteolysis mediated by cytosolic m-calpain. A mechanism parallel to the ubiquitin-proteasome pathway of nuclear factor-κB activation. *J. Biol. Chem.* **274**: 787-794.

Hanahan, D. and Weinberg, R.A. (2000). The hallmarks of cancer. *Cell* **100**: 57-70.

Hideshima *et al.* (2002). NF-κB as a therapeutic target in multiple myeloma. *J.Biol. Chem.* **277**: 16639-16647.

Higashitsuji, H. *et al.* (2002). A novel protein overexpressed in hepatoma accelerates export of NF-κB from the nucleus and inhibits p53-dependent apoptosis. *Cancer Cell* **2**: 335-346.

Hu, Y. *et al.* (2004). Requirement of Src kinases Lyn, Hck and Fgr for Bcr-Abl1-induced B-lymphoblastic leukemia but not chronic myeloid leukemia. *Nat. Genet.* **36**: 453-461.

Investigational Drugs database (www.iddb3.com).

Kalled, S.L. *et al.* (2003). BAFF: B cell survival factor and emerging therapeutic target for autoimmune disorders. *Expert Opin. Ther. Targets* **7**: 115-123.

Karin, M. *et al.* (2002). NF-κB in cancer: from innocent bystander to major culprit. *Nat. Rev. Cancer* **2**: 301-310.

Kitano, H. (2004). Cancer as a robust system: implications for anticancer therapy. *Nat. Rev. Cancer* **4**: 227-235.

Kucharczak, J. *et al.* (2003). To be, or not to be: NF-κB is the answer – role of Rel/NF-κB in the regulation of apoptosis. *Oncogene* **22**: 8961-8982.

Kuo, M.T. *et al.* (2002). Induction of human MDR1 gene expression by 2-acetylaminofluorene is mediated by effectors of the phosphoinositide 3-kinase pathway that activate NF–κB signaling. *Oncogene* **21**: 1945-1954.

Lashinger, L.M. *et al.* (2005). Bortezomib abolishes tumor necrosis factor-related apoptosis-inducing ligand resistance via a p21-dependent mechanism in human bladder and prostate cancer cells. *Cancer Res.* **65**: 4902-4908.

Leaf, C. (2004). Why we're losing the war on cancer (and how to win it) *Fortune* March 22: 77-92.

Levesque, H. and Lafont, O. (2000). L'aspirine a travers les siecles: rappel historique. *Rev. Med. Interne* **21** Suppl. 1: 8s-17s.

Li, Q. *et al.* (2005). Inflammation-associated cancer: NF-κB is the lynchpin. *Trends Immunol.* **26**: 318-325.

Lombardo, L.J. *et al.* (2004). Discovery of N-(2-chloro-6-methyl-phenyl)-2-(6-(4-(2-hydroxyethyl)-piperazin-1-yl)-2-methylpyrimidin-4-ylamino)thiazole-5-carboxamide (BMS-354825), a dual Src/Abl kinase inhibitor with potent antitumor activity in preclinical assays. *J. Med. Chem.* **47**: 6658-6661.

Loop, T. and Pahl, H.L. (2003). 'Activators and target genes of Rel/ NF-κB transcription factors – from bench to bedside.' in Nuclear factor κB. Regulation and role in disease. Rudi Beyaert (ed.). Kluwer Academic Publishers. Dordrecht. The Netherlands.

Losi, L. *et al.* (2005). Evolution of intratumoral genetic heterogeneity during colorectal cancer progression. *Carcinogenesis* **26**: 916-922.

Markmann, M. (2003). Are we winning or losing the war on cancer? *Cleveland Clin. J. Med.* **70**: 632-633.

Mayo, M.W. *et al.* (2003). Ineffectiveness of histone deacetylase inhibitors to induce apoptosis involves the transcriptional activation of NF-κB through the Akt pathway. *J. Biol. Chem.* **278**: 18980-18989.

McCarty, M.F. (2004). Targeting multiple signaling pathways as a strategy for managing prostate cancer: multifocal signal modulation therapy. *Integr. Cancer Ther.* **3**: 349-380.

Mercurio F. *et al.* (1997). IKK-1 and IKK-2: cytokine-activated IκB kinases essential for NF-κB activation. *Science* **278**: 860-866.

Mitsiades, N. *et al.* (2003). The proteasome inhibitor PS-341 potentiates sensitivity of multiple myeloma cells to conventional chemotherapeutic agents: therapeutic applications. *Blood* **101**: 2377-2380.

Munshi *et al.*, (2004). Inhibition of constitutively activated nuclear factor-κB radiosensitizes human melanoma cells. *Mol. Cancer Ther.* **3**: 985-992.

Nakano, H. *et al.* (1998). Differential regulation of IκBkinase alpha and beta by two upstream kinases, NF-κB-inducing kinase and mitogen-activated protein kinase/ERK kinase kinase-1. *Proc. Natl Acad. Sci USA* **95**: 3537-3542.

Nencioni, A. *et al.* (2005). Cooperative cytotoxicity of proteasome inhibitors and tumor necrosis factor-related apoptosis-inducing ligand in chemoresistant Bcl-2-overexpressing cells. *Clin. Cancer Res.* **11**: 4259-4265.

Neshat, M.S. *et al.* (2001). Enhanced sensitivity of PTEN-deficient tumors to inhibition of FRAP/mTOR. *Proc. Natl Acad. Sci. USA* **98**: 10314-10319.

Nimmanapalli, R. and Bhalla, K. (2002). Mechanisms of resistance to imatinib mesylate in Bcr-Abl-positive leukemias. *Curr. Opin. Oncol.* **14**: 616-620.

Nutton, V. (2004). Ancient Medicine. Routledge, London.

O'Hare, T. *et al.* (2005). *In vitro* activity of Bcr-Abl inhibitors AMN107 and BMS-354825 against clinically relevant imatinib-resistant Abl kinase domain mutants. *Cancer Res.* **65**: 4500-4505.

Orlowski, R.Z. and Baldwin Jr., A.S. (2002). NF-κB as a therapeutic target in cancer. *Trends Mol. Med.* **8**: 385-389.

Palanki M.S. *et al.* (2003). The design and synthesis of novel orally active inhibitors of AP-1 and NF-κB mediated transcriptional activation. SAR of *in vitro* and *in vivo* studies. *Bioorg. Med. Chem. Lett.* **13**: 4077-4080.

Perkins, N.D. (2004). NF-κB: tumor promoter or suppressor? *Trends Cell Biol.* **14**: 64-69.

Porter, R. (1997). The greatest benefit to mankind. A medical history of humanity from antiquity to the present. Fontana Press, London.

Pukac *et al.* (2005). HGS-ETR1, a fully human TRAIL-receptor 1 monoclonal antibody, induces cell death in multiple tumour types *in vitro* and *in vivo*. *Br. J. Cancer* **92**: 1430-1441.

Rachid, Z. *et al.* (2005). Synthesis of half-mustard combi-molecules with fluorescence properties: correlation with EGFR status. *Bioorg. Med. Chem. Lett.* **15**: 1135-1138.

Rayet, B. and Gelinas, C. (1999). Aberrant rel/nfkb genes and activity in human cancer. *Oncogene* **18**: 6938-6947.

Regenstein, L.G. (2002). Are we facing an epidemic of cancer? in Chiras, D. Human Biology. Fourth Edition. Jones and Bartlett, Sudbury MA.

Reuther, J.Y. *et al.* (1998). A requirement for NF-κB activation in Bcr-Abl-mediated transformation. *Genes Dev.* **12**: 968-981.

Rocha, S. *et al.* (2003). p53 represses cyclin D1 transcription through downregulation of Bcl-3 and inducing increased association of the p52 NF-κB subunit with histone deacetylase 1. *Mol. Cell Biol.* **23**: 4713-4727.

Rundall, B.K. *et al.* (2004). Combined histone deacetylase and NF-κB inhibition sensitizes non-small cell lung cancer to cell death. *Surgery* **136**: 416-425.

Russo, S.M. *et al.* (2001). Enhancement of radiosensitivity by proteasome inhibition: implications for a role of NF-κB. *Int. J. Radiat. Oncol. Biol. Phys.* **50**: 183-193.

Ryan, K.M. *et al.* (2000). Role of NF-κB in p53-mediated programmed cell death. *Nature* **404**: 892-897.

Sayers, T.J. and Murphy, W.J. (2005). Combining proteasome inhibition with TNF-related apoptosis-inducing ligand (Apo2L/TRAIL) for cancer therapy. *Cancer Immunol. Immunother.* in press.

Schmidt, C. *et al.* (2003). Mechanisms of proinflammatory cytokine-induced biphasic NF-κB activation. *Mol. Cell* **12**: 1287-300.

Senftleben, U. *et al.* (2001). Activation by IKKα of a second, evolutionary conserved, NF-κB signaling pathway. *Science* **293**: 1495-1499.

Shah, N.P. *et al.* (2004). Overriding imatinib resistance with a novel Abl kinase inhibitor. *Science* **305**: 399-401.

Shi, Y. *et al.* (2002). Enhanced sensitivity of multiple myeloma cells containing PTEN mutations to CCI-779. *Cancer Res.* **62**: 5027-5034.

Shishodia, S. and Aggarwal, B.B. (2004). Nuclear factor-κB: a friend or foe in cancer? *Biochem. Pharmacol.* **68**: 1071-1080.

Smith, C. *et al.* (2001). NF-κB inducing kinase is dispensable for activation of NF-κB in inflammatory settings but essential for lymphotoxin β receptor activation of NF-κB in primary human fibroblasts. *J. Immunol.* **167**: 5895-5903.

Sorlie, T. (2004). Molecular portraits of breast cancer: tumour subtypes as distinct disease entities. *Eur. J. Cancer* **40**: 2667-2675.

Stewart, B.W. and Kleihues, P. (2003). World Cancer Report. IARC Press, Lyon, France.

Strausberg, R.L. and Schreiber, S.L. (2003). From knowing to controlling: a path from genomics to drugs using small molecule probes. *Science* **300**: 294-295.

The History of Cancer. American Cancer Society (www.cancer.org/docroot/cri/content/cri_2_6x_the_history_of_cancer_72.asp?sitearea=cri).

Thevenod, F. *et al.* (2000). Up-regulation of multidrug resistance P-glycoprotein via nuclear factor-κB activation protects kidney proximal tubule cells from cadmium- and reactive oxygen species-induced apoptosis. *J. Biol. Chem.* **275**: 1887-1896.

Tergaonkar, V. *et al.* (2002). p53 stabilization is decreased upon NF-κB activation: a role for NF-κB in acquisition of resistance to chemotherapy. *Cancer Cell* **1**: 493-503.

Tergaonkar, V. *et al.* (2003). IκB kinase-independent IκBα degradation pathway: functional NF-κB activity and implications for cancer therapy. *Mol. Cell Biol.* **23**: 8070-8083.

Uetz, P. and Finley Jr., R.L. (2005). From protein networks to biological systems. *FEBS Lett.* **579**: 1821-1827.

Velcade, new science and new hope: a case study. National Institutes of Health Office of Technology Transfer. September 2003.

Vermeulen, L. *et al.* (2003). Transcriptional activation of the NF-κB p65 subunit by mitogen- and stress-activated protein kinase-1 (MSK1). *EMBO J.* **22**: 1313-1324.

von Hoff, D.D. (2002). Patterns. Patterns. Patterns. The future of cancer research. Oncology Issues. November/December: 38-40.

Voorhees, P.M. *et al.* (2003). The proteasome as a target for cancer therapy. *Clin. Cancer Res.* **9**: 6316-6325.

Wang, Y. *et al.* (2004). Synthetic lethal targeting of Myc by activation of the DR5 death receptor pathway. *Cancer Cell* **5**: 501-512.

Watters, J.W. and McLeod, H.L. (2003). Cancer pharmacogenomics: current and future applications. *Biochim. Biophys. Acta* **1603**: 99-111.

Waxman, S. and Anderson, K.C. (2001). History of the development of arsenic derivatives in cancer therapy. *Oncologist* **6** Suppl. 2: 3-10.

Wolmark, N. and Fisher, B. (1985). Adjuvant therapy in primary breast cancer. *Surg. Clin. North Am.* **65**: 161-180.

Yin, M.J. *et al.* (1998). The anti-inflammatory agents aspirin and salicylate inhibit the activity of IκB kinase-beta. *Nature* **396**: 77-80.

Yu, C. *et al.* (2003). The proteasome inhibitor bortezomib interacts synergistically with histone deacetylase inhibitors to induce apoptosis in Bcr/Abl$^+$ cells sensitive and resistant to STI571. *Blood* **102**: 3765-3774.

# Index